LIVING WITH
HEPATITIS C

A SURVIVOR'S GUIDE

Fifth Edition

D0018991

LIVING WITH HEPATITIS C

A SURVIVOR'S GUIDE

Fifth Edition

GREGORY T. EVERSON, M.D., F.A.C.P.

www.hatherleighpress.com

DISCLAIMER
This book does not give legal or medical advice.
Always consult your doctor, lawyer, and other professionals.
The names of people who contributed anecdotal material have been changed.

The ideas and suggestions contained in this book are not intended as a substitute for consulting with a physician. All matters regarding your health require medical supervision.

Library of Congress Cataloging-in-Publication Data

Everson, Gregory T., 1950-
  Living with hepatitis c : a survivor's guide / Gregory T. Everson, Hedy Weinberg. — 5th ed.
     p. cm.
  Includes bibliographical references and index.
  ISBN 978-1-57826-305-9 (pbk. : alk. paper)
  1. Hepatitis C—Popular works. I. Weinberg, Hedy, 1939- II. Title.
  RC848.H425E95 2009
  616.3'623—dc22
                                    2009030499

    ISBN: 978-1-57826-305-9

All Hatherleigh Press titles are available for special promotions and premiums. For more information, please contact the manager of our Special Sales department.

Designed by Dede Cummings Designs
10 9 8 7 6 5 4 3 2 1

DEDICATION

The first edition of Living with Hepatitis C: A Survivor's Guide *was published in 1998. Now, over 10 years later, we are still at it, trying to refine, improve and keep our book current with the rapidly evolving medical knowledge and treatments for hepatitis C. Maintaining quality and accuracy have been our goals—to do so takes time, a lot of time! And, most importantly patient loved ones. I wish to thank my family for tolerating my "late hours" of work, absence from home, and long periods at the computer. Special appreciation and thanks go to my wife, Linda, and sons, Brad and Todd. You truly are my inspiration. To all my friends and colleagues, I hope you get a chance to read this work and let me know if it is worthy of your readership.*

Gregory T. Everson, M.D., F.A.C.P.

To my husband, Michael, my love, a truly good person who stands up for what's right, yet keeps a sense of humor, warmth, and openness. Your support, encouragement, and belief in this book made its creation possible. And to our children — Ben and Yael, Shira and David, and Adam, who offered help and cheered me on —I'm proud of you, your values, and your strong sense of family.

Hedy Weinberg

We also thank our editor, Heather Ogilvie, for her guidance and valuable suggestions in the preparation of previous editions of *Living with Hepatitis C,* and our editor for this edition, June Eding.

In memory of Fred Kern, Jr., M.D., the authors and the publisher will contribute a portion of the profits from this book to the Kern Research Foundation for the Understanding and Treatment of Gastrointestinal and Liver Diseases to further hepatitis C research.

Kern Foundation
7500 East Dartmouth Avenue, No. 30
Denver, Colorado 80231-4264
Telephone (303) 750-5509
Fax (303) 750-4688

The authors would like to thank all those who have contributed to the Kern Foundation to further our research into hepatitis C and liver disease. We especially wish to acknowledge our publisher, Hatherleigh Press, for matching our own contributions of a portion of the profits from *Living with Hepatitis C: A Survivor's Guide* and *My Mom Has Hepatitis C.*

These contributions, supplemented by the Liver Disease Fund at the University of Colorado Medical School, have underwritten the cost of a fully automated high-pressure liquid chromatograph (HPLC). This chromatograph analyzes compounds in blood and saliva that are used to measure liver function. The research goal is to develop tests that more accurately measure liver function and predict a patient's clinical course of disease. These tests are currently being used in HALT C, the NIH-sponsored trial of maintenance interferon to prevent disease progression in patients with chronic hepatitis C.

CONTENTS

PREFACE

L IVING WITH HEPATITIS C: *A Survivor's Guide* grew out of a need I saw at the University of Colorado Health Sciences Center. When the first test for the virus became available around 1990, newly diagnosed patients asked questions but, unfortunately, we physicians had relatively few answers. As the years went by, our knowledge grew, and so did the task of educating the rapidly growing number of people diagnosed with hepatitis C.

To meet the public's need for information about hepatitis C, I began to give lectures specifically targeted to patients and their families. After one lecture, Hedy Weinberg, a hepatitis C patient and writer, approached me and suggested that we turn the lecture series into a guidebook for our patients at the clinic. What began as a simple pamphlet quickly turned into a long-term project that resulted in the publication of the first version of this book in 1997.

As we wrote and rewrote the text, we tried to create a useful guide that would take the patient step-by-step through the process of diagnosis and ongoing care. We tried to anticipate questions, translate medical jargon, and reduce the fear of the unknown. Therefore, we also presented overviews of emotional, financial, and nutritional issues that accompany this chronic illness. In subsequent editions, we added new chapters dealing with liver cancer, co-infection, and children. In these pages you will hear the voices of patients and staff at the University Hospital and the University of Colorado Health Sciences Center who generously contributed their knowledge and experiences and encouraged us to complete the work.

Our third edition (2001) continued to update information and resources while trying to maintain our goal of presenting complex medical terms in language that patients can understand. And, in our fourth edition a new standard of care, the combination of pegylated interferon with ribavirin had emerged (Chapter 9, Pegylated Interferons, The

Emerging Standard-of-Care). We also enlarged the scope of the co-infection chapter to include hepatitis B, as well as HIV/AIDS.

As we prepare each new edition, we note the advances in our knowledge and treatment of hepatitis C. This, our Fifth Edition of "Living with Hepatitis C: A Survivor's Guide" has added a 15th Chapter to the saga — the new and emerging advances in treating hepatitis C — protease inhibitors, polymerase inhibitors, immune modulators, maintenance therapy, and other key issues. We still have a long way to go to eradicate the virus, but the future looks hopeful.

We continually update this guidebook to help people cope with a disease that affects over four million Americans. In a short clinical visit, people often keep a "stiff upper lip." But for this book, patients shared their experiences—the funny and hopeful times, as well as the frightening, sad moments. I gained a new appreciation and insight into my patients' lives.

Throughout the book we emphasize the need for thoughtful well-controlled clinical and basic research of hepatitis C.

One last word: Although *Living with Hepatitis C: A Survivor's Guide* is a detailed reference guide, it does not replace the advice and care of your physician, nor does it give legal advice. Instead, it is designed solely to educate patients and their families about hepatitis C and how it affects their lives. Consult appropriate specialists and always work closely with your doctor when making medical decisions.

ACKNOWLEDGEMENTS

We appreciate and gratefully acknowledge the hard-working, dedicated members of the Liver Team at the University of Colorado Health Sciences Center, who are always generous with help and support: Igal Kam, M.D., Chief of Division of Transplant Surgery; Susan Mandell, M.D.; Cathy Ray, R.N., B.S.N., M.A., Jennifer DeSanto, R.N., Shannon Lauriski; Tracy Steinberg, R.N., M.S., C.C.T.C.; Michael Talamantes, M.S.S.W., L.C.S.W.

Dr. Everson wishes to further acknowledge the support of the staff at University Hospital and the University of Colorado Health Sciences Center in the care and management of patients with hepatitis C.

From The Children's Hospital in Denver, we thank Michael Narkewicz, M.D., Medical Director of the Pediatric Liver Center and Liver Transplant Program, Associate Professor in Pediatrics at the University of Colorado Medical School, Hewit/Andrews Chair in Pediatric Liver Disease, who once again gave generously of his time in reviewing Chapter 13. We also thank Ronald Sokol, M.D., Director of the Pediatric General Clinical Research Center, Professor of Pediatrics at the University of Colorado Medical School, Associate Medical Director of the Pediatric Liver Center; Marjanne Claassen, R.N., M.S., C.N.S., Clinical Nurse Specialist, Pediatric Liver Center Nurse Coordinator; and Nancy Butler Simon, M.S., R.N., C.N.S., C.P.N.P., Advanced Practice Nurse, Pediatric General Clinical Research Center; and the Pediatric Transplant Team, including Fritz Karrer, M.D.

We thank Steve Potter, Public Affairs Specialist, Social Security Administration, Denver, for reviewing our information on Social Security issues; and Meredith Pate-Willig, M.S.W., L.C.S.W., for her invaluable help with the emotional challenges of chronic illness.

Special thanks to Anne Jesse, Executive Director, The Hep C Connection, and to Hep C Connection support group members; the University Hospital Transplant Support Group; Kathy Kinch, Executive

Director, Rocky Mountain Chapter of the American Liver Foundation; and all the hepatitis C patients across the country who shared their stories and touched our lives.

FOREWORD

SECOND EDITION (1999)

SINCE THE DISCOVERY of the hepatitis C virus (HCV) in
1989, there has been an explosion of knowledge related to both
the virus and the disease it causes. Indeed, over 9,000 medical arti-
cles on hepatitis C have been published, and newspapers and magazines
have highlighted hepatitis C with increasing frequency. The rapid evolution of knowledge as well as the development of therapies and accurate
diagnostic tests have overwhelmed most practicing physicians and their
patients.

For individuals who have hepatitis C, the diagnosis often engenders
strong emotions, ranging from fear and denial to depression and anger.
The reactions of loved ones and close friends, whose support is so cru-
cial for people with hepatitis C, are often constrained by their own fear
of contagion and ignorance of the disease. Too often, patients and families find little comfort or confidence in the varied, and often conflicting,
information received from their health care providers, friends, newspapers, magazines, or the Internet. There is little wonder that for many
people the "C" in hepatitis C has come to stand for "confusion."

Fortunately, Gregory T. Everson, M.D., a noted hepatologist, and
Hedy Weinberg, a writer and proactive patient with hepatitis C,
responded to this need for information with the first edition of their
book *Living with Hepatitis C: A Survivor's Guide* in 1997. The title accurately captured the intent of the book to educate patients and their families about HCV, the disease hepatitis C, the variability and complexity
of its natural history and manifestations, the therapeutic options, and the
strategies for coping and living with a chronic illness. Combining solid
medical information with the perspectives, insights, and experiences of a
patient resulted in a particularly appealing and readable book. Sensitivity

to patients' perspectives and an emphasis on both scientific and psychosocial aspects of hepatitis C were the right prescription for a diverse audience—patients, families, support groups, nurses, and physicians—who has enthusiastically embraced *Living with Hepatitis C: A Survivor's Guide* as an invaluable resource.

The exponential increase in knowledge about hepatitis C over the past three years clearly mandated a second edition of *Living with Hepatitis C: A Survivor's Guide* to provide a comprehensive update on its natural history and transmission, and advances in therapy. The agreeable synergy of science and humanity that characterized the first edition has been sustained in the second edition with careful revision of the original text and addition of three notable chapters. These new chapters address the significant relationship between hepatitis C and primary liver cancer, the special concerns of patients coinfected with HIV and HCV, and the distinctive issues of children who are infected with HCV. The second edition of *Living with Hepatitis C: A Survivor's Guide* admirably achieves its goals and testifies to the authors' commitment to all the patients, families, nurses, and physicians who are challenged by hepatitis C on a daily basis.

John M. Vierling, M.D., F.A.C.P.
Director of Hepatology and Medical Director
of Liver Transplantation,
Cedars-Sinai Medical Center
Professor of Medicine, UCLA School of Medicine
Chair, Board of Directors
American Liver Foundation
1999

1

WHAT IS HEPATITIS C?

An Introduction

I work for a city agency, and we're required to take annual physicals. This year the doctor asked me to come back for more blood tests. My liver counts were high, he said. That's how I found out I had hepatitis C.

I'm managing. What else can I do? But my wife—she's having a tough time. It's hard to believe, but I had never even heard of hepatitis C before.

Barry

IF YOU'VE JUST BEEN DIAGNOSED with hepatitis C, you have a lot of questions: "What is hepatitis C? How did I acquire the infection? Is there treatment? If I tell them at work, will they fire me?"

Hepatitis C is a viral infection that causes inflammation, injury, and ultimately scarring of the liver. That sounds frightening, but try not to panic. You're not alone. Current estimates indicate that nearly four million people living in the United States have hepatitis C. Although hepatitis C is a serious problem, the infection usually progresses slowly over years or decades. You have time to consider your options.

Take a look at the bottom line. Hepatitis C can be dangerous if it damages your liver to the point of cirrhosis. According to the Centers for Disease Control and Prevention (CDC), for every 100 people infected with hepatitis C about 25 will clear the virus, and 75 will develop long-term infection. Five to 20 people might develop cirrhosis over a period of 20 to 30 years, and one to five people might die from the consequences of long-term infection—liver cancer or cirrhosis.

As you can see from these mortality figures, it's far more likely that you will have to learn to live with the virus until scientists find a cure. Success rates of current treatments have climbed dramatically in the last few years, and researchers anticipate exciting breakthroughs. Nevertheless, dealing with hepatitis C is a challenge. That's what this book is about: how to live with and survive hepatitis C.

Hepatitis C is a newly discovered disease. Researchers didn't develop a screening test until 1990—long after the hepatitis C virus had infected millions of people. Before this time, it was impossible to detect hepatitis C in donated blood. As a result, the nation's blood supply became contaminated.

That's what happened to Hedy Weinberg, who's writing this book with me. She was exposed to hepatitis C through an emergency transfusion. Let me introduce you to Hedy, who will tell you her story—a story you'll hear throughout the book, because it's typical of what most people face:

> In 1967, I gave birth to a stillborn baby girl. My uterus ruptured, I almost died, and they gave me five pints of plasma. Twenty-six years later, I found out I had hepatitis C. Looking back, it explains some symptoms I've had over the years: a thyroid condition, a slight blood clotting problem, some depression, and fatigue. The transfusion saved my life—but it gave me hepatitis C.

A Word of Caution: Information in this book does not substitute for the advice of your physician. If you have hepatitis C, you should be under a doctor's care.

In this chapter we'll discuss some basic facts and statistics about hepatitis C, its history and discovery, and information about viruses and other forms of viral hepatitis. Here are the topics we'll cover:

- You Are Not Alone
- A Silent Epidemic
- The Discovery of Hepatitis C
- Understanding Hepatitis C
     What Is Hepatitis?
     What Is a Virus?
     What Is the Hepatitis C Virus (HCV)?
- The Hepatitis Viral Alphabet
     Hepatitis A
     Hepatitis B
     Hepatitis C
     Hepatitis D
     Hepatitis E
- Hepatitis C: How Close Is a Cure?

You Are Not Alone

If you, or someone you love, has hepatitis C, know that you're not alone. The U.S. Centers for Disease Control and Prevention (CDC) estimate that 1.6 to 1.8 percent of the population, 3.9 million Americans, have been infected; 2.7 million of them are chronically infected. Hepatitis C is also a global problem. The World Health Organization estimates that hepatitis C infects three percent of the world's population: 8.9 million people in Europe and more than 170 million chronic carriers worldwide (see Figure 1A).

It's hard to relate to numbers this big, so let's make the statistics more real. The number of people in the United States currently infected with hepatitis C is triple that of HIV/AIDS, more than five times that of Parkinson's, and more than ten times the number of Americans with multiple sclerosis.

In my state of Colorado, which is quite typical, about 20,000 to 40,000 people have hepatitis C; that's roughly three out of every 350 residents. Although the public doesn't realize it, chronic hepatitis C is the most common reportable infectious disease in the state.

But numbers and statistics don't tell the whole story. When you're diagnosed with hepatitis C, all of a sudden, you feel as alone as you can possibly feel. It's as if an invisible fence has gone up between you and all the other people who don't have hepatitis C. You have an infectious ill-

FIGURE IA.   GLOBAL PREVALENCE OF HEPATITIS C
WORLD HEALTH ORGANIZATION 2001

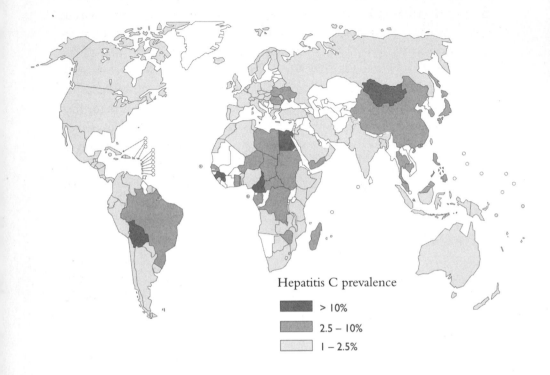

Hepatitis C prevalence

> 10%

2.5 – 10%

1 – 2.5%

ness; they don't. You're worried about yourself, and you're worried about the people you love. You're angry. Perhaps you even feel ashamed.

Hepatitis puts a heavy strain on relationships. Mothers and fathers hesitate to cook for their families. Friends who used to hug and kiss you pull away. People don't tell their bosses and co-workers because they fear losing their jobs. Lovers are afraid to touch one another.

> *My wife moved into the other bedroom. The doctor explained that it's okay for us to have sex—that if we're married and we're not sleeping around, there's almost zero risk that she'll get infected.*
>
> *But I don't know. It's like she hears the word "virus," and she freaks out. When I try to hug her, I feel her tense up. It hurts.*
>
> Tony

A healthy dose of facts about hepatitis C helps people deal with their fears. You can touch people; you can cook for them. Tell your family, friends, neighbors, and bosses that to get infected, they'd have to have their skin punctured with contaminated blood. Hepatitis C primarily is a blood-to-blood virus. People get it from transfusions, shared drug needles, tattoos, body piercing, borrowed razors, and so on.

Patients such as hemophiliacs and people on dialysis are at risk because of their exposure to blood and blood products. They make up about 10 percent of the hepatitis C population. Patients with a prior history of blood transfusion account for 20 percent (now, of course, tests screen donated blood for hepatitis C, and the risk of getting hepatitis C from a transfusion is exceedingly low); intravenous drug users represent 20 to 50 percent of cases; and 20 to 40 percent don't know how they came into contact with contaminated blood.

A Silent Epidemic

Hepatitis C is called the silent epidemic because you can have the virus and not know it. It's unusual to have severe symptoms until the end-stages of liver disease—a process that, if it occurs, may take decades. So it's hard for people to believe they're infected. Here's Hedy:

> In December of 1992, I went to my family doctor for a regular checkup. I didn't feel sick, just tired, but that's not unusual for me because I have a thyroid condition. Blood tests showed my liver enzymes were a little above normal. I agreed to stay off alcohol and repeat the tests every month for three months. No change. A specialist ordered more tests and a liver biopsy.
>
> My family doctor called with the results: "Inactive hepatitis C—the best outcome we could hope for." The next day, he phoned again. "There's been a mistake," he said in a sad, tentative voice. "The pathologist reread your slide, and it's mild chronic active hepatitis C."
>
> My stomach clenched. I felt a cold rush of fear, even though I didn't know what hepatitis C was or what to expect.

Hepatitis C usually progresses slowly, with peaks and valleys of activity. Although it's a serious illness, it's important to keep perspective. We now believe that hepatitis C becomes chronic in 55 to 85 percent of infected people.

While it's true that one-third of patients with chronic hepatitis C may develop cirrhosis (scarring of the liver), two-thirds may not. One of five people with cirrhosis may also get hepatocellular carcinoma, a form of liver cancer, but four out of five will not. The frustrating problem is that we can't precisely predict outcomes for individual patients.

A time bomb, the virus can lurk in the body for decades, silently injuring your liver and setting the stage for complications from liver disease.

> *I had a high-detail, difficult job managing a department store, so at first I thought it was too much stress. I felt foggy, confused. I forgot appointments, couldn't concentrate on the paperwork. Finally, I called a doctor. Maybe I was cracking up. I figured he'd give me an anti-depressant.*
>
> *Two days before my appointment, my eyes turned yellow, my stomach was out to here, and I itched all over. The diagnosis? Cirrhosis, end-stage liver disease caused by hepatitis C. My life narrowed down to two choices: die or get on a waiting list for a liver transplant.*
>
> *Jim*

We need to get the word out that hepatitis C is a major public health problem. Many people have no idea they're carrying the virus, but it's the most prevalent form of chronic hepatitis in the United States. When did this silent epidemic begin?

The Discovery of Hepatitis C

In the 1970s, researchers developed blood tests to identify the viruses that cause hepatitis A and B. However, it became apparent that many blood samples responsible for cases of post-transfusion hepatitis tested negative for A and B. For lack of a better term, scientists called this virus non-A, non-B hepatitis.

Then, in the 1980s—breakthrough! After many years of work, investigators under the direction of Daniel W. Bradley and Michael Houghton at the CDC and Chiron Corporation finally identified the virus in non-A, non-B infected blood. They used specialized genetic chemistry to identify the virus, and with this discovery, they were able to give it a name: hepatitis C.

In 1990 the first test for the hepatitis C virus (HCV) became commercially available. Routine physical examinations and blood bank screens uncovered an explosion of cases.

> *In my mail yesterday was a letter from the blood bank. They had refused my blood because it showed up positive for hepatitis C. What a shock! I couldn't believe it. I've never been sick a day in my life. What is hepatitis C?*
>
>   *Tom*

Understanding Hepatitis C

To understand hepatitis C, it helps to define three terms:
- hepatitis
- virus
- hepatitis C virus or HCV

What Is Hepatitis? Hepatitis simply means inflammation of the liver. Many injurious agents can cause hepatitis, including alcohol, medications, drugs, toxins, or viruses.

Unfortunately, the public hears so many stories of celebrities who injured their livers with substance abuse that they tend to lump all forms of liver disease together. As anyone with hepatitis C can tell you, it's not uncommon (although extremely unfair) to be labeled an alcoholic, even if you've never taken a drink.

> *When I finally tell someone I have hepatitis C, the atmosphere changes. I've had people give me this airbrush handshake because they don't want to touch me. Or they'll say, "Isn't that what that baseball star had? Didn't he drink himself to death?" Suddenly, there's this invisible wall.*
>
>   *Sara*

During the past 30 years, scientists have discovered hepatitis viruses A through E. Each virus has its own ways of infecting people, but it's hard for the public to see the differences.

It's an awkward moment when you let friends know you have this disease. They don't know what to say, and most of what they know about viruses has to do with AIDS, so you get a lot of weird stares and silences. You can see the stereotypes running through their heads. I'm so tired of explaining that the virus is almost never passed sexually, that it's a blood-to-blood thing.

Bob

What Is a Virus? The name virus evokes fear in people, fear of the unknown, the invisible. Viruses are not visible to the human eye or by standard microscopy; you need an electron microscope to see them. Despite their small size, viruses carry genetic material with enough punch to injure our organs and bodies and even cause death.

Viruses are as old as humankind—possibly older. Archeologists have unearthed an Egyptian mummy that bears pockmarks, evidence of the smallpox virus thousands of years ago. Among other diseases, viruses cause polio, mononucleosis, rabies, herpes, yellow fever, influenza, measles, rubella, chickenpox, mumps, the common cold—and new plagues, such as Ebola and AIDS.

"A virus," said Nobel Laureate Sir Peter Medawar, "is a piece of bad news wrapped in protein."[1] And that about sums it up. A virus contains a center of nucleic acid (the viral genes) surrounded by a protein coat.

When a virus's coat attaches to a cell in the body, the virus's genes enter the cell. It orders the cell to stop its own work and to make more viruses instead. In time, the virus multiplies to infect other cells.

Alerted to danger, the body's immune system sends out antibodies, special types of proteins, to stick to the invading virus and neutralize it. Viruses, however, are able to change and mutate to evade these antibodies.

Unfortunately, the hepatitis C virus is particularly good at mutating, which makes it difficult for scientists to create a vaccine. It's been hard to hit this moving target.

What Is the Hepatitis C Virus (HCV)? HCV is a single-stranded ribonucleic acid (RNA) virus organized like the RNA of flaviviruses, a family of viruses that produce yellow fever, dengue, and Japanese encephalitis. To complicate the hepatitis C picture even more, at least six distinct genetic strains (or genotypes) of the HCV virus have been identified.

The Hepatitis Viral Alphabet

When you tell someone you have hepatitis C, you usually end up fielding a lot of questions that have to do with other forms of viral hepatitis: "Do you get it from sex? From dirty food?" It helps to know the facts about the hepatitis alphabet—from A to G. Take Hedy's situation:

> For a long time, I didn't talk about hepatitis C except to my husband and kids. When I finally told a couple of good friends, I don't know what I expected—sympathy, horror. I didn't expect my friend to make light of the whole thing. "Maybe you ate in a dirty restaurant," she said. "No big deal. You'll be fine." I explained how hepatitis A spread.
>
> When I told a second friend, she looked so uncomfortable, I knew she thought I had been infected sexually. I finally convinced her that she was thinking of hepatitis B.
>
> Neither understood, and I felt frustrated and annoyed. I don't know why I was so upset. Before I knew I had hepatitis C, I didn't know what the differences among hepatitis viruses were either. It doesn't make sense, but it took me a long time before I felt ready to talk to a friend again.

As you now know, hepatitis means inflammation of the liver. The most common cause of hepatitis is viral. Hepatitis viruses primarily attack the liver, while other viruses (such as the herpes or mononucleosis viruses) injure the liver as part of a generalized infection.

We know at least five distinct hepatitis viruses, identified by the letters A through E. Blood tests distinguish and diagnose the different forms, but the public tends to lump them all together.

Hepatitis A. Outbreaks of this virus occur because of poor hygiene—a contaminated water supply or, for example, inadequate hand washing in a day-care facility. Hepatitis A, excreted in feces, is the most common cause of food or waterborne epidemic hepatitis. Areas of high prevalence include Mexico, Central America, Sub-Saharan Africa, Southeast Asia, and the Middle East.

People who contract hepatitis A typically develop flu-like symptoms within 10 to 40 days of exposure (the acute stage). They experience low-grade fever, muscle aches, joint aches, headache, malaise, anorexia, and mild abdominal pain. Often, but not always, these symptoms are rapidly followed by jaundice, a yellowing of the whites of the eyes and skin. In the vast majority of cases, the patient recovers completely with lifelong immunity against re-infection.

Hepatitis A never persists after the acute infection, so people don't develop chronic hepatitis, cirrhosis, or liver cancer. Rarely, in approximately one out of 1,000 cases, does the patient have severe acute hepatitis leading to liver failure and urgent need for transplantation.

An effective vaccine that prevents hepatitis A is available. It is currently recommended that patients with chronic hepatitis C receive hepatitis A vaccine.

Hepatitis B. Hepatitis B spreads primarily through blood inoculation: transfusions of blood or blood products, intravenous illicit drug use, hemodialysis, cardiac bypass surgery, or accidental needle-stick. It also spreads readily by sexual contact, both heterosexual and homosexual, and close personal contact, and can easily be transmitted from mother to infant at delivery.

Ninety to 95 percent of adults infected with hepatitis B clear the infection and maintain lifelong immunity. Rarely, a patient may develop liver failure from severe acute hepatitis B. The remaining 5 to 10 percent do not clear the virus. They become carriers or develop chronic hepatitis and risk progression to cirrhosis or liver cancer.

Untreated newborns who acquire hepatitis B from their mothers often develop lifelong infection. The good news is that treating the newborn with HBIG (hepatitis B immune globulin) and hepatitis B vaccine immediately after delivery prevents transmission in more than 95 percent of cases.

People with acute hepatitis B have the same symptoms as people with any other form of acute hepatitis. Chronic sufferers may not have symptoms or may complain of chronic fatigue, malaise, poor energy, and episodic jaundice.

Current FDA-approved medical therapies for chronic hepatitis B are interferon alfa-2b, peginterferon alfa-2a, lamivudine, adefovir, and entecavir. A highly effective vaccine that prevents hepatitis B is available. It is currently recommended that patients with chronic hepatitis C receive hepatitis B vaccine.

Hepatitis C. Hepatitis C is transmitted by blood, like hepatitis B. However, unlike hepatitis B, it seems to be poorly transmitted by sexual contact and is infrequently passed (6 percent) from an otherwise healthy mother to her newborn.

We've been married 15 years. I told my wife—and the doctor told my wife—that she doesn't have hepatitis C after sleeping with me all these years, and that it would be extremely rare to get it from sex.

We could use protection if that would help her feel safer. But it's pretty lonely. She doesn't even hug me anymore.

Ralph

Most infected people may not be aware that they had a past episode of acute hepatitis. In general, symptoms of acute hepatitis C are mild and liver enzyme elevations in the blood are modest. Two chronically infected patients may have identical symptoms and liver enzyme tests but very different results from a biopsy—from mild, benign histology (the study of the liver tissue under the microscope) to advanced injury with cirrhosis. Patients may be candidates for interferon-based therapy; the current, most widely used is the combination of pegylated interferon plus ribavirin.

Today, hepatitis C is the leading indication for liver transplantation. Twenty to 40 percent of patients on liver transplant waiting lists have hepatitis C. The virus recurs in the transplanted liver, and treatment may be necessary.

Hepatitis D. Hepatitis D, or delta hepatitis, is an incomplete virus that requires the presence of hepatitis B in order to complete its life cycle. For this reason, delta is typically found only in patients who have hepatitis B. Most patients with chronic hepatitis B, however, are not co-infected with hepatitis D.

Risk factors are the same as for hepatitis B. Hepatitis B patients co-infected with delta have a greater chance of developing fulminant hepatitis (a sudden, severe attack), more severe chronic active hepatitis, and an increased rate of progression to cirrhosis. The virus does not seem to have a major effect on hepatitis B patients' response to interferon therapy or on their survival or on the recurrence of hepatitis B after a liver transplant.

Hepatitis E. Symptoms are the same as hepatitis A. It is only acute. Cases in the United States appear to be imports from Central America, Mexico, and the Indian subcontinent. In most instances, patients don't become chronic carriers, and the virus is not associated with hepatocellular cancer.

Currently no vaccine or specific medical therapy exists. Acute hepatitis E acquired during pregnancy has been associated with high rates of maternal and fetal mortality. The Centers for Disease Control in Atlanta, GA, offer testing.

Hepatitis C: How Close Is a Cure?

Viruses are so complex, they can be a frustrating experience for patients who want to know more about them. Here's Hedy's experience:

> I'm a p.k.—a preacher's kid—and I'd always been taught that it was good to study and learn and understand. So when I knew I had hepatitis C, I ran to the library.
>
> As a writer, I've done medical research before, but I couldn't make sense out of the numbers and initials and blood types and medical jargon. It was really frustrating. It took a while for me to relax and admit that it was beyond me. It took even longer to realize that part of the problem was that scientists didn't have the answers either.

Researchers have grown the HCV virus in the laboratory and are studying the details of how the virus reproduces. The results could lead to a better understanding of how the virus gains entry to our liver cells and how it reproduces. This knowledge will be instrumental in developing new drugs and therapy to fight hepatitis C.

Recently, several laboratories isolated special enzymes of the hepatitis C virus called helicase and proteases. Researchers have developed specific drugs that will inhibit these enzymes and are currently testing them in patients. The future holds much promise.

Interferon-based treatment has also shown remarkable improvement with progressively increased rates of viral clearance. Ten to 15 percent of patients treated with standard interferon monotherapy cleared the virus. Combination therapy with ribavirin was the next big step in treatment with interferon. Sustained rates of viral clearance were 38 to 47 percent. Here's Hedy:

I was hesitant to try interferon when I was first diagnosed because I was worried about the side effects, leery of giving myself injections, and concerned about the low rates of success. A second biopsy showed my liver was getting much worse, and that gave me the push I needed to commit to treatment. I started with interferon monotherapy, responded—much to my surprise—then relapsed.

Combination therapy had just become available, and my doctor put me on that right away. I stayed on for a year—a long, hard year—but the results were worth it. Even though I was genotype 1b, I cleared the virus. It's been six years now since I finished treatment, and I'm grateful every day!

Hedy

The current standard of care is the combination of pegylated interferon plus ribavirin, resulting in sustained viral clearance of approximately 55 percent. Ninety-nine percent of patients who have a sustained viral clearance by six months post-treatment remain free of virus. Therefore, more than 50 percent of patients treated today may be "cured" of hepatitis C.

As a doctor, I'm excited when a patient conquers and clears the hepatitis C virus. Many patients fail to clear the virus but still have other victories along the way. Any illness, especially a chronic one, tests a person's limits. My hope is that the following chapters will help you learn more about hepatitis C and make you more comfortable with your choices and challenges from day to day.

The beginning of wisdom is to call things by their right names.

Chinese proverb

Reference
1. Peter Radetsky, *The Invisible Invaders: Viruses and the Scientists Who Pursue Them* (Boston: Little Brown and Co., 1994) p. 8.

2

WHEN YOU HAVE HEPATITIS C

Understanding the Diagnosis:
Blood Tests and Biopsies

For two years I knew there was something wrong. I was tired all the time. In a weird way it was almost a relief when my doctor came up with a diagnosis. Finally, I knew I wasn't crazy or a hypochondriac.

But hepatitis C? My skin wasn't yellow, and I didn't feel that bad. I blurted out the first thing that came into my head: "Did you make a mistake?"

Kevin

"BUT I FEEL FINE!" many of my patients say when I tell them that blood tests show they have hepatitis C. They often follow with, "Are you sure?" All of us, when we hear upsetting news, have the same reaction. A layer of protective denial shelters us from absorbing the news too quickly. We feel almost numb. Then, as our bodies adapt to the increased stress, we start to question. Could there be a mistake?

This chapter answers that question and many others about the testing process for hepatitis C from the time you are diagnosed through the years of ongoing care. It covers the following topics:

- Can Diagnostic Tests Be Wrong?
  ELISA
  Testing Limits
  HCV RNA Assays
   1. Quantitative PCR Assay
   2. Qualitative PCR Assay
  Genotyping and Quasispecies
  Liver Imaging Tests
   Ultrasonography (US, Ultrasound)
   Computed Tomography (CT Scan)
   Magnetic Resonance Imaging (MRI)

- Liver Biopsy
  Biopsy Procedure

- Interpreting Biopsy Results

- Liver Blood Tests
  Liver Enzymes
  Bilirubin
  Albumin
  Clotting Factors
  Alpha-Fetoprotein
  Complete Blood Count

- Noninvasive Testing
  Testing, Testing

Can Diagnostic Tests Be Wrong?

Although current tests for hepatitis C are very good, none are perfectly accurate. Every test has a low rate of both false positives and false negatives. To understand why, you have to learn a little bit about the way these tests work. Most of the tests for hepatitis C measure antibodies that your body produces against the virus. Other tests can actually measure the virus itself (RNA), quantitate levels of the virus, and determine the viral subtype.

When hepatitis C invades the body, your immune system, which is like an army, sends protein "soldiers" into your bloodstream. These proteins are antibodies, and they shape themselves to match molecules (called antigens) on the surface of the virus. The antibodies attach themselves to the hepatitis C virus, and your body's white blood cells then move in to destroy the invader.

The two primary blood tests used to detect hepatitis C, ELISA and RIBA assays, work by reacting to hepatitis C antibodies.

ELISA. Early tests produced many false-positive results and did not detect the virus in about one-third of cases. If you were diagnosed from 1989 to 1992, and you were never treated or retested, you may want to ask your doctor about repeat testing.

Let's go back to the original question, "Can my diagnosis be wrong?" The rate of false-positive reports is very low with current ELISA assays. Therefore, a positive test usually indicates infection.

The Food and Drug Administration approved a home testing kit for measuring hepatitis C antibodies in 1999. Initial studies suggest that results with this test are similar to standard blood tests.

Resource: The Hepatitis C Check, made by Home Access Health Company of Hoffman Estates, Ill., contains a lancet for obtaining a sample of blood, filter paper, and a mailer. Results are available anonymously by phone through a unique identification number.

Testing Limits. The above diagnostic tests measure your antibody response to the hepatitis C virus. They don't measure the virus itself. Antibodies may stay in your body even after you've cleared the virus. A positive result, therefore, means one of the following:

1. You've got an ongoing infection with hepatitis C.
2. You've been exposed to hepatitis C but you're not currently infected. (Some lucky people apparently do fight off HCV on their own, as many as 15 to 45 percent; others may respond to interferon and clear the virus.)

I found out I had hepatitis C when I donated blood and got a letter from the blood bank. What a shock! I didn't go to a doctor right away because I had recently changed jobs and I was waiting for my new insurance papers to arrive. So I joined a support group to find out what the heck I had.

They were all talking about a test that measured the amount of virus in your blood. After my insurance papers came, I had the test done and it came back negative—zero—nothing. Do I have hepatitis C or not?

Karen

HCV RNA Assays. Karen tested positive for hepatitis C antibodies. But when she took a test that directly measured the virus in her blood, called the quantitative HCV RNA assay, she tested negative. Does she have hepatitis C or not?

1. **Quantitative Assay.** This method measures the amount of hepatitis C and is used for monitoring people on interferon therapy to see if they are clearing the virus.
2. **Qualitative Assay.** Qualitative assays are so sensitive that they can detect as few as 50 virus particles per milliliter of blood. Modifications, such as Transcription Mediated Amplification (TMA) will make these tests even more sensitive.

Getting back to Karen's case, a quantitative assay can give different results at different times. Sensitivity and reproducibility of assays vary among laboratories, and viral levels in your body may fluctuate. Perhaps Karen had only a small amount of virus in her blood, so small the test cannot detect it. If she is retested for HCV RNA using the more sensitive qualitative test and is still negative, she had been exposed to hepatitis C and cleared it. The positive antibody reflects her immune response to the virus.

Here's Hedy's experience:

The first time I had a PCR test, the results were mathematical gobbledygook: 5.5 x 10^6 viral particles per milliliter of blood. What does that mean? Is that high? Low?

I wanted to hear that I had a low level of virus. For days, I was quietly depressed. Many months later, I had another PCR. I was prepared to hear I had the same or higher results. To my surprise, the viral count was down, way down. I was glad, but it also made me begin to accept how little control I have over this virus.

What do the numbers mean? What's high and what's low? Anything less than 2×10^6 is low. A number greater than 2×10^6 is considered high.

Genotyping and Quasispecies. After you've gone through these tests, you may want to know your genotype (genetic strain). The hepatitis C virus is really a whole family of viruses with six major genotypes. In the United States, types 1a and 1b account for 70 to 75 percent of cases. Different genotypes are more common elsewhere in the world.

Why is this important? We've learned that the genotypes respond differently to therapy. Genotypes 1a and 1b are relatively resistant to antiviral therapy. By contrast, genotypes 2 and 3 seem to respond better. However, we still can't accurately predict success or failure of therapy in an individual based on the HCV genotype. I've seen patients with all genotypes respond to therapy. Here's Hedy:

> When I learned that my genotype is 1b, I became even more leery of treatment. Other statistics also worked against me. I was older, I'd been infected for more than 30 years, and my latest biopsy was worse.
>
> I felt pretty sorry for myself until my sense of humor kicked in. So what if I wasn't a risk-taker? So what if I wasn't lucky, and the only lottery prize I ever won was an ugly crocheted hat at a charity bazaar? It was way past time to start treatment. I'd do whatever I had to do—and give it my best.
>
> Combination therapy worked for me. Six years later, I'm still in remission.

Another predictor of response to therapy may be the number of quasispecies of hepatitis C circulating in the patient's blood. Because the virus mutates so freely, patients often have multiple copies of the hepatitis C virus that vary genetically. This phenomenon is called quasispecies, meaning that the hepatitis C infection actually exists as a diverse set of hepatitis C RNAs within a given genotype.

Patients with the largest number of quasispecies may have more aggressive liver disease and a higher failure rate when treated with antiviral therapy. Patients who have had hepatitis C infection for longer periods of time are more likely to have a greater number of quasispecies. Currently, there are no commercially available tests to establish the degree of quasispecies within a given patient. These studies have been conducted primarily by research labs.

Liver Imaging Tests. Don't be alarmed if your doctor orders an ultrasound or a CT scan. The tests give information about the size and shape of your liver.

Ultrasonography (US, Ultrasound). Ultrasonography is a safe and painless way to investigate the size, structure, and the vascular (blood) supply of the liver. It's the preferred radiologic technique for an initial assessment for liver tumors.

Ultrasonic waves penetrate the body tissues and a recording device picks up reflected sound waves that yield an image of the liver. You can compare it to exploring for oil by using seismographic recordings of the earth's formations.

Ultrasound helps find out liver size and texture and the size of bile ducts and blood vessels. Doppler probes added to ultrasound can detect direction and rates of blood flow in vessels going to and from the liver. Your physician may order ultrasound to pinpoint the liver's location just before a biopsy.

Computed Tomography (CT Scan). Unlike ultrasound, computed tomography (CT scan) uses a highly sophisticated X-ray machine to scan the internal organs with minimal radiation. CT scans are used to confirm the findings of ultrasound and to get a clearer view because, unlike ultrasound, CT scans aren't blocked by air in the bowel. The scans are also more standardized and much less dependent on the expertise of

FIGURE 2A. CT SCANS OF NORMAL LIVER, CIRRHOTIC LIVER, AND LIVER TUMOR (HEPATOMA)

| NONCIRRHOTIC | CIRRHOTIC | LIVER CANCER (HEPATOMA) |

LEGEND 2A: CT scans are specialized radiologic tests that allow one to peer inside the abdomen. The image on the left demonstrates a normal liver and spleen. The middle panel depicts a liver with a knobby irregular surface and an enlarged spleen (⇨) in a cirrhotic patient. The image to the right shows a liver cancer (hepatoma) in the middle of the liver (➡). The patient with the cancer was treated by chemoembolization of the tumor and liver transplantation and is currently alive without evidence of tumor.

the technician performing the test. CT scans define the size and texture of the liver and can detect an early liver tumor (see Figure 2A).

Magnetic Resonance Imaging (MRI). Unlike ultrasound and CT scans, MRI measures special signals from the body's water molecules. Images are created from these signals. Magnetic resonance imaging is used mainly to diagnose liver cancers.

Liver Biopsy

Just the word "biopsy" strikes fear into people's hearts, but it's an essential part of your treatment. Only a biopsy can give your doctor a true idea of the condition of your liver. You need a biopsy for two reasons:

1. It confirms the diagnosis and rules out other disorders, such as granulomatous liver disease, infections, or biliary tract disorders. Liver biopsy along with ultrasound or a CT scan can be used to pinpoint the site of a lesion and rule out liver cancers.
2. It establishes the stage and degree of activity of hepatitis C. Typically, chronic viral hepatitis passes in sequence from a mild inflammatory stage to fibrosis and, later, cirrhosis. Biopsies may be done over many years to record the progression. Once cirrhosis has developed, there is little reason to continue the biopsies.

Biopsy Procedure. Years ago, liver biopsies were often performed under general anesthesia and required a short hospital stay. Today it's an outpatient procedure that literally takes seconds. In fact, you'll spend most of your time getting ready for the biopsy. However, it is invasive, and you will be asked to sign an informed consent form. It's a good idea to select a doctor who frequently performs this procedure and is very familiar with it. Biopsies may be performed every three to five years.

I didn't tell my wife I tested positive for hepatitis C; I didn't want to worry her. When my doctor ordered a biopsy and explained what it was, I figured "piece of cake."

I took the afternoon off from work and drove myself to the hospital and back, but we had tickets to a play that evening. I got back home with no time to rest. The play was a bad idea. We had to leave early, and the whole story came tumbling out. That was the end of my macho phase.

Kevin

As you can see from Kevin's story, it's helpful to plan a quiet, restful period after a biopsy. In my experience, most patients' fears come from not knowing what to expect. Here's how the procedure goes:

Your physician examines you carefully to decide exactly where to place the biopsy needle and cleanses the skin with iodine or an antiseptic solution. Then you'll get a local anesthetic, as you do at the dentist's, at the spot where the biopsy needle will be placed. Some doctors also prescribe intravenous benzodiazepine with a narcotic to lessen the anxiety and discomfort.

You'll feel strong pressure when the needle is inserted, but the whole procedure takes only a few seconds for a small core of tissue to be obtained. Then you'll be rolled onto your right side to help control any bleeding from the surface of the liver. You'll stay in the procedure area for two to four hours for observation. If you're stable, with no symptoms, you'll be discharged. Otherwise, you may be admitted to the hospital for observation.

After performing biopsies on hundreds of patients, I've seen very few complications. Reported rates vary from 1 percent to 0.1 percent. If the most common complication occurs, bleeding from the surface of the liver, the patient may require transfusions or even an operation. In rare cases, the biopsy needle may pierce another organ, such as the bowel, gallbladder, kidney, or lung. Death occurs very rarely, in less than one in 1,000 cases.

Interpreting Biopsy Results

Your doctor will tell you the results of your biopsy in terms of histologic stages. Histology means the examination of tissue under the microscope. There are four histologic stages in liver injury due to hepatitis C:

- **Stage I** is characterized by inflammation without the development of any scar tissue.
- **Stage II** features include inflammation with early scarring (fibrosis) in one zone (portal) of the liver.
- **Stage III** shows bridging of the fibrosis between adjacent portal tracts.
- **Stage IV** is cirrhosis (advanced scarring with loss of normal liver architecture).

Histologic stages don't correspond very well to the duration of infection. For example, a patient with slowly progressive disease may maintain

FIGURE 2B. HISTOLOGIC STAGES OF HEPATITIS B

STAGE I   STAGE II   STAGE III   STAGE IV

LEGEND 2B: This figure demonstrates the progressive microscopic changes that may occur in livers infected with viral hepatitis. Stage I shows only mild inflammation in the portal tract; stage II exhibits more inflammation with spread of fibrosis (scar tissue) into adjacent liver cells; stage III implies that fibrosis has spread between portal tracts; stage IV is cirrhosis with formation of nodules.

an early histologic stage for many years or even decades. Another patient may progress to cirrhosis in less than a decade. The stages of liver damage are distinctive under the microscope (see Figure 2B).

Physicians use certain specific terms when interpreting liver biopsies from patients with hepatitis C. Here's a quick translation:

Stage of Disease	Terminology
Early stage, mild activity (I)	Chronic Persistent Hepatitis C or Mild Chronic Active Hepatitis C
Intermediate stage (II or III)	Chronic Active Hepatitis C with Fibrosis
Advanced stage (IV)	Cirrhosis

Liver Blood Tests

Life with hepatitis C means lots of blood tests to monitor your condition. Have you ever wondered what the numbers really mean? Read the next few pages to review and understand the warning signals of five basic blood tests:

1. enzymes
2. bilirubin
3. albumin
4. clotting factors
5. complete blood count

Doctors frequently test blood in viral hepatitis patients because blood tests warn of changes. The most informative tests "dip" into the bloodstream to measure liver injury (enzymes) or assess liver function (bilirubin, albumin, clotting factors, complete blood count). At first, you may feel intimidated by medical terminology, acronyms, and numbers, but learning about these basic tests will help you understand your doctor's interpretation of results (see Table 2A). Hedy says:

> *Who ever heard of this complicated stuff before hepatitis C? At first, I kept track of my liver enzymes religiously, writing each ALT and AST score on a yellow legal pad. I ignored the other numbers on the lab report.*
>
> *Now I understand that the other function tests let me know how my liver is coping with the infection—like looking into the liver without a microscope. I always ask for a copy of my test results, and I keep my own file. It helps me feel as if I'm doing all I can on my end.*

Liver Enzymes. A liver cell produces proteins, called enzymes, that live within the cell or its membranes. In a way, you can think of your liver as a powerful chemical factory; it changes raw materials into the substances your body needs. Enzymes are catalysts that help a liver cell do its job of creating the specific chemical changes that give your body fuel to live. Here are the names of the enzymes you need to remember:

• ALT (SGPT)—alanine aminotransferase
• AST (SGOT)—aspartate aminotransferase
• GGT—gamma-glutamyl transferase
• alkaline phosphatase

By measuring their level in your blood, doctors can monitor ongoing liver injury. Why? Under normal conditions, the level of these enzymes in your bloodstream is relatively low. But when liver cells are injured, destroyed, or die, the cell becomes leaky, and the enzymes escape into the blood that's circulating through the liver. When the cell is injured, liver enzyme levels in the blood rise.

Massive liver injury is associated with marked increases in ALT; mild injury may be associated with mild—or even no—increase in ALT. The correlation is strongest at earlier stages of hepatitis C, before the

TABLE 2A. NORMAL AND ABNORMAL VALUES FOR LABORATORY TESTS

Test	Normal Range	Abnormal Range	
		Mild to Moderate	Severe
Liver Enzymes			
AST	< 40 IU/L	40–200	> 200
ALT	< 40 IU/L	40–200	> 200
GGT	< 60 IU/L	60–200	> 200
Alkaline Phosphatase	<112 IU/L	112–300	> 300
Liver Function Tests			
Bilirubin	< 1.2 mg/dL	1.2–2.5	> 2.5
Albumin	3.5–4.5 g/dL	3.0–3.5	< 3.0
Prothrombin Time	< 14 seconds	14-17	> 17
Blood Count			
WBC	> 6000	3000–6000	< 3000
HCT	> 40	35–40	< 35
Platelets	> 150,000	100,000–150,000	< 100,000

KEY:
IU = International Units
L = liter
dL = deciliter
mg = milligrams
AST (SGOT) = aspartate aminotransferase
ALT (SGPT) = alanine aminotransferase
GGT = gamma-glutamyl transferase
WBC = white blood count
HCT = hematocrit (percentage of blood occupied by red blood cells)

development of cirrhosis. However, once cirrhosis occurs, ALT levels may not be high; therefore, ALT is no longer a good indicator of further liver damage.

What do the numbers mean? Table 2A shows normal and abnormal test values. Blood test patterns relate somewhat to the type of liver injury. Typical hepatitis C patients show increases in ALT and AST but little or no increase in GGT and alkaline phosphatase. Those with cirrhosis or who have an underlying disorder of the biliary tract (the ducts that drain bile from the liver into the intestine) may have modest elevations in GGT and alkaline phosphatase. In some unusual cases of hepatitis C, I have even seen a predominant elevation in GGT.

Patients tend to focus on their ALT and AST counts, but other tests are more important in measuring the health of your liver.

Bilirubin.

After the birth of my second child—a cesarean delivery that required blood transfusions—I learned I was infected with hepatitis C. My AST and ALT counts were only slightly elevated. The most important thing to me was raising my little boys as best I could for as long as I could. I wanted them to know their mother. So I decided to delay treatment and watch my bloodwork every three months.

I made it to my youngest son's ninth birthday when the test pattern changed. "Your bilirubin is up," my doctor said. "It's time to start interferon."

There went the PTA and baking cupcakes—but I did respond to interferon. A good trade.

Jill

When red blood cells complete their life cycle and break down naturally in your body, they produce a yellow pigment that's passed to the liver and excreted into bile. Bile helps your body digest food, but the pigment, which has no digestive function, is called bilirubin. Blood levels of bilirubin tend to fluctuate in patients with hepatitis, although a prolonged persistent elevation in bilirubin usually means severe liver dysfunction and possibly cirrhosis.

Here's why. Most of the time, the body produces as many red blood cells as it breaks down, so you produce a constant amount of bilirubin. However, if your blood cells break down more rapidly (hemolysis) or your liver function becomes impaired, the bilirubin levels in your blood rise.

Your liver has to go to work to take up the excess bilirubin into the liver cell, metabolize it to make it more water-soluble for excretion into bile, and send it through special passages and ducts into the intestine. Microbes in the gut continue to metabolize the bilirubin until you expel it. (Stercobilin, a brown pigment derived from bilirubin, creates the dark brown color of feces.)

When the liver fails to eliminate bilirubin from the blood, the skin and whites of the eyes turn yellow (jaundice), urine darkens, and the color of the bowel movement lightens. In case you've wondered, now you know why your doctor asks you probing questions about the color of your feces.

Albumin. Albumin is another protein synthesized (manufactured) by the liver. Liver cells secrete albumin to maintain the volume of blood in arteries and veins. When albumin levels drop to extremely low levels, fluid may leak out of the blood vessels into the surrounding tissues. This causes swelling, known as edema. Normal albumin levels range between 3.5 to 4.5 grams/deciliter. Usually, edema occurs when levels drop below 2.5 grams/deciliter.

Unlike liver enzyme increases, which occur within hours to days of the liver injury, albumin levels don't fall unless there has been chronic progressive liver injury for at least one month or more. This is because albumin has a long residence time in the plasma; its half-life is approximately 30 days. A decrease in serum albumin, therefore, reflects a slowly progressive, ongoing reduction in the liver's ability to synthesize this protein.

Be aware that there are non-liver reasons for albumin to decrease and your physician will take these into account when interpreting test results. Nonetheless, a significant sustained decrease in serum albumin may mean poor liver function and cirrhosis of the liver. Patients with very low albumin counts may need to be considered for liver transplantation.

Clotting Factors. Remember our comparison of the liver to a chemical factory? The liver also synthesizes many proteins that maintain normal blood clotting. Prothrombin time (PT) is the name of the most common test that measures a combination of blood clotting factors. If your prothrombin time increases, it means your liver isn't creating enough factors, so it takes your blood longer to clot.

Unlike albumin, clotting factors can decrease rapidly—within days, or even hours, of a severe liver injury. In severe cases, clotting disturbances may signal the need for an early transplant. In patients with chronic hepatitis and chronic liver disease, a prolonged prothrombin time can be a warning that the liver is having trouble with its synthetic functions.

Typically, doctors will administer vitamin K, a vitamin essential for normal clotting factors, to determine whether the clotting disorder is reversible. Patients who have persistent, prolonged elevations in prothrombin time that don't respond to vitamin K may need to be considered for liver transplantation.

Alpha-Fetoprotein. This is a protein that regenerative cells or cancer cells secrete into blood. Increased blood levels of alpha-fetoprotein may indicate the development of liver cancer (see Chapter 11).

Complete Blood Count. The complete blood count test can be a detection system for liver scarring. Blood from your spleen flows through your liver via the portal vein. When the liver becomes scarred, it creates resistance to this blood flow (called portal hypertension), and the blood may back up into the spleen. When this happens, the spleen enlarges and traps blood elements, removing them from circulation and lowering blood counts.

Although all components of the blood count may decrease, those most sensitive to this condition are the white blood cell and platelet counts. Patients with portal hypertension from cirrhosis of the liver often have low counts. Similarly, patients may have an enlarged spleen, resulting from severe cirrhotic disease, and may need to be considered for liver transplantation.

Noninvasive Testing

There are two FDA-approved commercially available blood tests, Fibrotest® and Fibrosure®. In addition, a noninvasive scanning device,

Fibroscan®, is under investigation. Finally, other tests using new technologies, including Hepquant®, are being developed. These new tests use blood samples or scanning to determine whether you have cirrhosis or varices.

Testing, Testing. In the past few years, I've seen the advancement of specific new tests that help monitor your health. But all too often I find that patients feel shut out by the complicated language of test results. Don't worry if you didn't absorb every detail. Use these pages as a reference guide.

Ask for copies of your tests. When you have questions, look up the explanations in these pages. Often, your physician can calm your fears if you voice them. Talk with your doctor.

Knowledge is power.

Francis Bacon

3

WHY ME?
WHAT ABOUT THEM?

How You Got Infected and
How to Avoid Infecting Others

When my doctor told me I had hepatitis C, I said, "No way! You've got the wrong blood test. It's got to be some kind of mix-up."

I've never had a transfusion or done drugs. Even when I had my ears pierced, it was with those disposable studs. I mean, I'm a really cautious person. What did I do to deserve this?

Juliana

WHEN YOU'RE DEALING with a serious illness, it's the most human thing in the world to ask, "Why me? What did I do to get hepatitis C?"

The answer is both simple and complex. Most likely you acquired hepatitis C when you came into contact with blood infected with the virus, and it gained entry into your bloodstream.

The complicating factor is that as many as 20 to 40 percent of people with hepatitis C fail to report the way in which they were exposed to infectious blood. And, unlike with hepatitis A or B, patients rarely recall a severe initial attack of the disease to mark the time of infection.

How did you get hepatitis C? And how can you avoid giving the virus to others? We'll discuss ways to protect your family and friends. In addition, we'll provide up-to-date summaries of documented ways that hepatitis C is transmitted, including:

- Intravenous Drug Abuse
- Intranasal Use of Cocaine
- Transfusion of Blood or Blood Products
    Surgery or Medical Treatment
    Hemophilia
- Needle-Stick Accidents
- Tattooing and Body Piercing
- Sharing Sharp Instruments
- Birth and Delivery (rare)
- Sexual Transmission (rare)
- Organ Transplantation (rare)
- How Can I Avoid Infecting Others?

Intravenous Drug Abuse

What's the most direct way to get hepatitis C? Inoculate the virus from infected blood into your own bloodstream. That's why one of the most common risk factors is a history of using intravenous illicit drugs. Many drug addicts share needles. They spread hepatitis among themselves and maintain a pool of infected people. Studies suggest that more than 75 percent of current or past users of intravenous drugs may have hepatitis C.

Although heavy drug abusers may be at greatest risk, many people who have hepatitis C report only rare experimentation in the distant past. Unfortunately, the wise decision to stop taking drugs doesn't erase the risk from prior use.

I'm a therapist. People come to me for help with drug abuse. But 20 years ago, when I was a college freshman, I went a little wild. For the first time I was away from home, and I did some drugs. And yes, I shared needles once or twice. If only I could go back and change what I did....

Jake

When I question patients about how they got the virus, they usually don't have a clue. I ask them if they've had transfusions or experimented with intravenous drugs. They're shocked. "Can that do it?" they'll say. "It was only once or twice."

When we don't know how the person got hepatitis C, we call it "sporadic" or "community acquired." Some doctors think that most of these cases are due to prior use of intravenous drugs. Patients who are otherwise healthy, employed, and raising their families are stunned to hear they have hepatitis C. They can't believe the diagnosis relates to a past, seemingly insignificant experiment so long ago.

"I don't know how I could get hepatitis C from sharing needles. I was always so careful about cleaning them," patients often say. But to understand how contamination occurs, you have to appreciate how concentrated the virus is in the blood of infected patients.

The average patient with chronic hepatitis C has a blood concentration of the virus of two million particles per milliliter of whole blood. That's equivalent to 2,000 particles of virus in the amount of blood that would sit on the head of a small stickpin. With this concentration it's easy to see that wiping or rinsing a needle with water or salt solutions won't remove all the virus particles. Indeed, a large amount of virus may remain on the needle.

A concentrated solution of hydrogen peroxide will kill or inactivate the virus, and cleaning needles with this solution may reduce the risk of transmission. It won't protect you, however, if cleaning is superficial, such as a quick rinse, or if the internal chamber of the needle is not irrigated and the syringe and all its external and internal parts are not cleansed. Some people rely on others to clean a syringe and don't realize that it's not done thoroughly.

We Americans face a tremendous public health problem from illegal drug use. According to the 2004 National Survey on Drug Use and Health, 19.1 million Americans age 12 and older were currently users of illicit drugs during the month prior to the survey interview. An estimated 2.0 million currently used cocaine, and an estimated 166,000 currently used heroin.

On a personal level, the risk factor rises each time you use drugs. If you shoot up once, you may or may not get hepatitis C. But if you shoot up many times, you can almost count on it. The best way to avoid the risk is to avoid illicit intravenous drugs and to teach the next generation to avoid this dangerous behavior.

Intranasal Use of Cocaine

Cocaine causes constriction of the blood vessels in the mucous membrane of the nose, leading to disruption of the lining and ulceration. A well-known consequence of chronic cocaine use is necrosis of the nasal septum, leaving a hole in the cartilage that separates the two nostrils. Sharing straws during cocaine use, therefore, can lead to blood-to-blood transmission of hepatitis C. A recent epidemiological study for risk factors for hepatitis C highly correlated hepatitis C with patients who were regular users of cocaine.

Transfusion of Blood or Blood Products

The risk of getting hepatitis C from the transfusion of blood or blood products has been steadily declining since the mid-1980s. Before 1986, there was virtually no screening of blood donors for hepatitis C (then called Non A/Non B), except for sporadic ALT testing. In 1986, blood banks throughout the United States began screening blood donors for hepatitis by measuring ALT (a liver enzyme) and hepatitis B core antibody. Use of these tests by blood banks reduced the risk of acquiring hepatitis C by transfusion one hundredfold.

Two recent, widely quoted studies (see Table 3A) reported the per unit transfusion risk for the screening procedures. As you can see, scientists developed a test for hepatitis C in 1990 and then improved it in 1992. As a result, the risk of contracting the virus from transfusions went way down.

Blood banks currently use both HCV antibody, version 3, and RNA tests and have done so since 2002. The stated risk for transmission is one

TABLE 3A. RISK OF POST-TRANSFUSION HEPATITIS C		
Era	Test screening	Cases per 10,000 units transfused
Prior to 1986	None	45
1986–1990	ALT, HBcAb (HIV-Ab, 1985)	19
1990–1991	HCV-Ab, EIA 1	3
1992–1993	HCV-Ab, EIA 2	0.4
Current tests	HCV-Ab and HCV RNA assays	0.001

transmission per 2 million units transfused. Statisticians estimate the risk of infection as extremely low, but there's no such thing as zero risk.

Surgery or Medical Treatment. Certain medical procedures and operations were particularly associated with risk of acquiring hepatitis C due to the large number of transfusions required. These included hemodialysis, coronary artery bypass or heart surgery, lung resection, and major abdominal surgery.

Hemophilia. People with hemophilia lack certain clotting factors in their blood. In the past hemophiliacs were treated with plasma from a large number of donors. The plasma was combined and treated to extract those clotting factors.

Until the mid-1980s, hemophiliacs were at extreme risk for getting hepatitis B and HIV. Therefore, scientists pasteurized the clotting factor for hemophiliacs and this treatment inactivated the hepatitis C virus. When tests for hepatitis C became available in 1990, studies showed that hemophiliacs treated with unpasteurized preparations had an 80 to 90 percent chance of having hepatitis C, while those who received the pasteurized preparation had an extremely low risk, approaching zero percent. Today, current therapy often uses synthesized or genetically engineered clotting products with a zero risk of transmitting hepatitis C.

Resource: For more information, contact the National Hemophilia Foundation at 800-424-2634; website: www.hemophilia.org.

Needle-Stick Accidents

Health care workers face an occupational hazard: needle-stick accidents. Because many hospitalized patients and people who frequent emergency rooms have hepatitis, medical personnel run high risks if they accidentally get stuck with an infected needle, which can easily pierce rubber gloves. Here's Hedy:

> I watched the lab tech tie a rubber band around my arm. "I have hepatitis C," I said, noticing that she wore only one glove, so she could probe my skin to check for a 'good' vein. "You might want to put on another glove."
>
> "That's okay," she said, smiling. "I've got hepatitis C, too."

In one study of an inner city emergency room at Johns Hopkins Hospital in Baltimore, MD, 24 percent of 2,523 patients over age 15 were infected with at least one of three viruses: HIV (6 percent), hepatitis B (5 percent), or hepatitis C (18 percent). Eighty-three percent of the intravenous drug users, 21 percent of the people who had transfusions, and 21 percent of the homosexual male patients had hepatitis C. Of all the patients who were bleeding and who had invasive procedures performed, 30 percent had at least one virus.

This study shows the potential exposure of medical personnel to hepatitis C infection. HIV testing alone failed to identify 87 percent of those who had hepatitis B and 80 percent of patients with hepatitis C.

When I started my career as a medical technician, I got a needle stick. They gave me gamma globulin, but the supply was tainted until 1990. Then two years ago, they detected hepatitis C. I was really sick with infected fluid in my legs, and I was hemorrhaging. They gave me 25 units of blood.

Out of five people in our lab, three ended up with hepatitis C, but mine is the only one that became active. My doctor calls it "a thief in the night."

Erica

Fortunately, the risk of acquiring hepatitis C after a needle stick is relatively low. In two studies with a total of 201 cases of needle-stick accidents involving hepatitis C patients, transmission occurred in only 5 percent.

The best measure of virus in the blood is HCV RNA (see chapter 2, PCR assays). None of the RNA-negative patients transmitted HCV to the staff, but seven cases (10 percent) of hepatitis C developed in medical personnel who got the needle stick from an RNA-positive patient. These limited results suggest that health care workers receiving needle sticks from RNA-positive patients are at greatest risk.

More and more state laws and recent Department of Labor Occupational Safety and Health Administration (OSHA) directives now require the use of safe needle technology. Worldwide, unsafe injection practices cause an estimated 2.3 to 4.7 million hepatitis C infections a year. The World Health Organization and other partners have formed the Safe Injection Global Network (SIGN) to tackle the problem.

Tattooing and Body Piercing

Tattooing and body piercing are ancient rites in many cultures. In this country, we're witnessing a recent surge of interest in "body art." The practice of tattooing is particularly common in the military and among gang members and prisoners. It's also becoming an accepted cosmetic practice.

Celebrities have popularized the trend. Comedian Roseanne and ex-husband Tom Arnold had each other's names tattooed on their backsides. Famous athletes have decorated their bodies, including Mike Peluso's tattoo of the Stanley Cup and Steve Everitt's bleeding dagger. Unfortunately, even the most benign-appearing tattooing may have its dark side (see Figure 3A). Viral hepatitis, mainly hepatitis B, is the best-documented infection transmitted by tattoos in the 20th century.

> *Here's a switch. I'm a tattoo artist, and last year I found out I have hepatitis C. I have antibodies to hepatitis B, too. My joints hurt so much I can't work. I feel like I'm sliding down the evolutionary scale, because I can't move my opposable thumbs.*

FIGURE 3A: HEPATITIS C PATIENT WITH TATTOO

LEGEND 3A: This seemingly innocuous tattoo may have been a source of transmission of hepatitis C to this patient.

I'm sure I got hepatitis from a needle stick. Fifteen years ago, who wore gloves?

Peter

Nine percent of males and 1 percent of females in the United States get tattoos—with peak ages between 14 and 22. And tattoos are common in certain groups at high risk for hepatitis C and other viral infections: intravenous drug abusers, gang members, prostitutes, and prisoners. In one study 65 percent of prisoners had tattoos.

This flag on my arm—I was young and in the Navy. What did I know? Now I'm told that there are certified tattoo artists, and if you go to someone reputable, everything is sterilized.
Well, too late for me. It wasn't like that in Hong Kong.

Jerry

Tattooing involves shaving the skin, placing ink on it, then pushing the ink through the skin with a needle gun. A small amount of bleeding is common. The problem is that sterilization techniques vary, and home-tattooing kits may contain inadequate methods for sterilization. Other problems encountered with tattoo techniques are lack of disposable needles and repeated insertion of tattoo needles into potentially contaminated ink, which is then re-used on other clients.

Body piercing of the earlobes, nose, lips, and other areas also breaks the skin. Therefore, the principles and risk of transmission of hepatitis C are the same as in tattooing.

Resource: The Alliance for Professional Tattooists (APT) has developed a set of infection control guidelines in association with the FDA for its members. For a copy of "Basic Guidelines for Getting a Tattoo," access its website: www.safetattoos.com.

Sharing Sharp Instruments

Family and friends who live with hepatitis C patients don't appear to have an increased risk of getting the virus. Nonetheless, you should take care to prevent your blood, which contains hepatitis C, from inoculating another person accidentally.

Yesterday I found my oldest son, a teenager, standing in front of the bathroom mirror and trying to shave for the first time. I got so scared. My husband has hepatitis C.

Why didn't we see how fast our son was growing? Why didn't we warn him not to borrow his dad's razor?

Jan

Talk to family members and explain why it's important to avoid sharing razor blades, nail clippers, scissors, and toothbrushes. These measures are just good hygiene; it's also sensible to bandage any cuts or abrasions and to safely dispose of menstrual pads and tampons.

In my clinical experience I have seen only one case where transmission of viral hepatitis (hepatitis B, in this instance) from brother to sister occurred because they commonly shared a shaving razor blade.

Birth and Delivery

If you have hepatitis C and you're pregnant or planning a family, of course you're concerned about giving birth to a healthy baby. The period of risk occurs at delivery when the mother's and baby's blood may become intermixed. Mothers with hepatitis C who are otherwise healthy rarely transmit the virus to their newborns. The chance of transmitting hepatitis C from mother to baby at the time of delivery is approximately 6 percent. In contrast, mothers with HIV who are also infected with hepatitis C may transmit hepatitis C to their babies 15 percent or more of the time.

Mothers with hepatitis C often ask whether they can transmit the virus to their baby through breastfeeding. Current studies do not allow us to draw a definite conclusion. However, existing information suggests that hepatitis C is rarely—if ever—transmitted to an infant through breast milk. Even though hepatitis C may be detected in breast milk, it's likely that the baby's digestive juices and enzymes would destroy the virus (see Chapter 13).

Sexual Transmission

This is one of the most sensitive and troubling topics for patients. The risk of getting hepatitis C through sexual contact is minimal, but some spouses are wary. Trust dissolves, the gap widens, and the couple can end up in divorce court.

It's just as hard for singles. How do you start an intimate relationship without being honest about hepatitis C? And how will the other person react?

I'm single, and I'm not the smoothest, slickest character around. It's always been hard for me to meet women. Now I have to tell them I have hepatitis C. When should I tell them? Will they want to have anything to do with me?

Russ

I'm feeling low, depressed. I was dating this guy, and the relationship was going well. It felt right. Then he broke up with me two days ago. I'm trying not to be paranoid—I mean it could have happened anyway—but he broke up with me a week after I told him I had hepatitis C.

Nancy

Perhaps some solid information will help you come to grips with this issue. Compared to hepatitis B, hepatitis C circulates in your blood at relatively low levels. It is either not detected or found in low concentrations in body fluids, such as saliva, urine, feces, semen, or vaginal secretions.

The vast majority of sexual partners of patients with hepatitis C tests negative for hepatitis C. When a sexual partner does test positive, in most cases this partner has had other risk factors for acquiring hepatitis C, such as intravenous drug use or exposure to blood or blood products. In a study of selected couples without other risk factors, no case of sexual transmission of hepatitis C occurred—even after a calculated 713 person-years of exposure. In contrast, epidemiological studies suggest a higher risk. In my opinion, heterosexual transmission of hepatitis C is rare in a stable, single-partner relationship.

Sally's diagnosis shocked us. We were completely naive. She worried about giving me hepatitis C until we learned more and got a pretty good handle on it.

We've been cautious, but it's not like I'm terrified to go near her. We've been together six years, and I saw no reason to treat her differently or to change our behavior, because I was already exposed.

Sally felt dirty. I did everything I could to diffuse that. It didn't affect the way I felt about her. I kissed her the day before the diagnosis, so why not kiss her the day after?

Ken

My husband got completely paranoid. When I first found out I had hepatitis C, I wanted him to say, "We'll get through this together," but he didn't. He was really nice for a week, then he started getting hostile. He couldn't handle it. I think a big part of it was that we were getting conflicting information about whether or not you can transmit the virus sexually.

We were having troubles before—and I guess the added strain was too much. During my fifth month of interferon, he left me and our three-year-old daughter.

Danielle

Sexual transmission of hepatitis C may be more frequent in homosexual males or highly promiscuous heterosexuals. Some sexual practices are more traumatic to body tissues. For example, anal intercourse may disrupt the lining of the rectum and allow blood, containing hepatitis C, to enter the blood of a sexual partner.

Organ Transplantation

Can a person get hepatitis C from a transplanted organ? Yes, if the donor has hepatitis C, the virus will infect the recipient of the donor organ. Two studies address this issue.

In one study, 28 percent of patients who received organs from donors with hepatitis C developed clinical evidence of liver disease during a follow-up period ranging from three months to six and a half years. In a second study, all the recipients who did not have hepatitis C before the transplant, and who received an organ from a hepatitis C donor, developed hepatitis C after the transplant.

In the University of Colorado liver transplant program, we restrict the use of organs from hepatitis C patients to two situations: recipients already infected with hepatitis C or recipients in desperate medical condition who are awaiting a donor organ at the highest urgency status (hospitalized on life support and not likely to survive seven days without a transplant).

Can you, as a hepatitis C patient, donate an organ for transplanting? Yes. Even though you have hepatitis C, you may still be able to donate your organs for transplant. The organs most commonly used are the kidney and liver, but only if the liver shows no active disease or scarring.

How Can I Avoid Infecting Others?

My patients often inquire about protecting friends and family from the virus. Here are some common questions people ask:

Is it okay to kiss and hug my kids? Yes, you can kiss and hug your children, and they can kiss and hug you back. There is no data to suggest that you could infect your children by these actions.

Should I have members of my family tested for hepatitis C? The risk of transmission from you to other family members, including your spouse, is very low through casual contact and heterosexual activity and, in general, testing is not necessary. If your spouse or child has elevated liver enzyme tests, then they should be tested for hepatitis C. Children of infected mothers should be tested. If family members had any blood-to-blood contact, they should be tested.

Can I cook for my family? What if I cut myself while I'm preparing food? Certainly you can cook for your family. Even if you cut yourself and get blood in the food, it's unlikely that anyone eating the food will get hepatitis C. The enzymes in the digestive tract will destroy or inactivate the virus.

What if my child or friend eats food off my plate or uses my fork? You don't transmit hepatitis C by sharing drinks or food. Hepatitis C is transmitted by contaminated blood entering your bloodstream—not your stomach.

In some Asian cultures, caregivers pre-chew food for babies. It is hypothetically possible to transmit hepatitis C through saliva if the chewer and baby have mouth sores or bloody gums. Sharing of toothbrushes and anything else that might come in contact with blood or body fluids can also expose people to the same hypothetical risks. Even though these are not common or likely infection routes, it makes good common sense to avoid such behaviors for hygienic reasons.

My teenager borrowed my manicure scissors. Is that a problem? I recommend that you avoid sharing sharp instruments. There is a possibility that if your teenager cut herself on your scissors, she could inoculate herself with blood you might have left on the scissors. It's best to avoid sharing all sharp instruments, such as nail clippers, razor blades, toothbrushes, etc.

We've been married for 15 years. Is it safe to have sex? The existing information indicates that sexual transmission between individuals in a stable, single partner, monogamous relationship rarely—if ever—occurs. In addition, people involved in a stable relationship do not need to alter their sexual practices.

I'm single. What should I tell my dates? If you're heterosexual and involved with one partner, my sense is the sexual transmission is so low that it may not be an issue. On the other hand, you have a trust issue that you have to resolve; that may require disclosing your hepatitis C infection. Place the disclosure in the context of knowing that your hepatitis C infection need not fracture or destroy an otherwise promising relationship. Infected males may provide additional protection for their female sexual partners by using latex condoms.

What about French kissing? Oral sex? The details of these types of sexual activity have not been scientifically investigated. If blood barriers (lining of the mouth, lining of the genitalia) are breached, then blood-to-blood transmission may occur.

Should I always use condoms? Latex condoms and safe sex practices are especially suggested for individuals who have multiple sex partners.

Can I have a baby? Nurse my baby? Yes. Mothers who ask these questions are worried about transmitting hepatitis C to their infants. First, the risk of transmission appears to be limited to the time of delivery, when the blood of the mother and infant may become intermixed. Approximately 6 percent of babies born of mothers with hepatitis C develop the infection.

As stated above, swallowing mother's milk is not likely to be harmful to the infant. (For more information, see chapter 13.) Always discuss these decisions with your doctor.

How do I clean up a blood spill? If you have gloves available, use them. If not, take precautions to prevent contact of the blood with your skin or any cuts, abrasions, sores, or wounds on your skin. Take a rag or paper cloth and wipe the spill. If household bleach is available, use diluted bleach at the site of the spill. Dispose of the rag or paper in a plastic bag, and throw it in the garbage. Wash your hands afterwards. The term "Universal Precautions" when dealing with potentially infectious matter means to wear gloves, avoid exposure to infection, and wash your hands.

Is it necessary to tell people like my dentist that I have hepatitis C? In my opinion, patients should inform dentists and other health care professionals who need to perform invasive procedures or operations.

Can I be an organ donor? Yes. Some organs from hepatitis C patients are used, particularly for recipients who are critically ill or who already have hepatitis C.

We learn geology the morning after the earthquake.

Emerson

4

LEARNING ABOUT YOUR LIVER: YOUR BODY'S CHEMICAL FACTORY

Liver Facts and Liver Disease Symptoms

from Oda al Higado (Ode to the Liver)[1]
by Pablo Neruda

> *. . . navigating*
> *the hidden mysteries,*
> *the alchemist's chamber*
> *of life's microscopic,*
> *echoic, inner oceans . . .*

Translated by Herberto Morales and Will Hochman

IMAGINE A MACHINE that converts food into energy; stores nutrients, fats, and vitamins; makes proteins for blood plasma; and detoxifies poisons. Your liver does all this and more—much more.

But no machine, no matter how powerful, is as versatile as your liver. Even if 75 percent of the liver's mass is taken away, it still functions. And it's the only internal organ that regenerates itself.

This chapter will discuss what the liver looks like, how it functions, and what happens to the liver when it's infected with hepatitis C—including ten warning signals your body sends you when liver function is compromised:

• Liver Facts from Mesopotamian to Modern Times
• A Look at Your Liver
    Appearance
    Under the Microscope
• How Your Liver Works
    Blood
    Bile
    Lymph
    Immune System
    Chemical Factory
    Bilirubin
    ALT, AST, GGT, Alkaline Phosphatase
    Albumin
    Clotting Factors
    Hormones
• Phases of Hepatitis C
    Phase I: Infection
    Phase II: Inflammation
    Phase III: Fibrosis
    Phase IV: Cirrhosis
• Ten Danger Signs of Liver Disease
    Early Warning Signs: #1 and #2
     Early Symptoms
     Changes in Liver Functions
    Later Warning Signs of Cirrhosis: #3–#10
     Compensated Cirrhosis
     Decompensated Cirrhosis
     Changes in the Appearance of the Skin: Jaundice, Spider Nevi
        (Telangiectasia), Palmar Erythema
     Fluid Buildup: Ascites

Bleeding: Variceal Hemorrhage
Mental Confusion: Encephalopathy
Weight Loss
Thinning of Bones (Osteoporosis) and Fractures:
    Metabolic Bone Disease
Blood Clotting Problems: Coagulopathy
Itching: Pruritus
• Beyond the Liver: Conditions Associated with Hepatitis C
Kidney Damage
Cryoglobulinemia
Thyroid Disease
Skin Conditions
Autoimmune Conditions

Liver Facts from Mesopotamian to Modern Times

- Mesopotamians didn't know anatomy, but they could see that the liver seemed to be the collecting point for blood, the source of life. Archeologists have found 5,000-year-old Mesopotamian clay models of livers with markings that may have helped priests perform religious rites.

- In ancient cultures, animals were sacrificed before battle and their entrails were examined; a healthy blood-red liver was a good omen. Pale livers foretold defeat—an expression that has entered the English language with the term "lily-livered," meaning cowardly.

- In Greek mythology, Prometheus stole fire from the gods and gave it to mankind. Zeus punished him by chaining him to a rock in the mountains. Each day an eagle gnawed at his body, feasting on his liver. Because the liver has such great regenerating capacity, it grew back each night, subjecting Prometheus to an endless ordeal.

- In 1987, a granite sculpture of the liver was unveiled in Ferrol, Spain. The city's coroner, who doubled as the mayor, said that over the years he saw "hundreds of these organs tortured by cocktails, wine, tranquilizers, and other medications . . . but every day, the poor little liver is at work neutralizing and purifying everything we take in."[2] As the monument was dedicated, a local poet recited "Oda Al Higado" (Ode to the Liver) by the late Nobel prize-winner Pablo Neruda.

A Look at Your Liver

Appearance. As a hepatologist, a doctor who studies livers, I sometimes forget that my patients usually don't have a clear idea of what this organ looks like. Here's Hedy:

> As a kid, I hated the sight of blood, never looked at body charts in encyclopedias, and avoided first aid classes. In short, I didn't know where my liver was. Right side or left? High in my chest or low in my gut?
>
> I worried about every ache and pain, sure my condition was getting worse by the minute. So I went to the library and took out some children's books with terrific diagrams and simple explanations.
>
> Finally, I believed my doctor. What I was feeling was heartburn, pure and simple. Learning more about my liver helped me reduce stress and, incidentally, the heartburn.

Learning more about your liver can give you a greater feeling of control and reduce stress, so let's examine this organ—the largest one in your body. The liver weighs about three pounds in an adult male and sits in the upper right of the abdomen, protected by the rib cage (see Figure 4A).

If you've ever gone to the supermarket or butcher, you've seen animal livers. They give you a pretty good idea of what the human liver looks and feels like. Reddish-brown in color, it's shaped like a flattened football with two lobes. The larger lobe lies closest to your right side. The liver is surrounded by vital organs: diaphragm and lungs above, kidney behind, intestine and colon below.

Major blood vessels serve as conduits to deliver blood to and from the liver. Your blood system transports food, oxygen, and waste. Because your liver is a central depot for so many body functions, it has the largest and most complex blood supply of any organ in the body. In fact, about 1.5 quarts of blood flow through the liver every minute.

Like other parts of your body, the liver has an artery to supply it with oxygenated blood (the hepatic artery via the abdominal aorta) and hepatic veins to take blood back to the heart. The hepatic veins join the inferior vena cava, the major vein just below the diaphragm.

In addition to the hepatic artery, the liver has a second source of blood, the portal vein. This vein is responsible for at least two-thirds of

FIGURE 4A. ANATOMIC LOCATION OF THE LIVER IN HUMANS

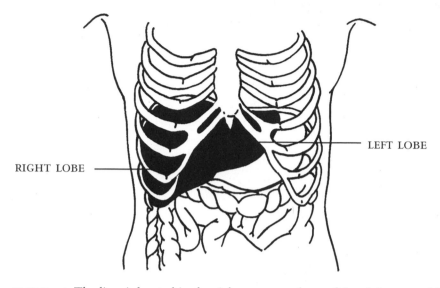

RIGHT LOBE

LEFT LOBE

LEGEND 4A: The liver is located in the right upper quadrant of the abdomen and is protected from external trauma by the rib cage.

liver blood flow and delivers nutrients and toxins absorbed by the intestine to the liver for processing.

Have you ever wondered why livers are a dull red color? It's because the portal vein transports nutrients to the liver in dark, deoxygenated blood.

Speaking of colors, your liver produces up to a quart a day of yellow-green bile, a liquid that looks like motor oil and breaks down fat in foods. Bile flows from the liver into the bile duct, which resembles the branches of a tree. The smallest branches are embedded in the liver while the common bile duct is the tree "trunk."

The common bile duct connects with the gallbladder (which stores bile and is attached to the underside of your liver) through the cystic duct. Then the bile duct continues through the pancreas, where it's joined by the pancreatic duct, and on to the intestine.

Under the Microscope. Tiny units, called lobules, are the building blocks of your liver tissue. Each lobule is a spheroid structure and measures about 0.2 inch across. Under the microscope, you see flat sheets of cube-shaped liver cells (hepatocytes) fanning out from a tiny central vein. Blood flows in the spaces (sinusoids) between the sheets.

Small branches of the hepatic artery (bringing oxygen from the heart) and the portal vein enter the lobule from the side and first deliver blood to the periphery of the lobule (portal area). Blood travels through the lobule toward its center, bathing the hepatocytes with nutrients, chemicals, and toxins carried from the intestine. Liver cells have special ways of extracting compounds from blood and metabolizing them—a topic I'll talk about in the next section.

The center of the lobule contains a very fine terminal branch of the hepatic vein. This vein then connects with other branches and "processed" blood flows through the hepatic veins to the inferior vena cava, returning to the heart.

In addition, each liver cell makes and secretes bile to its own tiny attached branch of the biliary system. The liver contains a whole network of these fine tubes that pipe bile to the bile duct and gallbladder.

How Your Liver Works

Knowing how the liver works will help you understand why things go wrong when a virus attacks it. Your liver affects your blood, bile, lymph, immune system, and chemical functions.

Blood. The liver greatly influences the makeup of blood in your body. Blood is composed of plasma (a liquid), red cells, white cells, and platelets. When the liver is diseased, all of these blood components may be affected.

Do you know how your body tissues get oxygen? Red blood cells deliver it. Do you know why wounds clot? Platelets plug bleeding capillaries and vessels. When you have an infection, white blood cells rush to the site as your first line of defense.

The liver receives blood from two sources: two-thirds from the portal vein (which comes from the intestine loaded with nutrients for the liver to process) and one-third from the hepatic artery. The hepatic artery, like all arteries, carries blood loaded with oxygen. About 15 percent of the blood pumped by the heart each minute runs through the liver.

As the liver becomes progressively injured, scar tissue builds up, making it difficult for blood from the portal vein and hepatic artery to flow through the liver. The blood tends to back up into other abdominal vessels and the spleen. As blood backs up in the spleen, cells become trapped and are destroyed—resulting in a decrease in platelets, red cells, and white cells.

Bile. Did you know that cholesterol is an ingredient in bile? Your liver makes bile from water, electrolytes (sodium, potassium, chloride, and others), proteins, organic salts (bilirubin), and lipids (cholesterol, among others). The liver turns compounds that don't dissolve in water into water-soluble substances that are secreted into bile. Toxins (poisons) absorbed from the intestine also circulate in blood to the liver, which extracts, inactivates, and secretes them into bile.

Back to cholesterol. A normal part of our diets, it's made by several cells in our bodies. When too much cholesterol accumulates, cells may alter their functions and even die. If too much cholesterol builds up in blood vessels, you may get hardening of the arteries (atherosclerosis). If it builds up in bile, you may develop gallstones.

Prevention of these complications depends on eliminating excess cholesterol. Your liver is the only organ that breaks down cholesterol into bile acid, secretes it in bile, and removes it from your body for good.

What else does bile do? Simply put, bile helps you absorb fat and vitamins that are dissolved in fat (A, D, E, and K). When disease interrupts this cycle, your body has trouble digesting and absorbing fats and fat-soluble vitamins and getting rid of pigments and toxins. Processing of medications may also be impaired if your liver is severely damaged, and your doctor may need to adjust the doses of your medications.

Lymph. Your liver produces about a quart of lymph a day. Filtered from plasma, it's a protein-rich fluid composed mostly of water and electrolytes. Lymph travels through channels next to the portal vein and joins other major lymph channels in the abdomen. Eventually, the lymph is dumped into the bloodstream.

Any kind of disruption, whether it's disease or congestion of the lymph channels, may mean that large amounts of lymph spill into the abdomen. Although this rarely happens, it may be one reason for swelling of the abdomen due to fluid (ascites).

Immune System. Here's a mouthful: lymphocytes, plasma cells, macrophages, fibroblasts, dendritic cells, and polymorphonuclear leucocytes. All types of immune cells, including these, are found in the liver. In fact, the liver is one of the major lymphoid organs of the immune system.

The immune cells in the liver protect against infections or toxins, but may also, in certain diseases, cause liver injury. In hepatitis C, liver damage is caused not only by the direct effects of the virus but also by the immune response to the virus.

Chemical Factory. Your liver acts as a chemical powerhouse—building the substances you need for life and neutralizing or safely dumping harmful material. In fact, your liver performs more than 500 complex chemical functions!

I hope you're beginning to see that your liver works overtime to help and protect you. Take your digestive system, for instance. The liver stores nutrients, then sends them out to the parts of your body that need them.

When you eat carbohydrates (potatoes, pasta, and other starches), your body breaks them down into glucose. You need glucose for energy, but because of your liver, you don't have to eat carbohydrates all day long. Instead, the liver stores glucose as glycogen. When you need a burst of energy, your liver turns glycogen back into glucose and sends it through the bloodstream to your body.

Some of the fats you eat build new cells. The liver sends extra fat into the blood and, eventually, your body stores it as fat cells (adipose tissue). If you run out of carbohydrates, the fat stored in your liver becomes a major source of body fuel.

Protein you eat is broken down in your gut into amino acids, which are absorbed and distributed via the bloodstream to your liver and body. Cells use the amino acids to make new proteins or burn the amino acids for fuel. Proteins made by the liver regulate your clotting system, transport fat and nutrients throughout your body, control hormone levels, and maintain your blood volume.

Bilirubin. Bilirubin is the yellow pigment responsible for jaundice. When red blood cells in your body break down, they release hemoglobin—a molecule that carries oxygen to your tissues.

Enzymes are proteins that make specific chemical reactions take place. One of these enzymes, called heme oxygenase, occurs in bone marrow and liver cells. It converts heme, the major component of hemoglobin, into bilirubin. The liver then removes the bilirubin from your blood and turns it into a water-soluble form that is excreted into bile.

Normally, the amount of bilirubin produced approximates the rate of red blood cell breakdown. Bilirubin levels rise when something goes wrong, such as the breakdown of too many red blood cells, the development of liver disease (such as hepatitis), a defect in liver metabolism, or a blockage of the bile system. Bilirubin accumulates in tissues, causing your skin and the white part of your eyes (sclerae) to turn yellow.

ALT (SGPT), AST (SGOT), GGT, Alkaline Phosphatase. Your liver creates all of these enzymes. When liver cells are injured, the enzymes escape and enter the bloodstream. If small numbers of cells are affected, there may be little or no increase in plasma levels of enzymes. When large numbers of liver cells are injured or die, the levels of these enzymes in plasma increase markedly.

Enzyme tests roughly reflect the level of ongoing injury, but they don't indicate how your liver is actually functioning. To do that, you need to look at the tests that measure your liver's ability to build and synthesize (albumin, clotting factors) or to excrete (bilirubin).

Albumin. The liver makes this protein. It is vital for maintaining body fluid balance, especially the volume of plasma in your blood.

Although albumin levels in plasma may be affected by other disorders, in liver disease the level of serum albumin is a good marker of your liver's ability to produce proteins. A sustained decrease below the normal range is one of the first signs of advancing liver disease.

Clotting Factors. The liver also makes many proteins that help the blood to clot. In contrast to albumin, which stays a long time in plasma, clotting factors have a relatively short survival period. Therefore, the liver must constantly work to produce enough coagulation factors to maintain normal clotting.

When the liver is injured and can't make clotting factors, plasma levels drop within one or two days. Soon patients notice that they're bruising or bleeding easily even after minor bumps and injuries. If liver failure occurs, patients may hemorrhage and often require plasma and blood transfusions.

Hormones. The thyroid is one of the main hormone-producing glands. Patients with chronic hepatitis C have a high occurrence of underlying thyroid disease. Interferon therapy may cause the thyroid condition to flare. Therefore, doctors commonly run tests for thyroid function before and after interferon treatment.

In late stages of liver disease (cirrhotic phase), patients may experience other hormonal imbalances, including altered ovulation or gonadal function and impairment of the pituitary gland (the main hormone control center). For example, men with cirrhosis often develop distressing enlargement of their breasts due to hormonal imbalance. In addition, pituitary hormones regulate functions such as sleep-wake cycles, appetite, and body temperature.

> *My wife kept nagging me to tell the doctor how sore the nipple was on my right breast. "But what if it's cancer?" she said. At my next office visit, I worked up the nerve to ask.*
> *"Hormones change in end-stage liver disease," my doctor said.*
> *"Are you telling me what I think you are?"*
> *"Yes," he said. "You're growing a breast."*
> *I couldn't believe it. Cowboys don't grow breasts!*
>
> *Larry*

FIGURE 4B. CONSEQUENCES OF HCV INFECTION

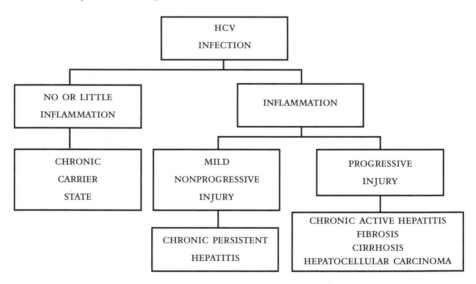

LEGEND 4B: Potential consequences of hepatitis C infection are shown. Some patients develop no or very little inflammation and co-exist with hepatitis C in a chronic carrier state. Others experience variable degrees of inflammation and liver damage. In the most severe cases, scarring becomes severe, resulting in cirrhosis or liver cancer (hepatocellular carcinoma—hepatoma).

Phases of Hepatitis C

Figure 4B diagrams the consequences of hepatitis C infection. We divide hepatitis C infection and disease into four overlapping phases:

I. Infection
II. Inflammation
III. Fibrosis
IV. Cirrhosis

Phase I: Infection. When the hepatitis C virus gets into the bloodstream, it attaches to liver cells, enters them, and starts to reproduce. The new virus, made within the infected liver cell, exits into the bloodstream where it attaches to and infects another liver cell. This process allows the infection to spread through the liver.

Patients often ask me, "Why do I have hepatitis C if I have antibodies against hepatitis C?" Although your body produces an immune response to the virus (antibodies form and immune cells called lymphocytes are recruited into the liver), it usually doesn't get rid of the infection. We now know that approximately 85 percent of patients become chronically infected. In other infections antibodies effectively fight the infection, but in hepatitis C the antibodies are ineffective and do not clear the infection. In fact, antibodies (when present) usually indicate active disease and ongoing infection.

Phase II: Inflammation. In this phase, liver inflammation (hepatitis) develops. Under the microscope, most liver cells appear relatively normal and uninjured. But in some areas there is liver cell injury and death. Inflammation in the liver is characterized by the presence of specific immune cells called lymphocytes. Lymphocytes are recruited to the liver to attempt to eliminate hepatitis C. However, they also release chemicals that damage liver cells and contribute to the liver injury.

In the majority of cases, the initial, acute phase of hepatitis C is mild in terms of symptoms. Most people don't realize they've had a first attack, and there are only a few cases of sudden, severe (fulminant) liver failure due to the virus. Most patients have no symptoms and only a fraction develop jaundice.

We now know that most patients with hepatitis C will develop chronic hepatitis. The chronic form, too, is usually mild and asymptomatic, although many patients complain of fatigue, poor stamina, and inability to concentrate.

Phase III: Fibrosis. Despite the mild nature of the inflammation and liver injury, the disease commonly progresses to fibrosis—the formation of scar tissue in the liver. If your liver biopsy shows significant fibrosis, it usually means you've had hepatitis C for more than 10 years.

Phase IV: Cirrhosis. When fibrosis increases, the fourth stage appears. With cirrhosis, the fibrosis is so severe that it affects how the liver functions and grossly distorts the architecture and blood flow of the liver.

Ten Danger Signs of Liver Disease

Warning symptoms fall into two categories: early and late. The liver sends few early warning signs. It's a large organ with great reserves; most people can lose three quarters of their liver without any change in function or development of symptoms.

In early hepatitis C, even though the liver is damaged, no symptoms appear. Symptoms early in the course of hepatitis C, such as muscle aches and headaches, are due to the virus itself and not to liver failure. Later in the course of hepatitis C, liver function diminishes and warning signs of advanced liver disease appear.

Early Warning Signs: #1 and #2

#1: Early Symptoms. Here's Hedy:

> At our hepatitis C support group, we compared notes. No one had serious symptoms like itching or mental confusion, even though one of us had cirrhosis. Almost everyone, however, complained of fatigue.
>
> It also turned out that four of us often experienced a kind of tender, achy feeling on our right sides. Doctors had dismissed the symptom by saying the liver didn't feel pain—not to worry. But of course, we did.
>
> So at my next medical appointment, I brought up the mystery symptom and got an answer. The liver doesn't feel pain, but the membrane around the liver and the liver itself may react to the inflammation from hepatitis.
>
> I reported back to the group, and we all relaxed. Nothing had changed, but the simple explanation helped. It kept us from imagining that we were sliding into liver failure.

Many people with hepatitis C, especially in the early phases, tell me they have no symptoms. I find, however, that if I question them closely, they complain of fatigue, feel less energetic, and are unable to work at their usual high level. Typically, appetite and weight are unaffected, but occasionally some patients report less enthusiasm for eating and so have difficulty maintaining their weight.

No one knows why these common symptoms occur. Some researchers think they're due to the viral infection itself, while others feel that the ongoing liver injury releases substances into the blood that produce these effects.

In my experience, these symptoms rarely, if at all, correspond to the severity of the disease. Some of my patients suffer extreme fatigue but have little injury to their livers, while others with aggressive hepatitis and cirrhosis may have no symptoms at all.

#2: Changes in Liver Functions. If you have hepatitis C, you need close medical supervision. Current recommendations call for an annual physical exam and liver blood tests every six months. Changes in blood tests usually indicate the first sign of deteriorating liver function.

Twenty-four years ago I had a really bad car accident, lost part of my liver, and had last rites. I received lots of blood transfusions. Afterwards, it was really weird. I got so tired I could barely mow my lawn.

Finally, I was diagnosed with hepatitis C. I was back in school, and right after graduation my blood tests changed. My bilirubin was up, so I was a little jaundiced. My platelet count was really low—one-third what it was supposed to be. Platelets coagulate your blood, so if I barely bumped something, my skin would tear, and I'd bleed. My nose was bleeding all the time.

Pete

At later stages of disease, albumin may decrease, bilirubin may rise, and prothrombin (a protein involved in blood clotting) time may increase. These changes occur because the liver is becoming less able to make its usual quota of substances the body needs. Another change that occurs is enlargement of the spleen. Platelets, white blood cells, and even red blood cells may drop because the enlarged spleen traps and destroys these cells. In my experience, a progressive buildup of fluid in the ankles and a low level of sodium in the blood are also common. These danger signs correlate with the cirrhotic stage. They indicate that the liver is less able to keep up with the amount of injury and often precede more serious symptoms of liver failure.

Later Warning Signs of Cirrhosis: #3 and #10

What does cirrhosis mean? Cirrhosis simply means the hardening of the liver due to a buildup of scar tissue and formation of nodules.

Compensated Cirrhosis. Patients who have early-stage cirrhosis, also known as compensated cirrhosis, may not have any symptoms or laboratory test abnormalities.

Decompensated Cirrhosis. Late-stage cirrhosis, or decompensated cirrhosis, is characterized by abnormalities in blood tests, complications (some of which are life threatening), and limited survival. Patients with any or all of the following signs may be potential candidates for a liver transplant.

#3: Changes in the Appearance of the Skin: Jaundice, Spider Nevi (Telangiectasia), Palmar Erythema.

Jaundice. Jaundice is the yellowing of the skin and whites of the eyes. It is due to an accumulation of the pigment bilirubin in the skin and other tissues of the body, such as the whites of the eyes. Jaundice commonly occurs in patients with hepatitis C when the liver disease is advanced and the hepatitis flares. In some cases, jaundice may disappear when the flare resolves.

> *I was like the walking dead. My skin was a poor color—gray. Other days, I was yellow, jaundiced. I didn't think I was going to make it, but I did. The transplant worked, and I'm grateful.*
>
> *Blaire*

Spider Nevi (Telangiectasia). Spider nevi are red spots, usually on the upper body and face. If you look at the spots closely, you will see a central red area with fine red lines emanating outward. These "spiders" are actually a collection of very small blood vessels caused by hormonal imbalance due to cirrhosis. The spiders disappear after transplantation.

Palmar Erythema. Palmar erythema is a reddening of the fleshy part of the palms of the hands. The condition occurs when blood vessels dilate because of hormonal imbalance due to cirrhosis. Palmar erythema and spider nevi often occur simultaneously.

#4: Fluid Buildup: Ascites. Ascites means that fluid builds up in the abdomen, so that the belly swells. Liver disease is the most common cause of ascites.

> *I didn't realize I was holding water. I thought, "What have I eaten that's made my stomach so bloated?" At one point the doctor figured I was carrying 30 to 35 pounds of water in my stomach.*
>
> *The swelling came and went, but in the last year it's been an acute problem. My fingers, knees, even my calves are swollen. My skin is so tight that my feet look like little porky pigs. The doctor gives me diuretics to make me go to the bathroom. It makes for a busy day!*
>
> *Jerry*

> *If I eat too much, the ascites gets worse. A huge meal does me in. Afterwards, I feel like I'm going to explode! The best thing is to eat in small amounts, a little bit at a time.*
>
> *Josie*

Physicians must remove and analyze the fluid to exclude other causes. To remove fluid the physician performs a paracentesis, which involves placing a needle through the abdominal wall and drawing out the fluid for a culture, cell count, biochemical tests, and a microscopic examination. If the ascites is due to liver disease, the fluid will be clear, yellow, and uninfected, and have a low cell count.

More than one problem, however, may be involved. Sometimes patients have a bacterial infection in the ascites (spontaneous bacterial peritonitis). In these cases, there are other signs of infection: fever, high white blood count, abdominal pain. It's important to recognize this condition right away and treat it early with antibiotics. We now have many treatments for ascites, including diuretics (drugs that increase the amount of urine excreted), paracentesis (drawing off fluid), or shunts (tubes that redirect the liquid), such as peritoneovenous shunts and transjugular intrahepatic portal-systemic shunts.

Muscle cramps are a common problem in patients with advanced liver disease. In particular, patients with ascites who are treated with diuretics commonly complain of severe cramping. This type of cramping may respond to reducing diuretics or administering magnesium, calcium, or possibly zinc.

Ascites is a serious warning sign of very advanced liver disease, and most patients with ascites will require a liver transplant for prolonged survival.

#5: Bleeding: Variceal Hemorrhage. The most dramatic and urgent complication of advanced liver disease is variceal hemorrhage. "Variceal" refers to varices, which are abnormally distended or swollen veins usually located in the esophagus, and "hemorrhage," of course, means bleeding.

Patients vomit large quantities of red blood, show signs of altered mental status, and have very low blood pressure. By the time they get to the emergency room, they may be in shock.

> *I didn't know I had hepatitis C until I went into the hospital with an esophageal bleed. It was in 1991. We were having a family picnic, and I had drunk lots of cherry Kool-Aid. I tried to convince myself the red stuff coming out of my mouth was the punch, but then I bled again. The doctors tubed me through my nose and stopped the bleeding.*
>
> *Chris*

It's urgent to get to an emergency medical facility when there's any sign of bleeding from the upper gastrointestinal tract. Variceal bleeding may be vomiting red blood, the passage of loose, dark, tarry feces, or the passage of a large amount of red blood through the rectum.

Doctors first must find the source of the bleeding before they can treat the problem. They insert a slender tube (endoscope) down the patient's throat to diagnose the cause or source of the bleed. Endoscopists have two treatments available: tying the bleeding veins with bands (ligation) or injecting a chemical into the vein to make it clot (sclerotherapy). Both therapies work well to control the initial bleed. But to eradicate the varices and avoid later hemorrhages, outpatient treatments must be repeated—usually two or three times.

Doctors may also give medications such as somatostatin, vasopressin, nitroglycerin, and plasma products to control the bleeding. Sometimes propranolol or related medicines are given to lower the risk of a rebleed.

Occasionally, varices are also found in the stomach, duodenum, intestine, and colon. It's harder to manage varices in these locations with endoscopic treatment. Doctors often will treat bleeding from these varices with either a surgical shunt (a tube that redirects the blood) or TIPS. Surgical shunts require major abdominal surgery and connect one of the portal veins to veins that bypass the liver (systemic veins).

TIPS is short for transjugular intrahepatic portal-systemic shunt. Radiologists put the TIPS in place, avoiding the need for risky abdominal surgery that might compromise a later liver transplant.

First, the radiologist places a catheter through a vein in the neck, then into the liver via the hepatic veins. A needle goes through this catheter into the liver and punctures a main branch of the portal vein. Once the portal vein and hepatic veins are connected, the radiologist dilates the tract and places an expandable cylindrical wire-mesh shunt across the liver to maintain the connection. When the shunt is in place, it relieves the back pressure on the portal veins, varices collapse, and the risk of further hemorrhage is greatly reduced.

Transplant surgeons welcome TIPS because it doesn't interfere with their surgery. However, occasionally, TIPS migrate into the portal vein and complicate a transplant operation, so most transplant doctors prefer that TIPS be placed by radiologists with a high level of experience with the procedure.

#6: Mental Confusion: Portal-Systemic Encephalopathy. The liver conducts many metabolic functions, including clearing or detoxifying the blood of harmful substances. When the liver fails, these substances may build up to toxic levels and impair the function of other organs, such as the brain.

Just before my liver transplant, my doctors had me take a mental test. They said there were no passing scores, and you couldn't fail—but I did. I flunked it. I know I did.

A year after my transplant, they asked me to take it again. This time I did well. In fact, I did so well, I scored higher than a third of the doctors who took the same test!

Jack

The brain reacts to altered liver functions, so patients with advanced liver disease commonly note changes in their mental abilities. These changes range from slight changes, such as decline in memory or reduced ability to perform complex calculations, to more severe changes, such as confusion, disorientation, blackout spells, or even coma.

It helps to understand four features of encephalopathy: (1) Encephalopathy is usually brought on by some other problem, such as gastrointestinal bleeding, infection, or electrolyte imbalance. (2) It's a completely reversible condition. (3) Effective medical therapy exists [lactulose (a non-absorbable carbohydrate); neomycin or rifaximin (antibiotics); a protein-restricted diet]. Early therapy may prevent the patient from lapsing into more advanced stages, such as coma. (4) A successful liver transplant completely reverses the condition.

This means that a patient experiencing encephalopathy must get urgent medical attention and evaluation, be treated promptly, and be considered for liver transplantation.

#7: Weight Loss. Because the liver acts as your body's metabolic factory and energy storehouse, advancing liver disease affects your nutrition. That's why your doctor looks for weight loss.

> *I had a lot of muscle because I was a physical therapist. When I look in the mirror now, I can see the wasting. I'm so much thinner in my arms, shoulders, and back. Then again, my stomach's out to here from fluid. So I've got this weird figure.*
>
> *Lila*

Patients need to eat an appropriate amount of calories. And because patients often are on a sodium restriction for ascites and a protein restriction for encephalopathy, that can be hard to do. I usually recommend supplements and a visit to a dietician.

Blood tests detect nutritional deficiencies. People with liver disease, for example, may have fat-soluble vitamin deficiencies (A, D, E, K) that can be at least partially corrected with oral supplements. I prefer retinyl palmitate (vitamin A), Calderol® (vitamin D-25-OH), tocopherol polyethylene glycol solution or TPGS (vitamin E), and Mephyton® (vitamin K). The TPGS formulation of vitamin E is an emulsified liquid that also aids the absorption of A, D, and K. A simple way to think of TPGS is that it's artificial bile. I recommend that all the fat-soluble vitamins be taken with the TPGS to improve absorption.

#8: Thinning of Bones (Osteoporosis) and Fractures: Metabolic Bone Disease. Did you know that as liver disease progresses, bone loss may accelerate? Bone loss is frequently observed in patients with advanced hepatitis C, especially those receiving steroid medication for other conditions.

In my whole life I had never broken any bones—pretty unusual. Then in the space of two years, I broke my toe twice. The first time, I fell off my bike; the second, I hit my toe against a floorboard. The final straw came when I fractured my kneecap. Two years later, my knee still aches when the weather changes.

Coincidence, growing older, hepatitis C—who knows? But my doctor wants me to take some tests.

Sheila

First, the doctor must exclude other causes of bone loss, such as vitamin D deficiency or hyperparathyroidism. Typically, patients with bone disease and fractures due to end-stage liver disease simply have a condition called osteopenia, which does not respond well to vitamin D, calcium, or fluoride. Recent studies suggest that a new drug, alendronate, may be of some benefit. To complicate matters, post-transplant use of steroids and the relative inactivity after surgery can make the bones more brittle. Most transplant centers now taper steroids sharply and encourage early walking to lower the risk of fractures.

#9: Blood Clotting Problems: Coagulopathy. People with end-stage liver disease have multiple defects in their blood clotting system that put them at risk for bleeding and hemorrhage.

Sometimes I just bite into an apple, and I see blood right there—on the fruit. Three times in the last month I woke up with blood in my mouth.

Also, I've been getting blood spots—like little red pimples—across my chest and arms. My wife says they look like spider veins. They don't hurt, but if I forget and scratch them, they bleed.

Gary

Coagulation proteins drop to such low levels that even minor trauma to skin, gums, lips or extremities causes marked bruising or prolonged oozing of blood. Major trauma, such as surgery, can result in excessive bleeding. In many cases your doctor may be able to administer clotting factors to reduce your risk of bleeding from these procedures. In addition, the spleen often holds and destroys platelets, reducing the body's other major clotting aid. If severe clotting disturbances develop, it's an ominous sign of advanced liver disease and means immediate consideration for a transplant.

#10: Itching: Pruritus. Although relatively uncommon in patients with hepatitis C, constant itching, day and night, may torment patients with severe jaundice or advanced liver disease. It's caused by a buildup of substances in the skin that are normally cleared by the liver, and it's not associated with hives or rashes (except what people get from scratching). Although generalized, itching may be peculiarly localized to the palms of the hands, soles of the feet, inside the mouth, and the external ear canal.

> *Excuse my language, but I call it "the bitchy itch." My symptoms began as a little itch. I hardly noticed it. I ignored it until it got bigger, and I started scratching. There was one spot the size of a quarter on my left leg. Creams did no good.*
>
> *Over a year and a half it got so bad I swore I'd never scratch—and I've got high will power. But I scarred my legs.*
>
> *Finally, someone in my support group told me to use cornstarch. So now I bathe, dry myself off, and apply the cornstarch. I've done it three times so far, and it helps.*
>
> *Saul*

The pruritus of liver disease does not respond to antihistamines, skin lotions, and creams, but improves with the use of medicines that promote bile flow, such as ursodeoxycholate, or that bind and inactivate substances in the intestine, such as cholestyramine.

Recent studies suggest that pruritus may be related to naturally occurring morphine-like compounds that build up in the patient and may respond to medications that block morphine effects (naloxone, naltrexone).

Some patients have severe, incapacitating pruritus that can't be helped by any of the therapies mentioned. A liver transplant successfully treats the condition.

Beyond the Liver: Conditions Associated with Hepatitis C

The ten danger signs of advanced liver disease and cirrhosis are common to all forms of liver disease, including hepatitis C. In addition, hepatitis C patients may find themselves dealing with other conditions associated with the virus. These conditions are called extra-hepatic (non-liver) manifestations of hepatitis C.

Kidney Damage. A specific type of kidney damage, called glomerulonephritis, can occur when immune complexes of the hepatitis C virus lodge in the kidney and cause inflammation. At first, there may be no symptoms. It's often detected when a routine urinalysis shows protein in the urine. As more protein is lost in urine, the blood albumin may decrease, and patients may notice swelling in the ankles or abdomen. Rarely, it can lead to kidney failure. Glomerulonephritis, complicating hepatitis C, may respond to treatment with interferon.

Cryoglobulinemia. The signs of this condition are skin rash, fever, kidney damage, and ulcerations on the fingers and toes. Cryoglobulinemia is caused by antibodies that the body manufactures against the hepatitis C virus. Management of cryoglobulinemia is complex but may involve interferon, steroids, cyclophosphamide, intravenous immunoglobulins, and plasmapheresis (passing blood through a filter to remove the antibody complexes).

Thyroid Disease. Thyroid disease is very common in the general population (2 to 3 percent) and even more common in hepatitis C patients (5 to 20 percent). Usually, it's an underactive thyroid causing the problem, but in rare cases, the thyroid can be overactive. The signs of an underactive thyroid include cold intolerance, sluggishness, dry skin, coarse hair, a change in voice, mental confusion. Signs of an overactive thyroid include palpitations, sweating, heat intolerance, jitters, tremor, poor concentrating ability, and hypertension.

An underactive thyroid is treated with thyroid hormone replacement, such as levo-thyroxine. Treatment of an overactive thyroid may involve radioactive iodine, beta-blockers, and propylthiouracil.

Skin Conditions. Skin conditions associated with hepatitis C include lichen planus, lichenoid dermatitis, and porphyria cutanea tarda.

The first two are usually best treated with dermatologic lotions/creams and may flare during interferon treatment.

Lichen planus is a reddish-brown raised round spot, typically less than one to two centimeters in diameter. Sometimes it appears scaly and may itch.

Lichenoid dermatitis looks like scaly, reddish flat areas, usually larger than two centimeters in diameter. It's occasionally itchy.

Porphyria cutanea tarda appears as blisters on sun-exposed areas or areas of trauma—usually on fingers and hands. Porphyria cutanea tarda responds to iron removal by taking blood (phlebotomy) and treatment of the hepatitis C.

Autoimmune Conditions. Case reports suggest that a number of autoimmune conditions may be associated with the hepatitis C virus or interferon treatment. These include idiopathic thrombocytopenic purpura (low platelet count), autoimmune chronic active hepatitis (inflammation in the liver caused by the immune system), arthritis, Sjögren's syndrome (dry eyes and mouth), Raynaud's syndrome (blanching and numbness of fingers and toes), vasculitis (inflammation of small blood vessels), and polyarteritis nodosa (inflammation of large blood vessels, particularly in the abdomen, liver, and kidney).

Disorders that may flare on interferon therapy include hemolytic anemia (red cells break down), pericarditis/pleuritis (inflammation of the lining of the heart and lung), psoriasis, rheumatoid arthritis, and systemic lupus erythematosis.

Reading this list of what can go wrong with your liver anticipates the worst that can happen. Remember that more than two-thirds of the people who develop chronic hepatitis C do not progress to cirrhosis over 20 to 30 years. Nevertheless, it's important to know what the symptoms are, so you can report any changes promptly to your physician.

In the next chapters, we'll take a look at ways you can help your liver with healthy eating habits and stress-reduction techniques. I'll contribute a medical perspective, we'll hear from experts who specialize in these areas, and we'll listen to patients as they share their personal stories.

The beginning of health is to know the disease.

Miguel de Cervantes

References

1. Neruda, Pablo. *Nuevas Odas Elementales.* Buenos Aires: Editorial Losada, p. 76–80.

2. "Sculpture in Spain Salutes the 'Silent, Unselfish' Liver," *Austin American-Statesman,* 28 June 1987:A2.

5

TAKING CARE OF
YOURSELF
NUTRITIONALLY
Guidelines for Healthy
Nutrition in Liver Disease

At first, when I was still in shock over the diagnosis of chronic hep-
atitis C, I was too scared to try interferon. So I decided to do all I could
with "natural" methods. I went to two dieticians who recommended a
low-fat diet to take a load off my liver. They also advocated intravenous
vitamin C and coffee enemas, which turned me off.

Then I saw a naturopath. He restricted my diet so much that I lost
ten pounds. I never looked so good! But I still felt tired, so I consulted a
nutritionist. She told me to keep a food journal, which made it possible
for us to review my diet and my eating patterns.

I had been skimping on protein because I thought that would help
my liver. Turns out that protein restriction is only for people in end-stage
liver disease who are mentally confused. The nutritionist suggested I eat

an appropriate amount of protein but divide it into smaller portions throughout the day.

Looking back, I can see what I was trying to do—control what I could in a world that suddenly seemed so out of control. I might not be able to stop the virus, but I could decide what I put into my body.

After a while, I found that all the junk food I used to love didn't taste so good anymore. It seems ironic to me now, but learning I was ill made me "healthier."

Hedy

M ANY PEOPLE, when they discover they have hepatitis C, become interested in improving their general health through good nutrition. I encourage patients to learn how to eat in a healthier way, but to avoid crash diets and food fads that promise more than they can deliver.

Caution: Always check with your doctor before making major changes in your diet or taking over-the-counter supplements and vitamins. Some seemingly harmless substances can injure your liver. (See "Herbs Harmful to the Liver," p. 77)

In the early, noncirrhotic stages of hepatitis C, people can maintain normal nutrition if they eat a well-balanced diet. It's rare for a doctor to recommend supplements beyond one multivitamin a day. However, as the disease progresses, malnutrition and vitamin deficiencies may develop.

Nutritional therapy includes the following goals:

- to maintain the appropriate balance between the calories you take in and the calories your body requires
- to avoid malnutrition or deficiencies in specific nutrients
- to use appropriate supplementation when needed

In this chapter, I'll discuss some general nutritional concepts, what happens when liver disease affects your nutrition, and some specific deficiencies and their treatments:

- • Nutritional Overview
    Ideal Body Weight
    Normal Diet

- Nutrition and the Liver
    - Carbohydrate Metabolism
    - Protein Metabolism
    - Fat Metabolism
    - Bile
    - Vitamins
- Nutritional Needs for Hepatitis C Patients without Cirrhosis
    - Caloric Requirements
    - Vitamin Supplements
    - Nutritional (Herbal) Therapies
    - Herbs Harmful to the Liver
    - Nutrition Tips from Patients
- Nutritional Needs for Hepatitis C Patients with Cirrhosis
    - Caloric Requirements
    - Protein Restriction
    - Vitamin Supplements
    - Mineral Supplements
    - Salt and Fluid Restriction

Nutritional Overview

The liver is your body's major digestive organ. When the liver receives nutrients from the intestines, it metabolizes*, packages, stores, and sends them to other organs where they are used for energy. Your liver's major nutritional jobs include:

- metabolizing carbohydrates, proteins, and fat for energy
- assimilating and storing vitamins
- manufacturing bile to aid in digestion and absorption of fats
- filtering and destroying toxins (including alcohol and drugs)

Ideal Body Weight. Most people worry about their weight with good reason. Two-thirds of American adults are overweight; about half of these are obese. With advanced liver disease, however, a major concern is the opposite problem, nutritional wasting.

---

*Throughout this chapter we use the term "metabolism," which we define as the body processes, including a whole host of chemical reactions that are necessary to maintain function and sustain life.

What, then, should you weigh? We have no exact measure of ideal body weight because the "norm" is based on population statistics, cultural perceptions, and the influence of genetically and environmentally determined differences in metabolism. In short, there are no absolute rules, only working guidelines:

- Men: 106 pounds for the first five feet, then add six pounds for every inch thereafter
- Women: 100 pounds for the first five feet, then add five pounds for every inch thereafter

Normal Diet. Food supplies us with carbohydrates, fats, and proteins that in turn supply energy. Energy is measured in calories. Carbohydrates and proteins provide approximately four calories per gram, and fat provides almost nine calories per gram—twice as much. People also need essential nutrients (such as certain vitamins, minerals, amino acids, and fatty acids) and other substances, such as fiber, from a variety of foods. Oranges, for example, are rich in vitamin C, bananas supply potassium, and a half-cup serving of cantaloupe contributes half of the daily requirement for beta-carotene.

I just read that lab tests at Cornell University show that natural chemicals in apples slow the growth rate of human liver cancer cells. The researchers said that they're not sure why, but it may be the antioxidants in fruits and vegetables—and it's best to eat a daily diet that includes five servings of a wide variety of fruits and vegetables.

Ha! "An apple a day" really does keep the doctor away.

Bonnie

A normal, healthy diet contains the amounts of essential nutrients and calories you need to prevent either a nutritional deficiency or excess and provides the right balance of carbohydrate, fat, and protein. What is a healthful diet? The U.S. Department of Agriculture (USDA) has updated the Food Pyramid to reflect the latest scientific information on diet and exercise. Called MyPyramid, the new symbol trades different color bands (shown here in shades of gray) for blocks and adds steps on the side to remind you to exercise regularly.

For a quick estimate estimate of what and how much you need to eat, enter your age, sex, and activity level in the MyPyramid Plan box on

MyPyramid.gov
STEPS TO A HEALTHIER YOU

1) Grain Group: Make half your grains whole
- Eat at least 3 oz. of whole-grain cereals, breads, crackers, rice, or pasta every day
- 1 oz. is about 1 slice of bread, about 1 cup of breakfast cereal, or 1/2 cup of cooked rice, cereal, or pasta

2) Vegetable Group: Vary your veggies
- Eat more dark green veggies like broccoli, spinach, and other dark leafy greens
- Eat more orange vegetables like carrots and sweet potatoes
- Eat more dry beans and peas like pinto beans, kidney beans, and lentils

3) Fruit Group: Focus on fruits
- Eat a variety of fruit
- Choose fresh, frozen, canned, or dried fruit
- Go easy on fruit juices

4) Milk Group: Get your calcium-rich foods
- Go low-fat or fat-free when you choose milk, yogurt, and other milk products
- If you don't or can't consume milk, choose lactosefree products or other calcium sources such as fortified foods and beverages

5) Meat & Beans Group: Go lean with protein
- Choose low-fat or lean meats and poultry
- Bake it, broil it, or grill it
- Vary your protein routine — choose more fish, beans, peas, nuts, and seeds

Find your balance between food and physical activity
- Be sure to stay within your daily calorie needs.
- Be physically active for at least 30 minutes most days of the week.
- About 60 minutes a day may be needed to prevent weight gain.
- For sustaining weight loss, at least 60 to 90 minutes a day may be required.
- Children and teenagers should be physically active for 60 minutes every day, or most days.

U.S. Department of Agriculture

Know the limits on fats, sugars, and salt (sodium)
- Make most of your fat sources from fish, nuts, and vegetable oils.
- Limit solid fats like butter, stick margarine, shortening, and lard, as well as foods that contain these.
- Check the Nutrition Facts label to keep saturated fats, trans fats, and sodium low.
- Choose food and beverages low in added sugars. Added sugars contribute calories with few, if any, nutrients.

the USDA website. Get a more detailed assessment with MyPyramid Tracker. Click on each color band to go "Inside the Pyramid" and learn more about the food groups: grains (orange), vegetables (green), fruits (red), milk (blue), meat and beans (purple), oils (yellow).

MyPyramid emphasizes that no diet is one-size-fits-all and encourages you to create your own customized nutrition plan. MyPyramid recommends a diet rich in fruits and vegetables, whole grains, lean meats, and low-fat or fat-free dairy products. Limit consumption of saturated and trans fats. Be physically active for a minimum of 30 minutes most days of the week. Take steps to a healthier you.

Resource: To personalize the Food Pyramid, enter your age, sex, and your amount of daily physical activity. My Pyramid Plan will display the amounts of each food group that you should eat daily. Website: www.mypyramid.gov

Resource: For a free copy of Dietary Guidelines for Americans, 2005, call the U.S. Government Printing Office toll free: 866-512-1800 or access the USDA website: www.usda.gov.

Resource: The American Dietetic Association's (ADA) Nutrition Information Line (to find qualified dieticians in your area) is 800-366-1655. Helpful books: *Complete Food & Nutrition Guide* by Roberta Duyff and the ADA, and *Dieting for Dummies* by Jane Kirby and the ADA. Website: www.eatright.org

Resource: The American Institute for Cancer Research provides practical tips on good nutrition with its newsletter, pamphlets (ask for "The New American Plate" brochure), and a toll-free AICR Nutrition Hotline staffed by a registered dietician: Call 800-843-8114 and ask for Nutrition Information. Website: www.aicr.org

Resource: *Nutrition Action Newsletter* (Center for Science in the Public Interest). Website: www.cspinet.org

Nutrition and the Liver

The liver is the major organ responsible for regulating and responding to your body's metabolic demands. Your liver must be functioning well to maintain normal metabolism of carbohydrates, fats, and protein; it is also responsible for processing and using several vitamins. This section deals with the role a healthy liver (and a healthy, well-balanced diet) plays in these nutritional processes.

Carbohydrate Metabolism. The most common sources of dietary carbohydrate are sugars, such as sucrose (table sugar), fructose (corn syrup), and lactose (milk sugar), and starches, such as breads, pasta, grains, cereals, fruits, vegetables, and potatoes. When you eat carbohydrates, specialized enzymes in the pancreas and gut process them to yield simple sugars (glucose, galactose, fructose, maltose).

These sugars are absorbed by intestinal lining cells, enter the portal circulation, and travel to the liver via the portal vein. During overnight fasting, blood sugar levels dip to a relatively low level, insulin secretion is suppressed, and blood insulin levels diminish. After a meal, blood sugar increases (stimulating the release of insulin from the pancreas), and insulin levels rise. Insulin, which rises in response to a meal, is the hormone that stimulates the liver to take in more glucose and to move the glucose into storage—mainly in the form of glycogen. The liver can then release glycogen to your muscles for energy during periods of fasting or exercise.

Although the liver can store considerable amounts of glycogen, it is the first energy source used during periods of prolonged fasting or caloric deprivation, and it can be depleted rapidly. After glycogen, the body taps other energy sources—including protein and fat.

Protein Metabolism. We take in dietary protein from dairy products, produce, and meats. Enzymes produced by the pancreas and intestine break down the protein into its amino acids and small peptides. The intestine rapidly absorbs the amino acids with specific transport systems within its lining cells and then delivers the amino acids to the liver via the portal vein.

When they reach the liver, they are used for energy or for making (synthesizing) new proteins. The newly synthesized proteins perform specific body functions (see Table 5A).

Fat Metabolism. In general, fats are neutral lipids (triglycerides), acidic lipids (fatty acids), and sterols (cholesterol, plant sterols). Triglycerides (dairy products, meats, oils, butter, margarine) are the most common type of dietary fat and represent a major source of energy. The liver is uniquely suited to regulate and process triglycerides.

Dietary triglyceride is digested in the intestine by lipase, an enzyme secreted by the pancreas in response to meals. Bile, secreted by the liver, makes the digested fat soluble and promotes its absorption. Absorbed fat is then repackaged and transported into blood, where the liver ultimately removes it from the circulation. Fat that reaches the liver is processed in three ways: (1) stored as fat droplets in liver cells, (2) metabolized as a

TABLE 5A. SOME COMMON LIVER PROTEINS AND THEIR
FUNCTION IN THE HUMAN BODY

Protein	Function
Clotting Factors (II, V, VII, IX, and X)	Maintain normal clotting
Albumin	Maintain normal blood volume
Renin	Regulate blood pressure
Binding globulins	Regulate hormone action
Transferrin	Transport iron
Ferritin	Store iron
Retinol binding protein	Transport Vitamin A to the eye
LDL receptor	Remove cholesterol from the blood
P-450 proteins	Metabolize drugs, chemicals, toxins

source of energy, and (3) repackaged, secreted back into blood, and delivered to other cells in the body.

The liver is also intimately involved with the processing of dietary cholesterol and is the main source of newly synthesized cholesterol in the body. Liver disease may be associated with both high or low blood cholesterol levels. In general, as liver disease progresses in patients with hepatitis C, the blood level of cholesterol drops.

Bile. The liver produces and secretes a fluid (bile) that enters the intestine to aid in digestion and absorption. Bile is clear yellow to golden-brown and contains water, electrolytes (salts), cholesterol, bile salts (detergents), phospholipids, and proteins. Bile helps to activate enzymes secreted by the pancreas and is essential for the digestion and absorption of fat or fat-soluble vitamins.

Vitamins. The liver plays a role in several steps of vitamin metabolism. I'll describe only a few of those steps. Vitamins are either fat-soluble (vitamins A, D, E, and K) or water-soluble (vitamin C and the B-complex vitamins).

Patients with advanced liver disease may become deficient in water-soluble vitamins, but this is usually due to inadequate nutrition and poor food intake. Vitamin B12 storage usually far exceeds the body's requirements; deficiencies rarely occur due to liver disease or liver failure. When dietary intake drops, however, thiamine and folate commonly become deficient. Oral supplementation is usually all that you need to restore thiamine and folate stores to the normal range.

Fat-soluble vitamins require not only adequate dietary intake but also good digestion and absorption by the body. That's why normal production of bile is essential. Bile in the gut is required for the absorption of fat-soluble vitamins into the body because these vitamins are relatively insoluble in water. Bile acts as a detergent, breaking down and dissolving these vitamins so they may be properly absorbed.

If bile production is poor, oral supplementation of vitamins A, D, E, and K may not be sufficient to restore vitamin levels to normal. The use of a detergent-like solution of liquid vitamin E (TPGS) improves the absorption of vitamin E in patients with advanced liver disease. The same solution may also improve the absorption of vitamins A, D, and K if the latter are taken simultaneously with the liquid vitamin E.

Nutritional Needs for Hepatitis C Patients Who Don't Have Cirrhosis

Caloric Requirements. In general, the noncirrhotic patient with hepatitis C has caloric needs similar to those of noninfected people of the same age and gender. For this reason we recommend the following:

- no salt restriction
- no protein restriction
- 30 to 40 calories per kilogram intake per day
- one multivitamin per day

Patients who drink excessive amounts of alcohol should stop drinking altogether. They may also need supplementation with thiamine and folate.

Patients often proudly tell me that they are restricting their protein intake to "help" their livers. I'd like to emphasize that moderate amounts of protein (as recommended by the Food Pyramid) should be a normal part of your diet. If you are concerned about fat content, choose low-fat sources of protein. Protein restriction is recommended only for patients with cirrhosis who have encephalopathy (mental confusion).

Common questions I'm asked are, "Will dietary fat harm my liver? Should I avoid fat? Can I digest fat?" Dietary fat (triglycerides) undergoes complex processing (see Chapter 4). In the setting of liver disease, fat may accumulate in the liver. However, dietary fat intake does not correlate with the degree of fatty accumulation. Nonetheless, liver fat (steatosis) may promote liver injury and fibrosis in patients with viral hepatitis. Therefore, we do recommend a diet relatively low in fat, particularly saturated fat.

On the other hand, viral hepatitis by itself does not alter fat digestion or absorption from the gut. Only patients with advanced liver disease (cirrhosis) with jaundice have altered fat digestion and absorption. Jaundice in the setting of cirrhosis indicates severe impairment of processing and secretion of bile. Reduced bile concentration in the gut limits fat digestion and absorption.

Vitamin Supplements. In general, noncirrhotic patients with hepatitis C do not require any additional vitamin supplementation other than that noted above. One concern is that if bile production drops, the patient may become deficient in fat-soluble vitamins during the course of hepatitis C infection. This deficiency rarely develops during the early stages of hepatitis C, but it may be fairly prevalent at later, cirrhotic stages of the disease. When detected, deficiencies of fat-soluble vitamins should be corrected by administering proper doses of the compounds.

I am frequently asked, "Is it okay to take iron?" The answer goes beyond a simple yes or no. Women who are actively ovulating tend to lose iron through menstruation. Some of these women may develop iron deficiency and anemia, and they may actually benefit from iron. Men and non-ovulatory or post-menopausal women typically are not iron-deficient, and supplementation is not necessary. In fact, inappropriate supplementation with iron-loaded vitamins may be harmful in patients with liver disease.

One theory of the development of liver disease is that oxidant stress promotes liver cell injury and also stimulates specialized cells in the liver (stellate cells) to produce the main fibrosis protein, collagen. Iron is a catalyst for oxidant injury by promoting formation of "free radicals" that can initiate injury and fibrosis.

Supplemental vitamin C may be of potential benefit because it has antioxidant properties. However, vitamin C may promote iron absorption and lead to excessive accumulation of iron in the liver. The latter effect could actually increase oxidant injury. A reasonable, middle-ground approach is to take in the daily FDA-recommended amount of vitamin C and to avoid excessive supplementation.

Nutritional (Herbal) Therapies. Patients with viral hepatitis have used a number of "nutritional supplements," such as echinacea, pycnogenol, dandelion root, silymarin (milk thistle), and a wide array of herbal remedies. Most of these have not been studied in controlled trials and, thus, are unproved therapies. Silymarin has been studied but has not demonstrated benefit.

Despite the lack of supporting data, the use of these therapies has gained widespread acceptance among patients with hepatitis C. Several factors seem to account for this phenomenon: a history of lack of effective therapies for liver disease in general; incompletely effective treatment for hepatitis C; a general attitude that, "It can't hurt me, and maybe it'll help"; and the relatively mild and slowly progressive nature of hepatitis C.

Herbs have been used to treat illness since time began. In fact, many modern pharmaceuticals were discovered in natural sources. Aspirin originally came from the bark of the white willow tree. Cyclosporin, the miracle drug that suppresses the immune system and makes liver transplants possible, was found in a fungus growing in the soil of a plateau in southern Norway.

I have no doubt that future controlled studies of herbs for liver disease will result in useful treatments. Saw palmetto, for example, has been studied in a controlled trial by New York University researchers and found effective in certain doses for prostrate conditions. Some "natural" substances are ineffective, and others may be as powerful as approved Western medicines. However, until we have proof of effectiveness and safety, I cannot endorse or recommend that patients undergo nutritional therapies.

Quality control of potency and contaminants is another problem. In 1998, California investigators found that "nearly one-third of 260 imported Asian herbals were either spiked with drugs not listed on the label or contained lead, arsenic or mercury."[1]

In addition, herbs can interact with other medications you may be taking. For example, St. John's wort, a popular herbal antidepressant, recently has been found to decrease levels of life-sustaining cyclosporine in heart transplant patients.[2]

I do not recommend using herbs, but if you are interested in them, become informed. And remember that it is vitally important to tell your doctor if you are taking any nutritional supplement.

Under current laws, herbs classified as food or dietary supplements are exempt from regulations governing quality control and proof of effectiveness. Often, people will take the recommendations of the clerk who sells the supplements.

> *I went to a health food store and asked them to give me anything that would help my liver. I got coltsfoot, comfrey, petasites, chaparral, and yohimbe.*
>
> *My enzymes shot up to 800. When the doctor asked me if I was taking anything new, I brought in the bottles and learned that these herbs were best avoided because they may be toxic for the liver. I stopped taking them, and my enzymes went back down. I never thought anything "natural" could harm me.*
>
> *Harold*

Why isn't more research done on herbs? In 1978, the German government set up Commission E. The agency doesn't conduct research, but it does review studies and other evidence of safety and effectiveness, including anecdotal reports, and publishes its findings. Congress responded to public interest and increased funding for the National Institutes of Health (NIH) Center for Complementary and Alternative Medicine/Office of Alternative Medicine. In 2005 NIH-NIDDK and NCAAM jointly sponsored the review and funding of proposals for investigation of silymarin.

In 1994 Congress passed the Dietary Supplement Health and Education Act (DSHEA) that gave dietary supplement manufacturers the freedom to market more products. The Food and Drug Administration (FDA) must review clinical studies of drugs to determine effectiveness, safety, dosages, and possible interactions with other substances. Under DSHEA, however, the FDA does not test dietary supplements.

Herbs Harmful to the Liver. After a dietary supplement is on the market, the FDA has the responsibility for showing that it is unsafe before it can take action to restrict use. In June 1997 the FDA proposed to limit the amount of ephedrine alkaloids in dietary supplements (marketed as ephedra, Ma Huang, Chinese ephedra, and epitonin, for example) and to provide warnings to consumers about hazards (including hepatitis) associated with use of these substances.[3]

In 1993 the FDA named before a Senate committee other supplements as possible hazards associated with illness and injuries to the liver.

The list includes chaparral, comfrey, germander, vitamin A (in doses of 25,000 or more International Units a day), and niacin (in slow-release doses of 500 mg or more a day or immediate-release doses of 750 mg or more a day).

Here's a list I give to my patients of herbs that have been documented to cause liver problems ranging from hepatitis to liver failure: *Atractylis gummifera, Azadirachza indica, Berberis vulgaris, Calliepsis laureola, Cassia angustifolia* (senna), *Crotaiaria, Corydalis, Hedeoma pulegoides, Heliotropium, Larrea tridentata* (chaparral bush, creosote bush, Greasewood), *Lycopodium serratum* (jin bu huan), *Mentha pulegoides, Sassafras albidum* (sassafras), *Scuteileria* (skullcap), *Stephania, Symphytum officinale* (comfrey), *Teucrium chamaedrys* [germander (mint family)], *Tussilago farfara* (peppermint), *Valeriana officinalis* (valerian, asfetida, hops, gentian), *Viscum alba* [mistletoe, margosa oil, maté tea, gordolobo yerba tea, pennyroyal (squawmint) oil];[4] *Senecio, Heliotropium, Chelidonum majus* (greater celandine), and "a variety of Chinese herbal mixtures (artemisia, hare's ear, chrysanthemum, plantago seed, gardinia, red peony root, etc.").[5]

In my opinion, if you have a chronic liver disease, such as hepatitis C, you should avoid herbs that have not been tested in controlled studies, especially if you are being treated with interferon. Any substance, such as herbs or over-the-counter medications, may interact with drugs you are taking. Always discuss medicines and herbs with your physician.

Resource: Food and Drug Administration, Office of Consumer Affairs, HFE-88, Rockville, MD 20857. Consumer Food Information Line (Center for Food Safety and Applied Nutrition Outreach and Information Center): 800-FDA-4010 (in Washington, D.C., call 202-205-4314). FDA Website: www.cfsan.fda.gov/~dms/supplmnt.html

Resources: Contact the National Institutes of Health (NIH) National Center for Complementary and Alternative Medicine (NCCAM)/Office of Alternative Medicine Clearinghouse at 888-644-6226. Website: http://altmed.od.nih.gov

Access the NCCAM website with links to thousands of scientific citations related to complementary and alternative medicine. Website: http://nccam.nih.gov

Access the NIH Office of Dietary Supplements website for more information on nutritional supplements. Website: http://dietary-supplements.info.nih.gov/

Resource: Tyler, Varro E. *The Honest Herbal: A Sensible Guide to the Use of Herbs and Related Remedies.* New York: Pharmaceutical Products Press. 1993.

Resource: Gruenwald, Joerg, Thomas Brendler, Christof Jaenicke. *PDR for Herbal Medicines.* Montvale: Medical Economics. 2000.

Nutrition Tips from Patients. People with hepatitis C who are interested in nutrition find many ways to work toward healthier eating habits. Here are some of their suggestions:

> *I think you're crazy if you have hepatitis C and you drink alcohol. It's like taking poison.*

> *I try to be kind to my liver. I've switched to eating more complex carbohydrates, like veggies, fruits, whole grains. If Olympic athletes train on complex carbs for energy, I guess it's good for me, too.*

> *I've given up caffeine. I figure it can't do my liver any good. So every morning I have hot water with a bit of fresh lemon in it. It was hard to switch at first, but I'm used to it now.*

> *I don't tolerate fats as well as I did. I can't handle the beans, chili, and tortillas I used to eat—too fatty and salty. I can't handle fried foods at all. When I cook at home, I use mostly olive oil—sometimes canola oil.*

> *Eating small meals several times a day works better for me than eating a few large meals because I don't have much appetite. I also keep unsalted nuts in the car, in case I need a quick protein snack.*

> *Hot oatmeal tastes good on a cold morning. To add a little protein, I sprinkle some unsalted nuts on top. Also—to avoid using too much sugar, I add just a little bit of maple syrup. It's sugar, too, but a little goes a long way.*

> *I used to drink 2 percent milk. Turns out that it is not low in fat. In fact, 35 percent of its calories comes from fat. So I switched to skim milk. Now I like it just as well, and it has almost no fat in it.*

I used to drink lots of soda, too, until I looked at the labels—lots of sugar and salt and preservatives. I stopped all soda about a year ago. The other day I took a taste of a friend's drink and almost spit it out. My taste buds have changed.

You should see my new juicer. I'm a little intimidated by it, but I made the sweetest, freshest tasting carrot juice today. I've also heard that a carrot, beet, and cucumber combo is good, too. I figured I'd drink some of my veggies.

A lot is attitude. If you think of a healthy, low-fat diet as a pleasure—not a burden—you can get into it. I take the time to shop in a really pleasant supermarket or health food store, and I try to add new fruits and vegetables to my meals or snacks.

I try to sit down and not eat on the run. My biggest problem is that I have to eat out a lot for business, but I've learned to order fish and rice more often.

Nutritional Needs for Hepatitis C Patients with Cirrhosis

Caloric Requirements. In general, the patient with early-stage or compensated cirrhosis still requires 30 to 40 calories per kilogram a day. You may need to alter your dietary habits to take in this number of calories, because as hepatitis C progresses to cirrhosis, you may begin to experience loss of appetite, increasing fatigue, reduction in physical activity, and alteration of your sleep-wake pattern. People commonly complain of loss of exercise tolerance ("I'm just too pooped out to get my work done"). In addition, these changes often precipitate a sense of despondency, anxiety, or depression. It helps to develop both a pattern of meals that allows you to use your diet for maximum energy and a rest pattern that reduces prolonged periods of physical activity.

No nutritional prescription is right for every patient. You need to address your specific nutritional needs with your physician. In my experience, patients with hepatitis C who develop compensated cirrhosis benefit by more frequent, smaller volume meals. Instead of one or two large meals, divide the equivalent amount of calories into four smaller meals. In addition, supplementation with one or two tablets of multivitamins is generally indicated, although the overall benefit is unclear. Despite this change in dietary habit, fatigue often persists. People benefit from "rest periods," usually 30 minutes or an hour in the mid-afternoon.

Caution: Please understand that advanced cirrhosis is associated with severe impairment of liver function and that specific dietary modifications may be necessary and could alter the general guidelines noted above. Your doctor may recommend a consultation with a dietician or provide you with a specific nutritional prescription.

Protein Restriction. It is important that the patient with cirrhosis take in enough protein to avoid excessive muscle wasting and energy depletion. However, if encephalopathy develops, rarely a doctor might prescribe a "protein-restricted" diet.

Encephalopathy is the alteration or cloudiness of mental function. When the condition is severe, the patient becomes disoriented, confused, combative, or even comatose. Encephalopathy may also cause altered sleep-wake patterns, altered personality, and lack of motor coordination.

Physicians treat encephalopathy with medications such as lactulose, neomycin, or rifaximin. If encephalopathy continues, the physician may restrict dietary protein.

While I was waiting for my liver transplant, I'd get in the car and forget if I was leaving or coming. If you've got too much protein, it can cause you to fall asleep at the intersection. The doctor told me to stop driving and put me on a protein-restricted diet. I watch the amount I take in, and if I feel too tired, I cut back. It took lots of modification to eat more vegetables. I eat them like medicine, but I'm getting better at it.

I'm from South Dakota. I was raised on meat and potatoes. In fact, my parents joke that I was 16 before I found out that gravy wasn't a beverage!

Bill

Vitamin Supplements. Most people with hepatitis C, even those with cirrhosis, have adequate intake and storage of water-soluble vitamins (C, B complex). To be sure, I recommend the addition of two tablets of multivitamins each day (one in the morning and one in the evening).

Patients who excessively use or abuse alcohol risk becoming deficient in these vitamins, particularly thiamine and folate, and they may benefit from taking supplements. As I have emphasized before, the hepatitis C patient should avoid alcohol. Those who avoid alcohol probably won't require either supplement.

There are few data on the overall extent of vitamin deficiencies in patients with hepatitis C. However, as part of our evaluation of cirrhotic patients for liver transplantation, we assessed the plasma levels of certain vitamins and found that approximately 20 percent of hepatitis C patients were deficient in vitamin A, vitamin D (25-OH), and vitamin E. Although few patients had symptoms that could be attributed to these deficiencies, it seems reasonable to monitor patients' vitamin levels as cirrhosis progresses and give supplements to those with low levels.

Mineral Supplements. Patients with cirrhosis may experience deficiencies in three minerals: calcium, magnesium, and zinc. Calcium deficiency may be related to a lack of vitamin D, poor nutrition, or malabsorption. Correcting the underlying abnormality may be all that is required to restore calcium balance. However, bone thinning may occur even without these specific problems, so I recommend 0.5 to 1.0 grams of calcium each day. Calcium may be taken in the form of dairy products or therapeutic supplements. When the patient can't take in enough dairy products because of protein, salt, or fluid restrictions (see next section), supplements are used.

Magnesium deficiency may occur due to inadequate dietary intake. However, it occurs more often when patients take diuretics to treat fluid retention because their kidneys flush out the magnesium as waste. Symptoms of magnesium deficiency include muscle cramps, fatigue, weakness, nausea, and vomiting. Often, it's not possible to modify or discontinue diuretics in cirrhotic patients, so magnesium supplementation (500 mg magnesium gluconate three times a day) may be required.

Zinc deficiency may cause the loss of the senses of smell and taste. Patients with these symptoms may benefit from supplementation with zinc sulfate (220 mg three times a day).

Salt and Fluid Restriction. Cirrhosis disturbs the regulation of body salt and water. Severe liver disease generates neural and hormonal signals to the kidney that cause the kidney to retain both salt and water. The salt acts like a sponge. As a result, fluid accumulates in certain tissues and body spaces, such as the ankles (peripheral edema), abdomen (ascites), and chest (pleural effusion).

TABLE 5B. 2–GRAM SALT DIET SAMPLE MENU*

Breakfast (352–765 mg)
  1-2 pieces toast (150-400 mg)
  1-2 tsp margarine (50 mg)
  1 tbsp orange marmalade
  1 boiled egg (62 mg)
      or 1 fried egg (162 mg)
  1 C cooked cereal with little or no salt (1 mg)
  ½–1 C milk (60-120 mg)
  6 oz brewed coffee (4 mg)/tea (5 mg)/herbal tea (2 mg)
  1 C cantaloupe (14 mg) or strawberries (2 mg)
  1 C orange juice (2 mg)

Lunch (503–611 mg)
  3.5 oz salmon patty (96 mg)
  1 slice tomato (½ mg) and ½ C lettuce (1 mg)
  1 oz. potato chips (about 10 chips) (170 mg)
  1 C fresh grapes (2 mg)
  1 C apple juice (7 mg)
  1 carrot (25 mg) and 1 stalk of celery (3.5 mg)
  1 piece angel food cake [161 mg (homemade); approx. 270 mg
      (packaged mix)]
  8 oz ice tea (5 mg) with lemon (less than 1 mg)

Dinner (431–601 mg)
  3.5 oz roast beef (63-73 mg) au jus with no added salt
      (if packaged gravy mix, 2 oz = approx. 160 mg)
  1 baked potato (16 mg)
  1 tbsp sour cream (6mg)/margarine (100 mg)
  ½ C frozen green beans (3 mg)
  1½ C tossed fresh salad (5 mg) with salt-free salad dressing
  1 piece apple (181 mg) with ½ C vanilla ice cream (53 mg)
  6 oz coffee (4 mg)

* *Sodium levels generally refer to fresh homemade items, are approximate, and vary with brand names of products used. Fast, pre-packaged, or canned foods usually contain much higher levels of sodium.*

The dietitian restricted me to 2,000 milligrams of sodium a day. That's one teaspoon! I try, but I really like salt. If I don't watch carefully, though—say I eat some broth, and it has salt in it—I pick up extra water. It takes days to flush it out.

I can get 11 to 14 pounds of fluid out every few days. Once I had 30 pounds of water on me. I had a belly like a pregnant rhino.

My wife says if I wouldn't cover everything with "white death," I'd do a lot better.

Randy

Treatment of fluid retention always requires dietary salt restriction, often requires diuretics (medicines that block the kidney and cause increased urination of salt and water), and sometimes requires fluid restriction. Patients need to understand that the major driving force behind the accumulation of fluid is the excessive retention of salt. Diuretics work because they cause the kidney to lose salt. If you take in too much salt in your diet, you'll cause more fluid to accumulate in your body. In other words, you can override the effects of the diuretics, and patients on diuretics can actually retain fluid if they don't comply with a salt-restricted diet.

The usual salt restriction is two grams per day (see Table 5B). Commonly used diuretics are Aldactone® (spironolactone), Midamor® (amiloride), Lasix® (furosemide), HCTZ® (hydrochlorothiazide), and Zaroxylyn® (metolozone). Aldactone® and Midamor® conserve potassium, while Lasix®, HCTZ®, and Zaroxylyn® waste potassium. Most of the time, a doctor will prescribe the two types of diuretics together to minimize any changes in blood potassium levels. Occasionally, potassium supplements are used to keep blood potassium in the normal range.

The physician usually orders fluid restriction only for edematous (swollen with fluid) patients with low levels of sodium in their blood. Fluid restriction means restriction of all fluids: water, tea, coffee, milk, etc. Patients with severe symptomatic low blood sodium may find it necessary to restrict their fluid intake to less than one quart a day.

Caution: Always consult with your physician regarding use of diuretics (doses and frequency) or dietary restrictions on salt or fluid intake. It is potentially dangerous to self-medicate or introduce dietary restrictions without physician consultation.

He who keeps on eating after his stomach is full
digs his grave with his teeth.

Turkish proverb

References

1. Gugliotta, Guy. "Supplements Aren't So Healthy," *Denver Post* March 19, 2000: 5A.
2. Breidenbach, T.H. M.W. Hoffman, T.H. Becker, H. Schlitt, J. Klempnauer. "Drug Interaction of St. John's Wort with Cyclosporine." *Lancet.* 27 May 2000; 355:1912.
3. Kurtzweil, Paula. "An FDA Guide to Dietary Supplements," *FDA Consumer* Sept.-Oct. 1998:29.
4. Larrey, D. G.P. Pageaux. "Hepatotoxicity of Herbal Remedies and Mushrooms." *Seminars in Liver Disease.* 1995; 15:183–188.
5. Schuppan, D. J.D. Jia, B. Brinkhaus, E.G. Hahn. "Herbal Products for Liver Diseases: A Therapeutic Challenge for the New Millennium." *Hepatology.* 1999; 30:1100.

6

TAKING CARE OF
YOURSELF EMOTIONALLY
Emotional Challenges
of Chronic Illness

As a person with hepatitis C, I live with the emotional highs and lows of this disease. Every blood test and biopsy report shakes me up. Every time I get tired and can't get through a job that I used to do easily, I get angry and discouraged. It's a struggle not to get obsessed with my health.

Some days, I get mad when my friends act too protective, and other times I get mad when they leave me alone. It's hard to shake off the sadness. And then there are those glorious moments—a crisp fall day, a family dinner—when life is a gift that's unbearably beautiful.

Hedy

IN THIS CHAPTER, Dr. Everson and I draw on the expertise of mental health professionals who work with hepatitis C patients. We also present the experiences of the patients themselves. Who else really understands?

Here are the topics we'll cover:

- The Emotional Challenge
- Phase 1: Diagnosis
- Special Problems with a Diagnosis of Hepatitis C
- Phase 2: Impact (Attitudes and Expectations)
- Phase 3: Reorganization
- Healing vs. Curing
- Warning Signs of Depression
- Understanding your Family and Friends (Family Systems)
  Boundaries
- Tools for Wellness: Some Practical Suggestions
  Medical Care and Psychological Help
  Exercise and Nutrition
  Feeling Useful/Having Fun
  Exploring Your Creative and Spiritual Sides

The Emotional Challenge

Hepatitis C is an emotional and physical challenge. Many researchers have tried to measure the health related quality of life (HRQOL) of patients in clinical trials. Recently, scientists examined the results of 32 such HRQOL studies and used various statistical methods to compare patients and control groups in eight categories: physical function, physical role, bodily pain, general health, vitality, social function, emotional role, and mental health.

The analysis found that patients with hepatitis C had a clinically significant consistently diminished health related quality of life compared with matched controls without hepatitis C. As one would expect, patients with a sustained viral response had an improved HRQOL compared with those who did not achieve it. The impact of hepatitis C was most pronounced on the vitality, general health, physical function, and social function scales.

Traditional measures, such as ALT levels and histological changes, did not correlate with HRQOL "suggesting that traditional outcomes may fail to capture the full spectrum of illness related to the hepatitis C virus." The data indicated that HCV itself may diminish health related quality of life in the absence of advanced liver disease, "perhaps as a result of extrahepatic symptoms related to HCV, cognitive dysfunction related to HCV, or a negative synergy between HCV and comorbid [other underlying] psychosocial disorders."[1]

As this analysis shows, hepatitis C may be the biggest emotional challenge you'll ever face. How do you deal with chronic disease without letting it take over your life?

"The goal is balance," says Meredith Pate-Willig, a licensed clinical social worker. Ms. Pate-Willig facilitates Denver support groups for the Hep C Connection and serves as a trainer for other support group facilitators.

How do you achieve balance and a "wellness lifestyle"? "There's no shortcut through normal, natural cycles of grief," says Pate-Willig. "Grieving is nature's way of helping us adapt to new information about our illness."

Too often, we're hard on ourselves as we grieve. In a world of instant cereal and microwave popcorn, we think we should be grieving faster, better. The truth is, each one of us goes through the process in our own time frame and in our own way—and the healing ingredient is kindness. Be patient with yourself. You will work it through, and you will come out of the crisis with a stronger sense of who you are.

According to Pate-Willig, it's helpful to think of these spiraling cycles of grief in three phases: diagnosis, impact, and reorganization.

Phase 1: Diagnosis

Diagnosis plunges you into a state of disbelief or shock.

> *I didn't realize it then, but it was the day my life changed forever. I was numb. I didn't even know that I was feeling shock and grief at what I had lost—my sense of health. When I walked out to the parking lot, the sun was still shining, but everything looked different. It felt unreal.*
>
> *Dave*

If you lose your sense of yourself as a healthy person, and you struggle or rebel against becoming a patient, how do you adjust? Some patients develop a sense of grief. Grieving is one way we work through loss, whether it's loss of our old selves ("I used to cook big family dinners. Now I'm too tired.") or loss of our dreams ("Will I ever marry now? Know my grandchildren? Launch a new business?"). According to Pate-Willig, "Grieving is normal—even necessary. It's the bridge between what was to what is. If you don't go across that bridge, you may face a continuing struggle."

In this first phase of diagnosis, you need your family and support system to pull together to help you adjust:

1. The diagnosis may make you feel uncomfortable or leave you with a numbing sense of shock and loss. You should understand that this response is normal.
2. Everyone needs psychological and social support—not just the person with hepatitis C. Other family members may be affected by the diagnosis. When one part of a system changes, everything in the system reacts in a "ripple" effect.

When I was first diagnosed, I went numb. The first person I told was my best friend. She broke down—a flood of tears. I was horrified to find that my inner reaction was rage. I wanted to yell, "Hey, just a minute. I'm the one with the problem here!"

Thank goodness, I didn't say anything out loud, but I was mad until I realized that she had her own grief about losing me, her best friend, as she's always known me. Her world was shaken up, too.

All I wanted, all I ever really want even now, is for someone to put an arm around me and say, "I'm here. I know this is hard. I care about you."

Estelle

People may not respond to you in the way that you anticipate or expect. You may process the information fast while family members take longer, or the reverse. How fast or how slowly people absorb the news affects the dynamics in a marriage or friendship—leaving everyone with the unconscious feeling that somehow the rules changed. In fact, just identifying these changes takes a while.

Sometimes, the patient or support system refuses to accept the new reality. "Denial," says Pate-Willig, "is a misunderstood defense. When it acts as a circuit-breaker, it keeps your system from overloading. That can be healthy. Denial becomes unhealthy when it keeps you from finding appropriate medical treatment."

Special Problems with a Diagnosis of Hepatitis C

Dealing with a diagnosis of any chronic illness is difficult, but patients with hepatitis C have special issues:

Feeling Low. You may be experiencing fatigue, low energy, loss of ability to concentrate, and a sense of inadequacy in doing daily tasks. These symptoms may make you more emotionally vulnerable and susceptible to periods of depression. Be sure to tell your doctor if you feel seriously depressed.

Feeling Contaminated. Although the virus is transmitted only by blood-to-blood contact, you may have questions and fears about who will avoid you. How will your friends or boss react? What do you tell your dentist?

> *I can't believe this guy at work. I left a can of pop on the table for a minute, and he drank it by mistake. He freaked out when he found out it was mine. Now he won't even talk to me if he can help it. When he passes my desk, he won't even look me in the eye!*
>
> *Bonnie*

How You Got Infected. When you try to figure out how this happened to you, your answer may affect how you deal with your diagnosis: (1) If you can point to a blood transfusion, you don't feel responsible for your illness; (2) if you've injected drugs, whether it was a minor episode or you're still involved, you have to process the painful idea that you did this to yourself; (3) people who don't know how they got infected may never figure it out, and that uncertainty creates its own dilemmas.

Looking Good. Strange as it sounds, people often have trouble offering comfort to someone who doesn't have a visible wound. In the early and middle stages of infection, you may suffer silent symptoms, such as fatigue and joint pains. Unfortunately, many people (including yourself) may have a hard time believing you're ill. Unless you explain the nature of hepatitis C, you may not get the support you need.

For years before I was diagnosed, I dealt with an energy level that seemed to be going downhill. I stopped playing tennis because I couldn't run fast enough to get to the ball. I had to give up biking when my knees ached so bad.

Now I just learned I have hepatitis C, but my wife doesn't listen. "You look fine," she says. "You're just getting older."

George

Fluctuating Nature of Hepatitis C. Who knows why a person's PCR assay shows a low viral load one month but a sky-high count the next? The fluctuating course of hepatitis C sometimes gives the patient the feeling of walking on shifting sand, never knowing what each day will bring.

Lack of Information. Uncertainty due to lack of information is a huge stressor. You have no way to answer the questions, "What am I dealing with, and how will it affect my life?" What facts your doctor offers you about your stage of illness, therefore, have a big influence on how you deal with the diagnosis.

What Can You Do to Help Yourself? "Be patient with yourself," says Pate-Willig. "Accept that this is a difficult time, and try not to beat yourself up for being normal, human."

The results of my second biopsy sent me into a tailspin. My liver was worse! It was like going back to the first day I was told I had hepatitis C. For days and weeks I struggled to control panic attacks and crying jags. I couldn't get on top of it.

Finally, a friend with hepatitis C told me not to stuff the pain and sadness. "The only thing that works for me," she said, "is to feel it all the way."

When I gave myself time to feel whatever it was—no matter how painful—I was able to move on with the rest of my day. I didn't get stuck.

Lani

"Remember to be kind to yourself. Patience, patience, and more patience. That's the key," says Pate-Willig. "Expect to feel emotional cycles, ups and downs, each time the activity of your disease changes or you experience a new symptom."

Phase 2: Impact (Attitudes and Expectations)

In Phase 1, the task for you and your support system is to pull together to confront and understand the new diagnosis. In the second phase, the question becomes, "How do we function now that we know that hepatitis C is a chronic condition? How do we gear up for the long haul?" It's a time of changing attitudes and expectations as you explore your options.

The challenge is how to connect with friends and family and still maintain the autonomy and space you need. Your questions may vary from large ("I'm a single parent with no one to care for me. Should I go back to my mom and dad's house or keep my own apartment?") to small ("My husband had a transplant. Should I play in my Thursday night bowling league or stay home with him?").

Families often have unspoken rules and myths about illness. Perhaps the message you got was, "Keep a stiff upper lip and don't show you're scared." Or maybe you grew up in a home where a cold meant deluxe pampering. What happens if you break these rules?

> *I finally told my older brother how scared and panicky I felt. It turned out that my brother had a friend who also had hepatitis C. "He doesn't make any big deal," my brother said. "In fact, he won't even discuss it. He believes in a positive outlook."*
>
> *Compared to my brother's friend, I was a big complainer. Of course, that was my secret fear all along—being the family wimp.*
>
> *Melissa*

Phase 3: Reorganization

As you move into Phase 3, you and your family begin to reorganize around the new reality. A sense of acceptance emerges, and you start to answer these questions: Who am I now? How am I going to make my life work?

At some point, things settle down. Perhaps you come to terms with a reduced energy level, make dietary changes, decide on a treatment plan.

It got to be too much for me. I couldn't even cope with a full work day. Cassie and I had planned a mountain climbing vacation in the Rockies, but we decided to spend a week at a bed-and-breakfast with a mountain view instead. Finally, I had to accept reality.

Jim

Anything that tips the precarious balancing act shakes the system. If you start interferon treatment, you and your family and friends may need to organize around the treatment. Suppose you decide to plan a nap each day, while someone else assumes your chores. What most people don't realize is that *any* change, positive or negative, alters the system. So, paradoxically, you may need to reorganize after you have finished interferon treatment. For example, you may still feel the need for a daily nap, but the people around you may now disapprove.

The cycle of confronting the diagnosis, feeling its impact, and reorganizing yourself to deal with hepatitis C may recur with each piece of health news. If hepatitis C moves into advanced liver disease and a possible transplant, the concept of death may come to the forefront.

"The first big breakthrough for most people is the realization of how physically fragile we humans are," says Pate-Willig. "It's a difficult task to process, reprioritize, accept your mortality, and—at the same time—plan for post-transplant living."

Healing vs. Curing

"We are all desperate for curing," says Pate-Willig, "but a physical cure may be years away. We need to shift to healing—a balance and wholeness of mind, body, and spirit.

"As we become more aware of our emotional responses, we learn how healthy it is to *lean* into the grief process and accept it. We learn how to tap into resources that can help, such as dietary changes and relaxation techniques. The goal is to come out of each cycle at a higher level, to feel better about ourselves, and to see more flexibility in ourselves and others as we learn how to cope."

Grief can be the great healer. Grief is to the psyche and the spirit what the physical process is to the healing of a wound.

So, you say, "That sounds great. But how do I grieve?"

"Talk about what's happening to you," says Pate-Willig. Talk to a friend, a support group, a journal. Get on the Internet. Help yourself by re-evaluating your feelings each time you tell and retell your story. As you do this, you fit your new self into your old idea of yourself.

"The Chinese symbol for crisis is both danger and opportunity. Chronic illness can give us the opportunity to become deeper, broader, more flexible, and to find meaning in our lives."

Warning Signs of Depression

While grieving and depression are normal, sustained depression is not. Fortunately, there are many ways to treat depression with medications and "talk" therapy, so it's important to tell your doctor, advises Robert House, M.D.

What are the signs of depression? According to Dr. House, be on the alert for some of these symptoms, if they are *changes* from your normal behavior pattern:

- low energy, fatigue, lack of interest in your usual activities
- withdrawn and/or irritable behavior
- sleep disturbances that show a change in your routine pattern (such as sleeping less or more, waking up a lot, or waking earlier or later than usual, not rested and ready to begin the day)
- significant weight loss over a short period of time
- loss of appetite, food doesn't taste good
- tearfulness, breaking into tears for no apparent reason, "out of the blue"
- forming and talking about ideas of suicide, or a sense that life is not worth living
- feeling of hopelessness, helplessness that things won't get better
- reluctance to resume activities of daily living after a transplant (such as not getting along with your family, if you've always done so before; not resuming sexual relations with your spouse after a reasonable length of time; not dating, if single; isolating yourself from others).

Understanding Your Family and Friends (Family Systems)

Chronic illness is a family illness. When one member of a family becomes sick, it affects everyone. Normally, a family stays in balance with its own set of unwritten roles and rules. Roles involve position (Who is the breadwinner? Who takes out the garbage?). Roles always change as the patient needs to do less and shifts tasks to others. Rules are values; they can be about communication (Who can say what to whom?), emotion (Who is allowed to be sad?), education, sex, religion, and parenting.

Most important for people with hepatitis C are the family rules and values about health and illness. Problems arise when your family rules (or the rules of the family you grew up in) clash. Can you take time off if you have a cold or only if you're deathly ill? How do you handle the medical system?

> *My husband and I are having a hard time about my hepatitis C. He's an exercise nut and overdoses on vitamins. I do what my doctor tells me, and that's enough. My husband is constantly after me to change my lifestyle, and I get exasperated. I want to shout at him, "Leave me alone. I'll do it my way!"*
>
> *Janice*

Boundaries. Families create different boundaries. Some are so enmeshed that it's hard to tell where one member begins and another ends. They know how to pull together but need to learn how to allow outsiders to help. At the other end of the spectrum is the disengaged family where members have a high degree of autonomy and very little strong communication with each other. They need to learn how to draw closer, so they can hear each other and support one another. Most families, of course, fall somewhere in between these two extremes.

> *My sister would say, "Come on, let's go shopping." I didn't want to go because the interferon treatment made me tired. I knew she'd get mad if I had to leave in a couple of hours. So I'd say no. Then she'd glare at me and preach to me. She was always trying to control me.*

We had a blowout. We had been inseparable, and suddenly we weren't speaking.

Sally

Chronic illness can cause disorganization, but this crisis can open more options and choices as the family modifies and changes its rules and values.

My mom always said it was hard to believe someone was sick unless you could see a bleeding wound. But she stuck up for me all through my interferon treatment. Even though she's 85, and you'd think it would be hard for her to change, she was—and still is—the one person who understands what I'm going through.

Pete

Families also go through life stages that have their own issues of separateness and connectedness, from the birth of a child to taking care of elderly parents. When illness occurs, it can disrupt the normal tasks of these life stages. Suppose, for example, that hepatitis C strikes a parent of a teenager. The teenager will feel pulled by conflicting forces: the need to separate and develop a life with peers versus the need to pull closer to the family. In this setting the adolescent must cope with developing separateness and freedom and providing more help with household or other chores.

Communication and openness are the keys to improving the level of understanding within your family. When family members talk about a problem in terms of shifts in roles, rules and life stages, it diffuses the personal element. Usually, people feel hurt when a conflict arises because they think the other family members don't care about them. When you define the problem as a conflict in family roles, values, or degree of separation/connection, you can work toward a resolution.

Suppose, for example, that George wants his wife, Susan, to come with him to all his medical appointments. Meanwhile, Susan has had to take a part-time job to help pay the bills. Even though it's no one's fault, she's angry. Susan can't do it all, and her former role as the family's primary emotional support needs to be modified. Instead of blaming each other and feeling unloved, Susan and George talk about the role changes and come up with a compromise. Susan will go to the important medical appointments, and George will ask his sister to accompany him to the routine ones.

Do people want to change a family system? No, but illness brings unavoidable changes and, therefore, a feeling of loss of control. You can choose to be angry, or you can decide what can be changed and what cannot. How can we figure out a new system that's fair to everybody? What roles and values can we let go or modify?

Tools for Wellness: Some Practical Suggestions

Life-challenging illnesses, like hepatitis C, present opportunities for rethinking priorities. We may not always be able to cure the disease, but we can improve the quality of our lives. We can nourish ourselves by getting good medical and psychological care, exercising, eating nutritional foods, trying to live meaningful and useful lives, deepening relationships, having fun, and exploring our creative and spiritual sides.

Adapt an open and curious attitude when exploring these areas, and don't try all of them at once. Make changes gradually. Here are some suggestions from Pate-Willig and others:

CAUTION: Specific recommendations regarding diet, nutrition, and exercise may vary and should be evaluated and discussed with your physician.

Medical and Psychological Help. Put together your medical team with care. The treatment of hepatitis C is evolving and requires knowledge of specialized tests and treatments. Many doctors don't have much experience with hepatitis C, so find a gastroenterologist or hepatologist who does. Most medical centers have doctors who specialize in liver disease (hepatologists) or can recommend appropriate community specialists.

Although credentials are important, effective therapy may also be dependent upon the doctor-patient relationship. Make sure that the two of you are a good fit. This is a very individual matter. Do you like your doctor to tell you exactly what to do, or do you prefer to have more input with decision-making? Does the doctor answer your questions fully, or seem anxious to exit? Do the nurses and receptionist seem friendly and supportive?

If you need to see a mental health professional (psychologist, psychiatrist, social worker, professional counselor), get names from friends you trust and interview a few practitioners. Ask about their backgrounds and qualifications. Make sure they have experience in dealing with issues of chronic illness. They should be graduates of an accredited master's or Ph.D. program and licensed by the state as an independent practitioner or supervised by someone who is licensed.

Keep abreast of developments in hepatitis C research. The more you know, the better your decisions will be. (See the "Resources" section at the back of this book.) And finally, look at your own beliefs and attitudes about illness. Otherwise, you can't decide what works for you and what doesn't. We don't choose to be sick, but we can choose how we try to handle the situation.

Resources:

Bridges, William. *Transitions.* Reading: Addison-Wesley, 1980.

Clarke, Peter & Susan H. Evans. *Surviving Modern Medicine, How to Get the Best from Doctors, Family & Friends.* New Brunswick: Rutgers University Press, 1998.

Flach, Frederic, M.D. *Resilience: The Power to Bounce Back When the Going Gets Tough.* New York: Hatherleigh Press, 1997.

Kushner, Harold S. *When Bad Things Happen to Good People.* New York: Avon, 1981.

Travis, John W., M.D. and Regina Sara Ryan. *Wellness Workbook.* Berkeley: Ten Speed Press, 1988.

Many studies prove the importance of support systems. The results of one well-known study, reported in 1989 by psychiatrist David Spiegel and colleagues, showed that women with metastatic breast cancer who attended weekly group therapy sessions lived significantly longer than those who did not.[2]

Most of us benefit from a network of informal supportive relationships. Effective support always includes a sharing of emotions and feelings—a quality of reciprocity. Each person feels heard and validated, and has a sense of being able to draw upon that support, if necessary.

Formal support groups are useful because they provide a common experience for hepatitis C patients, information-sharing, a sense of not being alone, and a safe place to share feelings.

Resources: The "Resources" section at the back of this book lists national organizations that can direct you to local support groups in your area, phone networks, and online support groups. Also, your local hospital might be able to refer you to a group.

Hepatitis magazine contains an updated directory of resources and organizations. Contact the magazine at 523 N. Sam Houston Pkwy. East,

Suite   300,   Houston,   TX   77060,   281-272-2744;   Email: editor@hepatitismag.com; Website: www.hepatitismag.com.

The Hepatitis Neighborhood offers a Support Group Search of almost 500 groups listed by state and a weekly Town Hall chat room (on specific topics) supervised by nurses. Website: www.hepatitisneighborhood.com.

Exercise and Nutrition. Physical movement not only strengthens your body, it helps your emotional state. If you can afford it, a personal trainer with experience in chronic illness is helpful. Hospitals often have cardiac or stroke rehabilitation experts who may be able to refer you to the right professional, but you don't need money to exercise. You can walk with a friend, rent yoga or tai chi videos, or try water exercise to avoid stress on painful joints. Be creative.

For information on nutrition, see chapter 5, Taking Care of Yourself Nutritionally.

CAUTION: Consult your doctor before you begin any exercise program or make dietary changes.

Feeling Useful/Having Fun. We need a sense of meaning and purpose in our lives. We also need to have fun and play. Look for activities that create joy, hope, and a sense of living fully.

> *I'd always been a workaholic, but I started to question that kind of life when I learned I had hepatitis C. I didn't even like my job!*
>
> *I started to try some new things like meditation. Then I got into art therapy and got really excited. One day I made a sand tray containing images of my life. In it, I put a house without a roof because my nice suburban dream had blown up. I made a monster in a cage, because I felt like a monster, and a treehouse with the goddess Diana, who was the powerful part of me. I made a bridge that meant I was trying to get somewhere—paradise, a stream, lots of unconscious images.*
>
> *I changed jobs. I played more. I ate healthier foods. As I look back now, I see that I'm in paradise. I crossed the bridge!*
>
> *Maria*

Ask yourself these questions: What is important to me? How am I acting on the important things in my life? How can I continue to have a meaningful existence within the limits of my health and energy levels?

Resources:

Anderson, Greg. *50 Essential Things to Do When the Doctor Says It's Cancer.* New York: Penguin, 1993.

LeShan, Lawrence. *Cancer As a Turning Point.* New York: Penguin, 1994.

Topf, Linda Noble with Hal Z. Bennett. *You Are Not Your Illness.* New York: Fireside, 1995.

Playing helps you recapture joy. "Like humor, a good joyful experience does as much for your sense of well-being as a good physical workout," says Pate-Willig. It requires flexibility and a commitment to explore options. If you can't climb mountains anymore, investigate handicapped-accessible trails or rent travel videos. Open yourself to new experiences. If you've never explored poetry, for example, now may be the time to visit your neighborhood library.

"Learn to live mindfully," says Pate-Willig. "Ask yourself: 'Do I notice the people chattering at my dinner table, and am I grateful for my family? Do I savor the vivid colors of the vegetables I'm cutting? Do I stop for a moment during the day to notice that I feel good?'"

Exploring Your Creative and Spiritual Sides. Using the mind's capacity for healing includes visualization, relaxation, guided imagery, meditation, journal writing, and creative arts. All of these are ways to help the mind create a quieter atmosphere and to improve your quality of life.

Visualization, meditation, and relaxation create a sense of relaxed alertness and counteract the stress of daily living. Visit a bookstore and look over the tapes and videos. There are more than 30 methods, so the important thing is to find what makes you feel comfortable.

Resources:

Benson, Herbert and Miriam Klipper. *The Relaxation Response.* New York: Avon, 1976.

Kabat-Zinn, Jon. *Full Catastrophe Living.* New York: Dell, 1990.

Journal writing lowers stress levels and can be your best friend in the middle of the night when there's no one else to talk to. Write quickly, don't censor yourself, and find a safe place to keep your journal.

Resources:

Capacchione, Lucia. *The Well-Being Journal.* North Hollywood: Newcastle, 1989.

Remen, Rachel Naomi, M.D. *Kitchen Table Wisdom, Stories That Heal.* New York: Riverhead Books, 1996.

Creative art forms (painting, drawing, music, dance, poetry) are healing because you work with symbols and images to express feelings.

Resource: Capacchione, Lucia. *The Creative Journal.* North Hollywood: Newcastle, 1989.

At first, after the diagnosis, I went a little crazy with therapies. I mean, I did it all—talk therapy, yoga, you name it and I did it. I ran myself ragged keeping up with all the appointments.

Finally, I decided it was too messy. I wanted to play. I took a dance weekend, and there it was. When I danced, I got to the stillness inside me. For me, dance relates to life and the creative process. Staccato movements, for example, meant I was having trouble with boundaries, with saying no. It became a metaphor for all of my life, and I began to feel healing on all levels.

Then we moved, and when I was going through boxes, guess what I found? A pair of little ballet slippers! I had completely forgotten that as a kid I had taken dance lessons—and loved them.

Sara

Guided imagery is a specific kind of relaxation and movement using the mind's own images. Most mental health professionals who deal with illness can assist you in creating an individual tape that works for you. A prerequisite is to practice relaxation so you can access guided imagery. The technique uses all five senses and works best when it's tailored to you. Not everyone sees images, for example. If that's the case with you, the therapist will use sounds or smells instead.

My ALT counts were high—in the 500s, so I went on interferon. It sounds a little far out, but I started to do this white light meditation. I visualized the interferon working on the hepatitis. Then my viral counts lowered to zero.

I visualized the interferon, like white knights assisting my immune system. B.I.S., Bill's Immune System. I saw a whole army of three million knights in shining armor!

Bill

Even if you don't hold formal religious beliefs, you can tap into your spirituality, says Pate-Willig. "Think back to your feelings at the birth of your child, or when you suddenly came upon a bed of glorious wildflowers. Spirituality connects you with a sense of something larger than the self."

If I had had to face death the year I was diagnosed, I would have felt I never lived. I was terrified, and I would have been angry with lots of regrets.

But as I got sicker, I had to go on disability. That gave me the time to explore, and I found out I could meditate, become still, and have a connection to a higher power. Now that I've had a chance to live fully, somehow I'm not as frightened of death.

Steve

Illness, however, can also present a theological challenge. According to Dr. House, some patients "go through a crisis of faith. People who've gone to church all their lives may suddenly feel rejected, alone and abandoned, angry with God, or feel this illness is punishment for some unknown sin. Their social network is centered on their church, so if they lose this, they lose a lot. I recommend that they talk to their clergy or to the hospital chaplain."

"Spiritual distress," says Rev. Julie Swaney, chaplain at the University of Colorado Health Sciences Center, "occurs when a person's faith or spirit is suddenly full of holes. Everything you believe in is gone. You've lost your value system, and you feel alone. But one of the gifts of illness is the way it opens us up to life. People reassess relationships, values, their sense of time, of what's important. Spirituality has to do with how we make meaning out of our experiences. Embrace what works for you."

Resources:

Benson, Herbert, M.D., with Marg Stark. *Timeless Healing: The Power and Biology of Belief.* New York: Scribner, 1996.

Byock, Ira, M.D. *Dying Well, Peace and Possibilities at the End of Life.* New York: Riverhead Books, 1997.

Frankl, Victor E. *Man's Search for Meaning.* New York: Simon & Schuster, 1984.

Kushner, Harold S. *When All You've Ever Wanted Isn't Enough*. New York: Simon & Schuster, 1986.

Finally, one last word on being good to yourself: Take small steps to wellness slowly, over time. There is no correct formula. You may move back and forth, concentrating first on one area, then another—whatever works!

> *There is no grief which time does not lessen and soften.*

> *Cicero*

Reference

1. Spiegel, Brennan M.R., Z. M. Younossi, R. D. Hays, D. Revicki, S. Robbins, F. Kanwal. "Impact of Hepatitis C on Health Related Quality of Life: A Systematic Review and Quantitative Assessment." *Hepatology*. April 2005; Vol. 41, No. 4: 790-800.
2. Spiegel, David. M.D. *Living Beyond Limits*. (New York: Random House, 1993), p. 79.

7

TAKING CARE OF
YOURSELF FINANCIALLY
An Overview

Hey, this hepatitis C thing is tough. I get so tired, I almost fall asleep driving my truck. I've learned to pull over and take a quick nap. Just a few minutes, then I'm okay again.

I told my bosses I had hepatitis C. They nodded and said all the right things, but hey, it doesn't matter. I still have to do my job or I'm out. And if I'm out, I don't have health insurance. Then I can't afford interferon. But if I'm on interferon, I'm tired and I'm having trouble doing the work.

It's a Catch-22 situation, all right.

Tim

LIKE TIM, you may feel too sick to work, but you can't quit because you need to hold on to your health insurance. Or you're getting so many medical bills, you're worried about paying the mortgage. Any chronic illness can put a dent in your budget.

Each one of you, however, faces a different situation. This chapter presents a general overview of financial issues and supplies you with resources to help you find your own solutions.★

We'll cover:

- Cost of Treatment
  Ongoing Medical Care
  Antiviral Treatment
  Transplantation Costs
- Private Health Insurance
  Selecting Health Insurance
  Types of Private Health Insurance: Managed Care or Fee-for-Service
  HMOs
  PPOs
  Fee-for-Service Plans
- Government Health Insurance
  Medicare
  Medicaid
  Veterans Administration (VA)
- When You're Too Sick to Work: Applying for Disability
  Short-Term Disability Leave
- Disability Insurance
  Social Security Disability Insurance (SSDI)
  Supplemental Security Income (SSI)

★*Note:* This chapter is an overview, not an exhaustive treatment of financial options and programs. It does not provide legal advice; always contact agencies and companies for specific information and consult a lawyer for legal advice in specific cases.

Cost of Treatment

Ongoing Medical Care Costs. If you have a chronic illness, like hepatitis C, you have to consider the cost of lifelong medical care. At the very least, you need regular exams and blood tests to monitor your liver functions. For stable patients, the minimum recommendation is an annual physical examination and blood tests twice a year. You may also need a liver biopsy every three to five years. Ask your doctor what he or she recommends.

In the past year I've had a liver biopsy and a blood clotting problem that landed me in the emergency room and intensive care unit overnight. That cost big time.

I've got health insurance, so I didn't worry until I heard at my hepatitis C support group that some insurance companies put a $1 million lifetime cap on their policies. It seemed like a fortune until I started to add up just this year's medical expenses. I finally called my company and found out my cap is $2 million. What a relief!

Susie

Antiviral Treatment Costs. Interferon treatment is costly. For information, you may contact Schering-Plough Corporation, the manufacturer of INTRON® A (interferon alfa-2b, recombinant), PEG-INTRON® (peginterferon alfa-2b), and REBETRON™ combination therapy; Hoffmann-La Roche, Inc., the manufacturer of ROFERON®-A (interferon alfa-2a, recombinant) and PEGASYS® (peginterferon alfa-2a); and Valeant, the current license holder for INFERGEN® (interferon-alfacon-1).

If you need help to pay for treatment, you, your doctor, or a family member may contact the pharmaceutical company's reimbursement search and financial assistance program to see if you qualify for aid.

Resource: For information about Schering-Plough's medications, call 800-222-7579. To enroll in the patient support program Be In Charge® with 24-hour access to a nurse counselor, call 888-437-2608. Website: www.schering-plough.com.

Schering's Commitment to Care℠ Program, 800-521-7157, offers help in finding coverage, cost-sharing, and the providing of drugs to indigent people.

Resource: For information about Roche's medications, call customer service at 800-526-0625. For questions about PEGASYS® or financial aid, call the Roche Patient Assistance Program at 866-247-5084. Website: www.rocheusa.com.

Resource: For information about Valeant's INFERGEN®, contact the INFERGEN® Patient Support Line, INFERGEN® Aspire, with 24/7 nursing support: 1-888-668-3393. The Reimbursement Hotline for patients who need financial help is the same number, but hours are 9 A.M. to 8 P.M. EST. Websites: www.infergenaspire.com; www.infergen.com; and www.valeant.com

You might also consider enrolling in a study. Pharmaceutical companies often sponsor studies of promising new treatments; in many cases, the sponsor covers all costs of treatment. Be sure you understand exactly what the study involves, before you sign up for it. Ask your doctor for information or call a major research center or medical school near you (see chapter 14, Research Trends).

Transplantation Costs. The hospital's financial coordinator will be on your transplant team to help you figure out how you can afford the procedure. There are many costs involved: tests and consultations before the operation, the transplant operation itself, hospitalization, and follow-up care and medications.

According to Fabi Imo, coordinator, transplant financial services at the University of Colorado Health Sciences Center, the charges for liver transplantation (from admission to discharge, but not including before or after care) vary widely, from $150,000 to more than $1 million. The average charge is approximately $250,000. Costs vary widely around the country.

"Transplantation and living donor liver transplantation are more accepted medical procedures now so they are covered by more insurance companies," says Imo. "Presently, Medicare and our state of Colorado Medicaid approve living donor transplantation because it is no longer considered an experimental procedure.

"Work with your hospital transplant financial coordinator to explore all your options. People often have insurance benefits they're not aware of. For example, some patients are covered for travel, lodging, and mileage costs."

According to Imo, sometimes patients who need financial help find themselves in a "Catch-22" situation. If you are disabled by liver disease and apply for Social Security Disability Insurance, a federal program, it takes 24 months (starting from the date you became eligible) for Medicare to become effective. Medicare does pay for liver transplants, but you may not be in a condition to wait two years.

"Another 'Catch-22' situation is the biggest problem I see," says Imo. "If the patient is over the minimum eligibility level, he or she will not qualify for Medicaid. And even if you have Medicaid, not all state Medicaid programs will cover a liver transplant."

Not all private insurance policies cover transplants, and both private and government health insurance impose certain criteria. For example, people who have additional medical problems, such as a heart condition or a malignancy, may find themselves excluded from coverage.

In addition to determining insurance coverage for the transplant procedure itself, it's also important to look at your prescription drug benefit and how it covers immunosuppressive drugs. According to Imo, "The medications probably are the largest financial expense out of the patient's pocket. Post-transplant immunosuppressive medicines can be thousands of dollars a month." If you need help with medication costs, talk to your transplant coordinator about possible resources, such as pharmaceutical companies or state-funded social service programs.

According to Imo, "A problem may occur when a patient is reassessed by the Social Security Administration and is no longer deemed disabled. Medicare is no longer effective, and the patient loses not only the Medicare coverage for insurance purposes but also, and most importantly, the immunosuppression coverage. It's a real dilemma."

Note: Medicare now pays 80 percent of immunosuppressive drug costs for the lifetime of the transplanted organ. The patient must already be covered by Medicare at the time of transplantation. This policy applies to all Medicare-entitled beneficiaries who continue to meet all of the other program requirements for coverage under this benefit.

According to *Medicare & You 2006,* Medicare coverage for immuno-suppressive drugs is available if the transplant was paid for by Medicare or by an employer group health plan that was required to pay before Medicare. You must have been entitled to Part A at the time of transplant and entitled to Part B at the time you get immunosuppressive drugs. The transplant must have been performed in a Medicare-certified facility.

Note: The area of government-sponsored drug benefits is changing rapidly with Prescription Drug Coverage (Medicare Part D). Consult your transplant financial coordinator and/or your transplant social worker to choose the plan that is best for you.

Adding to direct costs are many indirect expenses. Patients some-times forget to allow for organ recovery costs or travel and lodging for family members, childcare, and so on. It's important to plan ahead.

Finally, cautions Imo, it's important for patients to be involved with insurance companies. Know the name and phone number of your case manager, and always inform your financial coordinator and your liver transplant team immediately if you change insurance companies.

Resource: A booklet by the United Network for Organ Sharing (UNOS) discusses a number of topics, including financing transplantation.

For a copy of *What Every Patient Needs to Know,* call 888-TXINFO1 (888-894-6361). The book also appears on the UNOS website: www.unos.org.

Resource: The National Transplant Assistance Fund website: www.transplantfund.org

Resource: The American Liver Foundation (ALF) has established a Liver Transplant Fund that provides professional administration, at no cost, for funds raised on behalf of patients to help pay for medical care and associated transplantation expenses. For information, call 800-GO-LIVER or 888-4-HEP-ABC.

Private Health Insurance

Selecting Private Health Insurance. When you have a chronic illness like hepatitis C, you must select your health insurance carefully:

- Read your policy before signing it. Ask questions. If there is any part you don't understand, get help.
- Make sure your plan allows you to see doctors who are experts in hepatitis C: gastroenterologists, hepatologists, and transplant physicians.
- Understand the restrictions and make sure they won't affect the quality of your care. For example, does the policy cover emergency rooms, experimental treatments, drugs like interferon? What happens if you're out of town and you need medical help?
- Is there a lifetime limit or cap on treatment or drugs? A million dollars may sound high, but is it too low for a chronic condition?
- Use common sense in assessing a medical policy. When you have hepatitis C, you have to plan ahead for extra medical care, even though you may never need it.
- Check to see if your policy pays based on "reasonable and customary" fee schedules. Policies that use fee schedules may not pay the entire bill if they feel that your doctor or hospital does not charge "reasonable" rates.
- Know any managed care provisions in your policy. Do you have any particular doctor or hospital that you are required to use? If you use a "preferred provider," will the insurance cover a larger share?

Types of Private Health Insurance: Managed Care or Fee-for-Service. Private health insurance policies fall into two categories:

(1) managed care, or (2) fee for service. Managed care plans limit your choice of physician, but usually cost less. Managed care options include Health Maintenance Organizations (HMO) and Preferred Provider Organizations (PPO).

Fee-for-service policies usually provide the freedom to choose your doctor, but they often are more expensive. Look at the following factors when comparing cost of fee-for-service policies:

- monthly premiums—what the insurance costs each month
- annual deductible—how much you have to pay out of your pocket each year before the policy will pay benefits
- coinsurance—what percentage you have to pay that your insurance will not cover, usually 20 to 30 percent
- out-of-pocket maximum—the amount that you pay in coinsurance before the insurance company will begin to pay at 100 percent
- policy maximum—the maximum amount that insurance will pay over the lifetime of the policy

Whether you choose a managed care or traditional fee-for-service plan, be sure you understand how your plan works and the appeal process. If you're dissatisfied with your insurance policy, you may always review these issues with your State Commissioner of Insurance.

HMOs. Under HMO plans you have a primary care physician, a gatekeeper, who coordinates your care and decides if you should be referred to a specialist. This plan is the least costly but the most limiting in terms of freedom of choice. Because the goal is to keep costs at a minimum, your access to specialists, tests, medications, or hospital care may be restricted. It's important to do a thorough check on limitations.

PPOs. You may choose a doctor within the provider network and get 90 to 100 percent coverage of your costs or choose a doctor outside the network and receive a smaller percentage of the cost, usually 70 percent.

Fee-for-Service Plans. Usually, the choice of doctor is totally yours, but these plans are typically the most expensive. Patients with chronic hepatitis C who are exploring fee-for-service plans should choose a major medical policy that offers subspecialty physician services and adequate hospital coverage.

The insurance company usually pays 80 percent of the bill, and you pay 20 percent up to a total amount designated by your policy. Hospital and physician fees that the insurance company deems unreasonable may not be fully reimbursed.

Resource: To help consumers with the process of choosing a suitable health-care plan, check out two government websites: the Quality Inter-agency Coordination Task Force at www.consumer.gov/quality-health/index.html and the Department of Health and Human Services at www.healthfinder.gov.

Resource: For help in evaluating health insurance plans, call the National Committee for Quality Assurance at 800-839-6487. Website: www.ncqa.org.

Resource: Another useful booklet is *Checkup on Health Insurance Choices,* AHCPR #93-0018, by the Agency for Healthcare Research and Policy: 800-358-9295. Website: www.AHRQ.gov

Resource: In 1996, Congress passed the Health Insurance Portability and Accountability Act (Public Law #104-191), sponsored by Senators Edward Kennedy and Nancy Kassebaum. This act includes many significant health insurance reforms.

Some highlights of the act include: (1) "portability" provisions, (2) increased availability of coverage, and (3) expansion of COBRA continuation coverage benefits. The "portability" provisions are designed to eliminate the fear that employees will lose their health insurance if they change jobs.

You may request a copy of the act and its accompanying conference committee report from your U.S. representative or senator. Also, as with other legislation of this type, government agencies, such as the Labor Department, the Internal Revenue Service, and the Department of Health and Human Services, issue regulations to implement the act's provisions. In addition, almost all states made changes in state legislation to comply with the act. For information, call your state legislators and your state insurance department.

For questions about the Health Insurance Portability and Accountability Act (HIPPA), contact the Centers for Medicare and Medicaid Services (CMS). Toll-Free Phone: 877-267-2323, TTY Toll-Free: 866-226-1819 HIPAA Hotline: 866-282-0659 Website: www.cms.hhs.gov/hipaa/

Resource: Some states have set up risk-sharing pools to enable people who are otherwise uninsurable to purchase health insurance. State insurance laws differ, so call your state insurance department for specific information. If you have difficulty locating your state insurance department, contact the National Association of Insurance Commissioners for the listing: 816-842-3600. Website: www.naic.org

For information on various states' high-risk insurance pools, access the National Association of State Comprehensive Health Insurance Plans (NASCHIP) website: www.naschip.org

Resource: Insure.com is a consumer insurance guide website that explains your COBRA rights and your rights to health insurance portability under HIPAA: www.insure.com/health/cobra.html and www.insure.com/health/hipaa.html

Government Health Insurance

CAUTION: Laws and regulations change over time. Double-check your facts with the agency involved. Only the agency itself can give you up-to-date, accurate material.

There are some situations when Medicare may eventually end, based on Social Security Disability Insurance (SSDI) eligibility. Also, the effects of work on benefits [SSDI and Supplemental Security Income (SSI)] and Medicare/Medicaid are complicated and different depending on what benefit you get. The best thing to do is to call the Social Security Administration before you or your spouse works to see what the specific effects will be on your cash benefits and/or medical coverage.

This chapter does not give legal advice and is not a substitute for the professional services of an attorney. Always consult a lawyer when legal issues are involved.

Medicare. At age 65, you may be eligible for medical insurance for hospital and other medical services. If you receive Social Security disability benefits for 24 consecutive months (see following section), you also may qualify for Medicare.

Hospital insurance (Part A) covers inpatient hospital care. You already paid for this as part of your Social Security and Medicare taxes when you were working. Medical insurance (Part B) pays for doctors' services, post-transplant immunosuppressants, and some outpatient facility and doctor visits. Part B is optional, and you'll be billed monthly for your premium. Prescription Drug Coverage (Part D) is an essential benefit. Consult your transplant financial counselor and/or your transplant social worker.

If you are not already getting Social Security benefits, sign up for Medicare at your local Social Security office three months before you become 65, and you'll receive your Medicare card. Ask about enrollment periods. If you are getting Social Security benefits, you will automatically be enrolled, and you will receive your card in the mail. You may also want to purchase a Medigap policy, or Medicare Choice Plan, or other Medicare supplement (private insurance that fills in some of the "gaps" in Medicare's coverage).

Resources: For more information, call 800-MEDICARE or access the website: www.medicare.gov.

If you have a low income and few resources, you may qualify for state aid to help pay for Medicare premiums and some other expenses; ask for *Guide to Health Insurance.* You may also call the Department of Social Services.

Medicaid. Medicaid is a federal-state health program for people with low assets and incomes. At present, state social services departments administer the program. To apply, call your county social services department.

Veterans Administration (VA). For questions about medical benefits and disability, veterans may call the Veterans Administration Regional Office. Dial this number and your call will be automatically directed to your regional office: 800-827-1000.

When You're Too Sick to Work: Applying for Disability

As hepatitis C progresses to the stage of cirrhosis, you may be less capable of functioning at home or on the job. In general, this occurs only in patients who have had the disease for many years and who have cirrhosis and signs of worsening liver function.

Our goal in this section is to provide you with a general overview of the available options for disability benefits and the process involved. For those who wish to consider applying for disability benefits, the process varies depending on your income, personal situation, and insurers or government programs.

CAUTION:

1. Laws and regulations change; unexpected circumstances arise. It's best to double-check your facts with the company, agency, or organization involved. Medical social workers can help direct you to the appropriate agencies or programs.
2. Keep a file with copies of all your medical records. Begin right now, if you haven't already done so. Always keep your EOBs (Explanation of Benefits) sent to you by your insurance company. The EOB is the

document that explains what the medical provider and/or hospital is paid and contains a description of payment procedures.

3. Start a journal. Keep track of your symptoms and how they affect your daily tasks. This documentation will help you explain your symptoms to your doctor and will be important later if you ever have to file for disability.

4. This chapter does not give legal advice and is not a substitute for the professional services of an attorney. Consider consultation with a lawyer when legal issues or hearings are involved.

Resource: Call the American Bar Association at 312-988-5000 for your state's lawyer referral service number or check your phone book. Attorneys specialize in different areas, such as disability or insurance, so explain your specific problem. If you can't afford a lawyer, contact your local Legal Aid Society or a law school that sponsors a student association offering free legal advice. Your local United Way may also direct you to possible sources of legal help.

Short-Term Disability Leave. Become familiar with your company's policies. Some companies offer paid short-term disability leave or allow you to use accumulated sick days. Companies usually require that a doctor accurately assess the nature of your symptoms and verify that you are disabled. The diagnosis of hepatitis C or treatment with interferon and other antiviral medications are not sufficient, in and of themselves, to necessarily justify disability.

I was exhausted when I started taking interferon. My sister had died recently, and I thought it was depression that had me so tired. My doctor told me I had beginning cirrhosis, and I was so sick I needed to take some time off from work.

I was incredulous. Taking time off was for operations! That was my own denial, my survival system. I was amazed that my company did approve leave—and I was paranoid. I expected surveillance cameras to sneak up on me. When I finally went back to work, it was part time, then full time. It was rough. I was achey; I had headaches. I just stayed in my cubicle and did what I had to do.

I was afraid of losing my job. I didn't know my rights. I thought if I had six absences in a row, I'd be out the door.

Joe

If you are an eligible employee and you or your family member (child, parent, spouse) becomes seriously ill from advanced hepatitis C, the Family and Medical Leave Act allows you to take up to 12 weeks of unpaid leave each year. Workers returning from leave must be restored to their original jobs or equivalent jobs with the same pay, benefits, and working conditions.

Resource: For more information and to find out if you are an eligible employee under the act, call the nearest office of the Wage and Hour Division, listed in most telephone directories under U.S. Government, Department of Labor, Employment Standards Administration.

Resource: The 1990 Americans with Disabilities Act (ADA) prohibits job discrimination against "qualified individuals with disabilities." Employers covered under the act must make a "reasonable accommodation" for such persons depending on the particular facts in each case and on whether or not it imposes "undue hardship" on the employer. "Reasonable accommodations" apply to the area of attendance and leave policies. To see if the ADA covers you and your employer and to get more specific information on the provisions of the act, call the President's Committee on Employment of People with Disabilities Job Accommodation Network at 800-ADA-WORK or 800-526-7234.; email: jan@jan.wvu.edu; website: www.jan.wvu.edu.

Disability Insurance

If you're self-employed, you may have paid for your own individual disability insurance. If you work for a company, find out if you are eligible to enroll in your company's group disability coverage. Read the terms of coverage carefully.

> When I went on disability, I was at my highest earning capacity. It's a good thing I couldn't take a less stressful job at my company for less money. I would have had to quit anyway, and then I would have shot myself in the foot because my disability was computed as a percentage of my paycheck. It's hard enough to live on what I did get—60 percent of what I was earning.
>
> *Arthur*

Two Social Security Administration programs offer assistance if you have to file for disability: Social Security Disability Insurance (SSDI) and Supplemental Security Income (SSI).

CAUTION: Brief descriptions of the programs follow, but only the agency itself can give you up-to-date, accurate material. *Call the Social Security Administration and ask them to send you information about disability programs:* 800-772-1213. You can speak to a service representative between the hours of 7 A.M. and 7 P.M. on business days. Hearing-impaired callers using TTY equipment can call 800-325-0778 during the same hours. Website: www.ssa.gov

Social Security Disability Insurance (SSDI). This insurance covers workers (and their children or surviving spouses). In order to qualify for this disability coverage on your own record, you must have worked long enough and recently enough to have made sufficient contributions to your Social Security account. You may also qualify on the record of a parent or as a disabled widow(er). Adults must have a physical and/or mental problem that prevents them from working for at least a year or that is expected to result in death. Benefits continue until a person is able to work and earn a certain amount of money again on a regular basis.

You may file a claim by phone or mail, or by visiting the nearest Social Security office. The claims process can take about 180 days while the agency obtains medical information and decides if the disability affects your ability to work. Call the Social Security Administration for the SSDI pamphlets that describe the program and for the medical and work information you will be asked to provide.

After my biopsy I had to acknowledge how sick I was. I had cirrhosis. I was so fatigued that I had no life outside of work. For the time I had left, this was not the kind of life I wanted. So I became more assertive. Instead of waiting for my doctor to suggest disability, now I suggested it.

As long as I was ambulatory, I thought I wasn't disabled. But when I put my symptoms on paper, I had to accept my feelings. I wrote about my inability to concentrate, my depression, the aches and pains, the constant headaches—and I presented the list to my doctor.

He said I was disabled, outlined restrictions, gave me a prescription, and I took it to my employer. The disability plan at our company required me to sign up for Social Security Disability Insurance also.

At first, Social Security denied my claim. I went to a lawyer for help. I wish I had gone to him earlier. He told me it wasn't unusual to be denied at first. Hepatitis C symptoms of fatigue are vague, subjective. We appealed.

Social Security asked for an independent medical evaluation. I was prepared. I had kept a log of activities I could do and those I could not do. I went armed with my biopsy report. I finally saw myself as an educator of what hepatitis C was all about. I got disability.

Nadine

The Social Security Administration recommends that you don't wait to file your claim, even if you don't have all this information right away. (There is a waiting period before benefits begin, so the sooner you apply, the better.) If you need someone's help, a family member, caseworker, or other representative can contact the agency for you.

If the claim is approved, you'll receive a notice showing the amount of your benefit and when payments start. The amount of your benefit is based on your lifetime average earnings covered by Social Security, but workers' compensation benefits can affect your disability check. Your case will be reviewed periodically to see if you remain disabled. After two years from the date of onset of disability, you will be eligible for Medicare benefits, regardless of your age. If your claim is denied, a notice will explain why, and you will have opportunities to contest the decision.

Resource: Call the Social Security Administration at 800-772-1213 (website: www.ssa.gov). Ask for all available SSDI pamphlets.

Supplemental Security Income (SSI). SSI is a Social Security Administration program that makes disability payments to adults and children with little or no income or resources. To get SSI, you must be 65 or older, blind, or disabled. Disabled means you have a physical or mental problem that keeps you from substantial work and is expected to last at least a year or to result in death.

The basic SSI payment is the same all over the country, but some states add money to your check. Any income you or your spouse has may affect the check amount. Call the Social Security Administration for information.

When I applied for SSI, it was as if I was fighting against my whole value system. I had dreams that I was a gunrunner in South

America. It felt as though I was doing something wrong or breaking the law.

I was barely making it before hepatitis C, and now that I'm exhausted all the time, I can't make it at all. What else can I do?

Sam

If you qualify for SSI, in most states you will be able to get other aid from your state or county, such as Medicaid (which helps pay doctor and hospital bills), food stamps, or other social services. Call your local social services department or public welfare office.

If you get Medicare and have low income and few resources, you may qualify for help with some Medicare premiums or co-pays under the Qualified Medicare Beneficiary (QMB) or Specified Low-Income Medicare Beneficiary (SLMB) programs. Only your state can decide if you qualify. Contact your county Social Services.

Whether your income meets SSI requirements depends on some very specific criteria defining what's included in income and what's included as assets. For more information, call the Social Security Administration.

Sometimes people can get both Social Security and SSI benefits. The rules that determine if you're disabled are the same for Social Security and SSI (refer to the previous section, Social Security Disability Insurance). You must be unable to do any substantial kind of work to be considered disabled under both programs.

If you think you are eligible for SSI, the Social Security Administration recommends that you file a claim right away, even if you don't have all the information at hand. The SSI pamphlets list the information you will need to supply.

Resource: Call the Social Security Administration at 800-772-1213 (website: www.ssa.gov). Ask for all available SSI pamphlets.

Riches serve a wise man but command a fool.

English proverb

EVOLUTION OF TREATMENT FOR HEPATITIS C

Improvements in Therapy from 1989 to 2006: The Interferon, Ribavirin, and Peginterferon Story

When I was diagnosed with hepatitis C, I panicked—especially when the doctor described interferon treatment to me. I had just read this book about how toxic our environment is, so I decided to try an alternative route: macrobiotic diet, vitamin supplements, changing my dental fillings from mercury to gold—the whole nine yards.

My ALT and AST levels went down some; the PCR test went down some. I thought I had hit the cure. But the next time I got tested, the scores crept up again. It turns out that hepatitis C spikes—up and down, high and low. I was into a much healthier lifestyle—and that was good—but I still had the virus.

I finally started interferon. My test levels went down and have stayed down. As far as I'm concerned, it's the only antiviral game in town.

Ted

THE FIRST TREATMENT for chronic hepatitis C, interferon alfa-2b given as monotherapy, was approved for the treatment of chronic hepatitis C in February 1991. Since then, substantial improvements have occurred, including the addition of ribavirin and chemical modification of interferon to a more effective long-acting form, peginterferon.

In this chapter I'll describe key features of the evolution of antiviral therapy of hepatitis C and cover the following topics about interferon, ribavirin, and peginterferon:

• What Is Interferon?
  Discovery and Identification
  Defining Criteria for Selection of Patients for Treatment with Interferon
  Alpha Interferons used in Treatment of Chronic Hepatitis C
  Pegylated Interferons
  Advantages of Pegylated Interferon
  Interferon Side Effects
• What is Ribavirin?
  Development
  Effect of Ribavirin when Used in Combination with Interferon
  Ribavirin Side Effects
• Measuring Response to Therapy
  Effectiveness
  Virologic Response
• Patients' Experiences with Interferon and Ribavirin
  Injections
• Treatment Tips from Patients

NOTE: The current standard of treatment, pegylated interferon plus ribavirin, is discussed in detail in chapter 9.

What is Interferon?

Discovery and Identification. Scientists identified interferon in 1957 by demonstrating that cells infected with a virus secreted a substance that had the ability to protect other uninfected cells from becoming infected. This substance, interferon, is a naturally occurring protein whose name is derived from its ability to interfere with viral replication.

Since these early studies, the interferon story has become increasingly complex. Three classes of interferons, alpha, beta, and gamma, are currently recognized. Gamma interferon is ineffective against hepatitis C. Beta interferon is less effective than alpha interferon. Alpha interferons are the most effective interferons in treating patients with hepatitis C. All of the current FDA-approved interferons, including pegylated interferons, for treatment of hepatitis C are alpha interferons.

Defining Criteria for Selection of Patients for Treatment with Interferon. The criteria for selecting patients for treatment were developed initially by investigators participating in the US Multi-Center and NIH trials and published in 1989. These criteria centered on three main issues: how long the patient had the disease (chronicity), confirmation of a diagnosis of hepatitis C, and absence of severe liver injury (compensated liver disease). Here is a listing of the criteria (see Chapter 2 for a full explanation of the terms used in the list below):

- persistently elevated ALT for at least six months
- liver biopsy compatible with diagnosis of chronic hepatitis
- no other serious underlying medical condition
- no evidence of hepatic failure (ascites, variceal bleed, encephalopathy)
- bilirubin <4 milligrams/deciliter
- albumin >3 grams/deciliter
- prothrombin time <3 seconds prolonged beyond control
- platelet count >70,000/microliter
- white blood count > 3,000/microliter, polymorphonuclear leucocytes (PMN) >1,500/microliter
- hemoglobin >11 grams/deciliter

Although these criteria still serve as general guidelines for selection of patients for treatment, we currently require that patients test positive for HCV RNA and that HCV genotype is defined. The initial studies of interferon were conducted in the most stable patients who had no other medical problems. In contrast, in recent years interferon and peginterferon, in combination with ribavirin, have been used in patients who are more "difficult-to-treat." The latter patients include those with African American heritage (see "Treatment of African Americans" in chapter 9), cirrhosis and more advanced liver disease (see "Treatment of Patients with Cirrhosis" in chapter 9), renal failure (see "Treatment of Patients with Renal Failure" in chapter 9), HIV co-infection (chapter 12), or those who have undergone liver transplantation (chapter 10).

Alpha Interferons Used in the Treatment of Chronic Hepatitis C. There are five FDA-approved alpha interferons that are effective in the treatment of chronic hepatitis C (Table 8A). All the alpha interferons are given by subcutaneous injection. The standard, non-pegylated, alpha interferons are interferon alfa-2b (INTRON® A, Schering-Plough), interferon alfa-2a (ROFERON®-A, Roche), and interferon alfacon-1 (INFERGEN®, Amgen, Intermune, and Valeant). Typically the standard interferons are administered three times a week or daily.

Interferon alfa-2b and interferon alfa-2a are produced by molecular cloning of the genes for the naturally occurring interferons. Interferon alfacon-1 differs in that the gene was synthesized from consensus sequences of genes of a number of alpha interferons and, as a result, does not exist in nature. Interferon alfacon-1 is slightly more potent against HCV genotype 1 compared to the two other standard, non-pegylated, alpha interferons. The frequencies and severity of side effects are similar among these three standard interferons.

Pegylation of interferon alfa-2b yielded the first FDA-approved pegylated interferon, PEG-INTRON®, Schering-Plough, and pegylation of interferon alfa-2a yielded PEGASYS®, Roche. Pegylated interferons are administered weekly. Pegylation of interferon slows the absorption from the subcutaneous tissues into blood and reduces the rate of elimination of the pegylated interferon from the blood; as a result, there is typically a delay in onset of side effects and a more prolonged antiviral effect. In the large registration trials of the pegylated interferons used in combination with ribavirin in treatment of chronic hepatitis C, side effects were less and clearance of hepatitis C was more frequent, compared to the non-pegylated parent interferons.

Pegylated Interferons. The "peg" of pegylation is an abbreviation for polyethylene glycol (PEG), a biologically inert compound. Researchers are using PEG, a substance that thickens lipstick and shampoo products, to improve the effectiveness of medicines. Your body basically ignores the inert PEGs so when PEGs are attached to other molecules (such as interferon) the molecules stay in your system longer before your body eliminates them.

TABLE 8A. FDA-APPROVED THERAPIES FOR THE TREATMENT
OF CHRONIC HEPATITIS C.

Drug Name	Trade Name	Pharmaceutical
ALPHA INTERFERONS		
Interferon alfa-2b	INTRON®A	Schering-Plough
Interferon alfa-2a	ROFERON®-A	Roche
Interferon alfacon-1	INFERGEN®	Amgen, Intermune, Valeant
Peginterferon alfa-2b	PEG-INTRON®	Schering-Plough
Peginterferon alfa-2a	PEGASYS®	Roche
RIBAVIRINS		
Ribavirin	REBETOL®	Schering-Plough
Ribavirin	COPEGUS®	Roche
COMBINATIONS		
INTRON + REBETOL	REBETRON®	Schering-Plough
PEGINTRON + REBETOL		Schering-Plough
PEGASYS + COPEGUS		Roche

The two FDA-approved pegylated interferons used to treat hepatitis C have different lengths and molecular weights. PEG-INTRON® incorporates a PEG molecule of 12,000 molecular weight (12kD), and PEGASYS® incorporates a PEG molecule of 40,000 molecular weight (40kD). Pegylation is a synthetic process whereby a molecule of PEG is bonded to a molecule of interferon. Scientists precisely control the process so that the active site on the interferon molecule is not covered or damaged by the PEG molecule.

Note: Hereafter, PEG-INTRON® will be designated in the text as Peg-Intron, PEGASYS® as Pegasys, and REBETRON™ as Rebetron.

Advantages of Pegylated Interferon. Why is pegylation important? The following discussion highlights the unique properties of pegylated interferons and their advantages over standard interferons.

Because pegylation converts interferon from a relatively short-acting medication to a long-acting one by reducing the rate at which the body eliminates interferon, the time between injections is extended. Instead of three injections of standard interferon a week, the patient injects pegylated interferon only once a week.

> *I like pegylated interferon best—better than monotherapy and standard combo (Rebetron). I hated three shots a week, so it's much easier once a week.*
>
> *Three times a week was a roller-coaster ride, and I had three after-shot bad days. Now I have one bad day. It might be a little worse, but it's just one.*
>
> *Anna*

Pegylation makes interferon more effective in clearing hepatitis C because the addition of PEG maintains consistent and prolonged levels of interferon in the body. In contrast, non-pegylated interferons are essentially cleared within 12 to 24 hours, and injections three times a week are associated with extreme peaks and valleys of interferon levels. Patients benefit by the increased constant level of interferon, which clears hepatitis C in a greater number of cases. This advantage has been well-documented in trials comparing pegylated interferons to standard interferons (see below).

Pegylated interferon reduces the body's immune reaction to interferon. Interferons are proteins. When injected into your body, they can induce an antibody response by your immune system. In general, these antibodies have not been associated with disease, illness, or inactivation of interferon. Nonetheless, it would be best to avoid production of these antibodies, if possible. Scientists designed and directed pegylation of interferon so that it reduces the antibody reaction.

Interferon Side Effects. All of the alpha interferons, including pegylated interferons, exhibit a similar profile of side effects. As noted above, side effects may be less frequent and less severe with the pegylated interferons. Each person reacts differently to interferon.

Flu-like Symptoms. The most common complaints are flu-like symptoms. Why? When you get an actual case of the flu, your body fights back by sending interferon to attack the invader. Interferon is at least partially responsible for the tired, achy, and feverish symptoms. Some people don't have many symptoms during interferon treatment; others experience chills, muscle aches, nausea, even diarrhea. These symptoms usually subside after the first few weeks. Weight loss is also a common side effect, but it tends to persist throughout the course of therapy. If you experience these side effects during treatment you may be able to maintain your weight and improve your energy by using supplements, such as Ensure Plus®, Resource®, and Suplena®.

Use of Acetaminophen. To help with side effects, I recommend two regular strength Tylenol® just before you take the injection. Currently most hepatologists limit use of Tylenol® to 6 regular-strength or 4 extra-strength pills total per day. If you are taking Tylenol® it is especially important for you to avoid use of alcohol, since alcohol may increase your risk of liver damage. Side effects may also be reduced if you're well hydrated before and after the injection (two glasses before an injection and about two and a half quarts of fluid a day).

Fatigue. For fatigue, it may help to have a daily nap or rest period. Paradoxically, some patients feel their fatigue is relieved by daily activity, including exercise. In some cases fatigue is not relieved by these measures and medications may be prescribed. Stimulants, such as Ritalin® or Adderall®, have been used but side effects are common and I tend to prescribe these medications sparingly. Provigil® is FDA approved for the treatment of fatigue in patients with multiple sclerosis and has been used by some hepatologists to treat the fatigue associated with interferon therapy of chronic hepatitis C. Although there are no controlled studies, anecdotal reports suggest benefit. If your appetite is poor, small-sized, more frequent meals may be more palatable and maintain your weight. To reduce skin reactions, rotate the injection sites.

Depression, Poor Concentrating Ability, and Mood Instability. Another very common side effect is disturbance of mood, concentrating ability, or other cognitive processes. Depression on interferon usually occurs in patients with a pre-treatment history of depression. However, it can occur in any patient, bears close supervision, and may require reducing the dosage or even stopping treatment. In some cases, in order to continue interferon, your physician may prescribe medication to control symptoms of depression (Zoloft®, Elavil®, Effexor®, Celexa®, Lexapro®, Prozac®). Paxil® has been particularly useful in managment of anger and irritability.

Thyroid and Autoimmune Disease. Less commonly, patients may experience weight loss, nausea, and hair loss. If hair is lost during treatment, it usually grows back after treatment stops. Rare reactions include thyroid disease (~1%), severe lowering of platelet count (ITP, less than 0.1%), or exacerbation of underlying autoimmune diseases (inflammatory bowel disease, psoriasis, rheumatoid arthritis, systemic lupus erythematosus). Your physician will monitor you closely to watch out for these rare side effects, including thyroid disease or the development of other autoimmune disorders (see Chapter 4).

WARNING: Be sure to tell your doctor if any of these symptoms appear:
  - **thoughts of suicide**
  - **thoughts of homicide**
  - **sustained fever (greater than 102° F) or other signs of infection**
  - **generalized rash**
  - **any symptoms that are interfering with your daily activity**

Infection. Interferon may affect your ability to fight infection. Do not undergo procedures, such as excessive dental work, without checking with your doctor first; your physician may decide to prescribe an antibiotic to protect you.

Low Blood Cell Counts. During interferon therapy you will need frequent blood tests. The main reason for doing these blood tests is to be certain your blood counts are adequate. Interferon reduces the white blood cell count and the platelet count. This effect of interferon is directly related to the dose used; higher doses cause a greater lowering of the counts. Sometimes the dose of interferon may need to be reduced or even discontinued. Interferon may also suppress red blood cell count, but rarely causes anemia, and compared to the effect on white blood cells and platelets the effect on red cells is modest.

Growth Factors. The depression of white cell and platelet counts is usually managed by reducing the dose of interferon. Because dose reduction may compromise sustained virologic response (SVR), some have advocated use of growth factors. In the case of low white cells an alternative strategy to dose reduction is subcutaneously injected granulocyte-colony stimulating factor (G-CSF). G-CSF is generally highly effective in raising white blood cell counts. Medical treatments to increase platelet counts are less effective. Interleukin (IL-11) stimulates platelet counts but the effect is highly variable and IL-11 is associated with significant side effects, including fluid retention and edema.

Generally, most people adjust well to interferon treatment. I tell patients to keep busy, exercise, drink lots of water, rest when they need to, and socialize. Focus on the positive—curing oneself of hepatitis C. Above all, don't let interferon isolate you.

What is Ribavirin?

Development. Ribavirin was initially synthesized decades ago, potentially to be used as a general antiviral compound. It is administered orally (taken by mouth) and is a nucleoside analogue of guanosine, active against a variety of DNA and RNA viruses. Ribavirin also modifies the immune response and enhances the antiviral activity of interferon. The exact mechanism of action of ribavirin against hepatitis C is unknown and under investigation. When used with interferon, it slightly enhances on-treatment virologic response, but its major effect is the prevention of relapse once treatment is discontinued. As a result rates of sustained virologic response to interferon therapy are markedly enhanced by the addition of ribavirin. Although ribavirin exhibits potent antiviral activity when used with interferon, it has very little activity against hepatitis C when used as monotherapy, without interferon. Blood levels of HCV RNA do not decline significantly in patients treated with ribavirin alone.

Effects of Ribavirin When Used in Combination with Interferon. Experience with interferon therapies over the last 10 years has taught us that the addition of ribavirin to interferon improves chances for sustained virologic response. At the time of the first edition of this book (1997) the standard of care was interferon monotherapy. Combination therapy with interferon plus ribavirin was under investigation and considered experimental. By the time of our second edition (©1999), large multi-center multi-national trials indicated that the combination therapy of Intron®A and Rebetrol® (Rebetron™, Schering-Plough) was significantly better than monotherapy with Intron® A. When the third edition was published (2002), Rebetron™ had been approved by the FDA and was the standard of care. The combination of pegylated interferon with ribavirin was emerging as the next treatment standard, because large registration trials were demonstrating improved virologic responses and reduced side effects compared to the previous standard combination. Now two combinations of pegylated interferon with ribavirin are FDA approved and these combinations are currently considered the standard of care in the treatment of chronic hepatitis C (See chapter 9 for a complete description of combination therapy with pegylated interferon plus ribavirin).

Ribavirin dramatically improves rates of sustained virologic response, whether used with nonpegylated or pegylated interferon. The first studies to clearly demonstrate this benefit of ribavirin used nonpegylated interferon and the results are depicted in Table 8B. The results with the combination of pegylated interferon plus ribavirin are discussed in detail in Chapter 9. As demonstrated in Table 8B, addition of ribavirin to interferon therapy increases the likelihood of sustained virologic response and this effect occurs regardless of genotype, viral load, or duration of treatment. Combination therapy is clearly superior to interferon monotherapy.

Side Effects of Ribavirin. The intensity of flu-like symptoms attributed to interferon is increased by the addition of ribavirin. Also, there are specific side effects of ribavirin that require monitoring.

Anemia. The most noteworthy is anemia which is mainly related to breakdown of red blood cells, but is also due, in part, to suppression of the bone marrow's production of red blood cells. Anemia from ribavirin can impair delivery of oxygen to the heart and other tissues. For this reason, patients with risk factors for underlying cardiovascular disease require stress testing of the heart and may also need vascular studies of blood vessels (angiography of abdominal vessels).

Rash. Skin rashes are also fairly common in patients taking ribavirin. The rash of ribavirin is generalized, covering most areas of the body, and responds to discontinuation or decrease in the dose of the drug.

Poor Taste, Mouth Soreness, Cough. Another troublesome side effect is irritation and soreness of the mucous membranes of the mouth and throat. Symptoms related to this include poor taste, loss of appetite,

TABLE 8B: EFFECT OF RIBAVIRIN ON SUSTAINED VIROLOGIC
RESPONSE TO NON–PEGYLATED INTERFERON THERAPY

| | % of Patients (Pts) with SVR | | % Improvement in SVR due to |
	Interferon	Interferon/Ribavirin	Ribavirin
Genotype 1			
24 Weeks	2	16	+14
48 Weeks	7	28	+21
Genotype non-1			
24 Weeks	16	69	+53
48 Weeks	29	66	+37
HCV RNA level, HVL			
24 Weeks	4	27	+23
48 Weeks	7	36	+29
HCV RNA level, LVL			
24 Weeks	9	42	+33
48 Weeks	29	43	+14

TABLE 8B. Abbreviations: HVL, high viral load (>2 million copies/ml); LVL, low viral load (<2 million copies/ml). In every comparison, there was improvement in SVR when ribavirin was added to interferon (far right column). Enhancement of SVR by ribavirin occurred independently of genotype, viral load, or duration of therapy.

mouth soreness, and cough. This side effect, like the skin rash, clears with discontinuation or reduction in dose of ribavirin.

Twenty to 26 percent of patients will require dose reductions in ribavirin related to any of the above side effects.

WARNING: Another very important issue regarding use of ribavirin is **avoidance of pregnancy**. Ribavirin has the potential to alter genes and its use during pregnancy could be associated with increased risk of stillbirth and birth defects in infants. Current recommendations are that women practice effective contraception (birth control pills or other similarly effective measure) and that both sexual partners use preventive measures (double contraception).

Measuring Response to Therapy

Effectiveness. How do you know when your treatment is working? We measure the effectiveness of treatment in three ways:

1. Clearance of hepatitis C from your blood as measured by assays for HCV RNA—the best response, called sustained virologic response (SVR), is undetectable HCV RNA in blood 6 months after the end of treatment. Long-term followup suggests that 99% of these patients have been cured of chronic hepatitis C.
2. ALT levels become normal. Hepatitis C is a liver disease, and the ALT reflects ongoing injury to the liver. Normalization of ALT implies that liver injury has stopped or is diminished.
3. A post-treatment biopsy of the liver demonstrates improvement in inflammation and fibrosis.

Figure 8A: The three main types of response of hepatitis C to antiviral therapy are shown. Sustained responders (solid black line), clear virus (HCV RNA) from blood during therapy, usually within 3 months, and virus is undetectable throughout the remainder of treatment and post-treatment followup. Relapsers (dashed line) clear virus (HCV RNA) from blood during therapy but HCV RNA re-emerges once treatment has been stopped. Nonresponders (dotted line) fail to clear virus both during and after treatment.

Virologic Response. Looking at experimental statistics gives us important information, but when you are the person who's taking interferon, you want to know how to measure success or failure. Physicians have a special vocabulary, mainly based on measuring HCV RNA, to describe response (Figure 8A):

- **End-of-Treatment Response:** The patient has no detectable HCV RNA in his or her blood during at the end of treatment.
- **Relapse:** Patients who are RNA negative at the end of treatment, are classified as relapsers when HCV RNA becomes positive after treatment is stopped.
- **Sustained Response:** Sustained responders are negative for HCV RNA six months after treatment has been discontinued. More than 98 percent of sustained responders remain free of hepatitis C after years of followup and are likely "cured."
- **Nonresponse:** These patients do not respond to current antiviral treatment. HCV RNA remains positive throughout therapy.
- **Histologic Response:** In most studies, interferon therapy is associated with improvement in the condition of the liver cells. This improvement occurs not only in those who clear HCV RNA but also in at least a proportion who remain positive for the virus. Improved histology is due mostly to reduced inflammatory activity. Studies of maintenance therapy with pegylated interferon, like the HALT C trial, are currently examining the ability of long-term treatment to halt disease progression and stabilize or reduce fibrosis. We await the results of these trials.

The Patient's Experience

Many patients are nervous about interferon injections and concerned about dealing with side effects of treatment.

Injections. In my experience, patients quickly learn how to give themselves injections. Most people think of the deep muscle injections they get for flu shots, and they panic about doing this to themselves. Interferon injections are much easier to administer because they are subcutaneous. Subcutaneous means you have to get the needle only under the skin and not deep into muscle.

I was really nervous about learning how to give myself a shot. When I came into the office, the nurse was looking all around for an orange to practice on. She never did find it. So we used the pad on the exam table, then a tissue box. It was funny, and it made me laugh—something I never expected to happen.

The first couple of times I did it myself at home, I put the needle in too horizontally. I was going push, push, push and nothing happened. I got awful bruises.

Back to the nurse. She told me to pinch my skin between two fingers, hold the syringe like a dart and go in straight at a 90° angle. That worked!

Marla

It's important that you ask questions and practice injections under a nurse's supervision until you feel comfortable. You should be taught about storing and preparing the drug for injection, sterile technique, how to pick injection sites, and how to dispose of needles. Be sure to ask for the helpful teaching material and videotapes that pharmaceutical companies give to physicians for their patients' use.

I recommend that the first shot be given in the office. Although it's highly unlikely for a patient to have an immediate adverse reaction, we observe the patient for a couple of hours.

Treatment Tips from Patients

Here are some tips from hepatitis C patients who've gone through treatment. Remember, what works for one person may not work for you. Once you become familiar with these drugs, you'll find your own comfort level.

For me, drinking lots of water helped. If I didn't stay hydrated, I felt worse.

When my husband started interferon, it changed our lives. We weren't prepared for it. Interferon can be hard on the spouse, too. To be supportive, I had to plan things at a slower rate.

My husband and I used to ski all day long—black and double-black runs. We used to take 10 to 15 mile hikes. During treatment, I would have to encourage him to take a half-hour walk on flat ground—just to get him off the couch and outside.

I dropped 20 pounds because I had no appetite—and I'm pretty thin as it is. My stomach was... I don't know, I just couldn't seem to eat. You really have to make sure you eat, even if you have to take several smaller meals throughout the day.

Now that I'm off interferon, I'm drinking two of those instant breakfast mixes each day, and I've gained back 12 pounds!

I'm on five million units, and I'm able to continue to ride my bike 200 miles a week. If I can't ride, the effects of the interferon seem stronger.

The people in my support group decided the two major things that helped were to get a lot of rest and to have a positive attitude. What's really interesting is that in spite of the side effects, no one was sorry they had tried interferon.

Here's a tip that works for me. Take your thumb and press hard for 10 seconds on the place where you're going to inject. It numbs the skin a little bit.

I'm a fair bit more irritable. So I apologize and say I'm not feeling well. It's me, not you. I do a fair amount of apologizing.

It's a peculiar kind of headache. I call it the interferon headache. Also, it seems as though I'm more forgetful. All my friends tell me they forget things, too, that I'm just getting older. But it seems different to me. Now I write everything—and I mean everything—down!

One night I took an early bath and really soaked. Then I did the shot. My skin was so soft, the needle went right in. Don't do the reverse, though. Don't take a hot bath after the shot.

In the morning and at night, I feel nauseous. If I eat, the nausea goes away. I have to concentrate on eating. And if I eat right before or after an injection, I don't have side effects.

My hairdresser told me my hair was thinning out, but not to worry because it was so thick in the first place. When I stopped interferon, it all came back.

For me, the fatigue is the tough part. I got over the slight fever and upset stomach in the first couple of days. But I do get tired, and I just have to rest more. About midway through the treatment, I had to go on an antidepressant, and that's helped me a lot.

I've had to learn to say no. It's amazing how you can simplify your work life if you have no choice. And I've learned not to schedule too many appointments in one day. If I'm running from one thing to another, I'm wiped out at the end of the day.

I had a breakthrough on interferon, so my doctor put me on rib-avirin right away. It took me weeks to adjust to the shortness of breath. When I walk fast—and I'm used to walking fast—I start to feel faint, like I'm going to pass out. Stairs are even worse.

My lower red blood cell count means I get less oxygen. I've learned to move slower, not to rush from one thing to another. Also, if I feel faint, I slow down and take deep breaths to get more oxygen in my system. On the plus side, my counts are down again!

This ribavirin really kicks my butt! I couldn't keep up at work. Finally, I told everyone what's going on. They still resent having to pick up some of the slack, but they're much more understanding.

I started combination therapy two weeks ago. I expected chills or something, but I didn't feel anything—maybe a little ache in my back. I notice I get winded easier, but I just ride my bike slower.

I've felt worse taking antibiotics for a sinus infection. Drinking a lot of water seems to help.

I had a hard time getting used to the ribavirin. I started to get nerv-ous, anxious. I was very ragged, emotionally. Also, I lost weight. If I had known I'd feel better after a couple of months, I could have taken it in stride. I thought it would go on forever.

I was brushing my teeth when I saw something black on my tongue. When I looked closer at the mirror, there were lots of black spots. "My gosh," I thought, "I've got the plague, the Black Death!"

Turned out the spots were prominent veins. My doctor reduced my ribavirin dose, and the spots went away. My cough got better, too. But

I've also noticed more dry skin, dry eyes, itching. I just keep putting oint-
ments on everything.

I was so discouraged when my doctor reduced my dose. I thought it
was all over. Then I found out that a woman in my support group went
down to only four pills a day—and she cleared the virus. It's six months
now, and she's still clear! That made me feel better.

I lost a lot of weight at first because the ribavirin made me queasy.
I don't know why, but I was taking the pills on an empty stomach. Now
I take them after I eat, and I drink lots and lots of water. I don't feel
nauseous anymore.

Where do these rashes come from, especially the dry spots on my
elbows? I get purplish bumps, like goose bumps—and they itch. Some-
times bathing in water with sea salts helps.

This chapter presented you some of the initial experiences with
interferon and ribarvirin in the treatment of chronic hepatitis C. Side
effects of medications and patient experiences with treatment and managing side effects were highlighted. In the next chapter, Chapter 9, I will
discuss the current standard of care, combination therapy with pegylated
interferon plus ribavirin.

A drug is a substance which when injected
into a guinea pig produces a scientific paper.

Anonymous

Reference

1. Table 8B was created using data from Table 4 in the following article:
McHutchison, J. G., S. C. Gordon, E. R. Schiff, M. L. Shiffman, W. M. Lee,
V. K. Rustgi, Z. D. Goodman, M. H. Ling, S. Cort, J. K. Albrecht for the
Hepatitis Interventional Therapy Group. "Interferon alfa-2b Alone or in
Combination with Ribavirin as Initial Treatment for Chronic Hepatitis
C." *New England Journal of Medicine.* 1998;339:1485–1492.

9

PEGYLATED INTERFERONS PLUS RIBAVIRIN

The Current Standard-of-Care

My first liver biopsy in 1998 showed cirrhosis, but I had no symptoms. When I asked my gastroenterologist what my life expectancy would have been if I hadn't found out I had hepatitis C, he told me five years—if I was lucky. That brought me up short!

I tried interferon monotherapy. Slowly, my liver functions went down, but not to normal, and my viral count never went down.

I realized I had to do something or by 50 I'd be dead. The hepatologist said I could try combination therapy. My liver enzymes went down to normal, but my viral load did not—and I had terrible side effects.

"It's not working. Take a break," the hepatologist said. "I've got some clinical trials coming up with pegylated interferon." I'm never doing this again, I thought. But when they called me for the HALT C study last year, I decided I needed to do something to stay alive.

I'm nine months into the study, and three months ago the virus was undetectable. Even if I don't hold the response, I'm glad I enrolled. I've had hepatitis C since 1980—21 years—and this is the first time my liver has gotten a rest!

Emma

THE COMBINATION of pegylated interferon and ribavirin is the current standard of care in the treatment of chronic hepatitis C. You should consider treatment with this combination if you have not previously been treated or if you had previously been treated with nonpegylated interferons and relapsed or did not respond. In this chapter I'll explain basic facts about treatment with the combination of pegylated interferons plus ribavirin. Here are the topics I'll cover:

- Getting Yourself Ready for Treatment
    Mood and Physical Activity
    Remember: Alcohol and Hepatitis C Don't Mix
    Co-Existing Medical Conditions
    Complementary and Alternative Treatments
- Treatment Regimens and Expected Outcomes
    Pegasys
    Peg-Intron
    Pegylated Interferon Monotherapy
    Pegylated Interferon plus Ribavirin
        Pegasys plus Ribavirin
        Peg-Intron plus Ribavirin
        Dose of Ribavirin and Duration of Treatment
- Early Treatment Effects that Predict Outcomes
        Rapid Virologic Response
        The 12-Week Guideline
- The Patient's Experience: Treatment with Pegylated Interferon Plus Ribavirin
- Treatment Tips from Patients on Pegylated Interferon Plus Ribavirin
- Special Considerations
    Nonresponders or Relapsers
    African Americans
    Patients with Cirrhosis
    Patients with Renal Failure
    Acute Hepatitis C
- Maintenance Therapy
    Definitions and Goals
    Criteria for Selection of Patients
    Outcomes

• After Treatment, What Next?
  If you are a Sustained Responder
  If you are a Relapser or Nonresponder
  Vaccination

Note: Refer to chapter 8 for additional information on pegylated interferon, ribavirin, definitions of treatment response, and patient issues related to side effects of treatment.

Getting Yourself Ready for Treatment

Mood and Physical Activity. As a patient with chronic hepatitis C, you may experience fatigue, loss of energy, loss of concentrating ability, and a sense of inadequacy in performing your daily activities. These symptoms, feelings, and attitudes may make you emotional or susceptible to periods of depression. It is important for you to do all that you can to address these issues and correct problems prior to embarking on a course of therapy with pegylated interferon and ribavirin. Some patients may require evaluation by a counselor, social worker, or psychiatrist or initiation of antidepressant therapy for two to four weeks prior to starting antiviral treatment.

I encourage you to continue to remain physically active, pursue your occupation, socialize, and maintain proper nutrition. I also recommend regular exercise and a well-balanced diet supplemented with one multivitamin per day. (See chapters 5 and 6 for more detailed suggestions on how to take care of yourself nutritionally and emotionally.)

Remember: Alcohol and hepatitis C don't mix. Undoubtedly you have been counseled to avoid excessive alcohol intake; the combination of alcohol and hepatitis C may accelerate your liver disease. In addition, your ability to respond to pegylated interferon/ribavirin combination therapy is impaired by use of alcohol. Your chance for sustained virologic response decreases with increasing alcohol use. For these reasons, I discourage the daily drinking of alcohol or taking large amounts at any time in all patients with chronic hepatitis C.

However, alcohol use is so common in our society that many patients ask me if they can take a drink once in a while. My first and foremost response is avoid alcohol. If you're not willing to abstain completely from alcohol, you should at least limit your alcohol intake to less than two ounces total per week.

Co-Existing Medical Conditions. Pegylated interferon and ribavirin are potent medications that can stress your body. Severe anemia from ribavirin has been associated with angina (heart pain) and even heart attacks. If you are over age 60 or have risk factors for coronary artery disease, such as smoking, high cholesterol, high blood pressure, diabetes mellitus, obesity, or positive family history, then cardiac stress testing may be indicated prior to therapy. Rare patients have experienced retinal hemorrhages on therapy, and risk factors for this complication are underlying diabetes mellitus or hypertension. An eye examination by an ophthalmologist may be warranted if you have diabetes or hypertension.

Complementary and Alternative Medicines (CAM). Patients also question me about alternative therapies. A number of herbal remedies, teas, potions, over-the-counter products, and even acupuncture claim to be effective in treating liver disease and viral hepatitis, but none have been adequately studied. I do not recommend CAM as an alternative to pegylated interferon and ribavirin to eradicate hepatitis C because the effectiveness is doubtful and the safety, in general, is unknown. Some have advocated use of CAMs in patients taking pegylated interferon and ribavirin in the hope that this approach will lessen side effects and improve adherence to the treatment regimen. But the effectiveness of CAM strategies remains unproven. Published reports implicate various CAM therapies in sporadic cases of severe liver injury. One example, Jin Bu Huan, marketed as a Chinese herbal sedative and analgesic was associated with severe liver injury in seven patients. Be sure to check with your doctor before taking any over-the-counter products, herbal remedies, CAM therapies, or other substances (see Chapter 5, section on Herbs Harmful to the Liver).

Treatment Regimens and Expected Outcomes

Two pegylated interferons, Peg-Intron and Pegasys, are FDA approved for the treatment of chronic hepatitis C either alone or in combination with ribavirin. (See chapter 8 for a discussion of the unique characteristics of these drugs, including a description of many of their side effects.) In the following discussion I will focus on what you can expect in terms of virologic response and commonly encountered side effects from treatment with pegylated interferon and ribavirin.

At first, I'd start to feel the side effects 24 to 48 hours after the injection. Now, five months later, the symptoms come on in 12 hours—instant flu.

I think pegylated interferon has more residual effects than the doctors originally thought, because you're piling it up all the time.

Ray

When I tried interferon monotherapy years ago, it felt as if I had the flu, but only for a week after the first injection. It wasn't so bad after that.
Pegylated interferon is different. There's a slow buildup. It's cumulative. But I got better at compensating for the side effects.

Dan

Pegasys. The usual starting dose of Pegasys is 180 micrograms per week. The compound is pre-mixed and is in solution in a preloaded syringe.

After Pegasys is injected, it slowly enters your bloodstream and takes 80 hours to reach peak concentrations in your blood. Your body slowly clears Pegasys; it takes 10 to 12 days to eliminate half of the drug. Most interferons are at least partially cleared from the body by passing through the kidneys into the urine. Pegasys is too large to be filtered by the kidneys and is not cleared by passage through the urine. Your body biodegrades the interferon and the inert 40,000 PEG passes from the liver into bile and is eliminated from your system.

Blood concentrations remain fairly constant over the course of the week between injections. With multiple doses, over the course of a year of treatment, Pegasys tends to accumulate in your body and blood levels tend to increase.

Peg–Intron. Dosage varies according to the patient's weight. For example, a 70-kilogram man who receives 1.5 micrograms per kilogram will inject 105 micrograms of Peg-Intron. Peg-Intron is stored as a powder in a special prefilled syringe; it must be dissolved by a vial of liquid within the pen prior to injection into the body.

After Peg-Intron is injected, it takes 20 hours to reach peak concentrations in your blood. Your body eliminates half a dose of Peg-Intron in two to two and a half days. In contrast to Pegasys, Peg-Intron is smaller, and approximately 30 percent is cleared through the kidneys. In addition, the interferon component is biodegraded by the body, and the 12,000 molecular-weight PEG is eliminated by passage from the liver into bile and from the kidneys into urine.

There is a six fold difference between the peak concentration and the lowest concentration achieved over the course of the week between injections. Compared to Pegasys, Peg-Intron accumulates less and has lower blood levels towards the end of the week prior to the next injection.

TO THE READER: On a personal note, Hedy and I realize that the following discussion of treatment with pegylated interferon and ribavirin is very technical and requires careful reading. Our goal has always been to translate medical jargon into everyday language without sacrificing accuracy. A full chapter focused on this treatment presents us with the challenge of reporting on the results of multiple trials (with a voluminous amount of information) while trying to keep the text readable. I try to summarize the data and studies to give you a general sense of what you may expect to achieve with your treatment. One key variable in this discussion is your genotype of HCV. The single most important determinant of your treatment prescription and outcome from treatment is HCV genotype. (If you are unfamiliar with HCV genotypes, please read chapter 2, "When You Have Hepatitis C.")

Pegylated Interferon Monotherapy. Monotherapy with pegylated interferon is rarely used, but may be necessary when ribavirin is contraindicated. Patients with anemia, kidney failure, advanced liver disease, or transplants may not tolerate ribavirin. Pegylated interferons when given as monotherapy are more effective than standard nonpegylated interferons in producing sustained virologic response. In addition, although the spectrum of side effects are similar, pegylated interferons tend to have lower frequency and severity of side effects. There have been no studies comparing the two pegylated interferons head-to-head as monotherapy. However, the reported improvement in sustained virologic response over standard interferon was greater for Pegasys (20 percent) than for Peg-Intron (13 percent). Thus, when combination therapy is contraindicated, pegylated interferon monotherapy is the treatment of choice.

However, I must emphasize that most patients treated today will be treated with the combination of pegylated interferon with ribavirin and not pegylated interferon monotherapy.

Pegylated Interferon Plus Ribavirin. Most physicians who treat chronic hepatitis C would agree that pegylated interferon plus ribavirin is the current standard-of-care for the treatment of chronic hepatitis C.

Data from three large clinical trials of the combination of pegylated interferon with ribavirin are highlighted below: two using Pegasys (Fried and Hadziyannis studies) and one using Peg-Intron (Manns study).

Pegasys Plus Ribavirin. A multi-center international trial of 48 weeks evaluated the combination of Pegasys plus ribavirin (Fried study). There were three arms to the study: 453 patients were treated with Pegasys plus ribavirin, 444 patients received Rebetron, and 224 patients were treated with Pegasys monotherapy. Patients in the three arms were similar in age (mean of 42 to 43 years), gender (mean of 68 to 73 percent were male), body weight (mean of 78 to 80 kilograms), genotype 1 (mean of 64 to 66 percent), and percentage of patients with cirrhosis (mean of 12 to 15 percent).

The sustained virologic responses at six months after discontinuation of treatment was 56 percent for Pegasys plus ribavirin, significantly higher than the 45 percent reported for Rebetron and 30 percent for Pegasys monotherapy (P < .001) (Figure 9A).

Figure 9A. Panel 1. The sustained virologic responses (%) in all patients treated for 48 weeks with either Pegasys plus ribavirin (RBV), Rebetron, or Pegasys monotherapy are shown. SVR was significantly higher with Pegasys plus RBV (56%) compared to both Rebetron and Pegasys monotherapy.

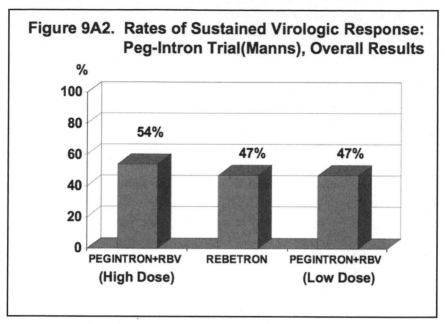

Figure 9A. Panel 2. The sustained virologic responses (%) in all patients treated for 48 weeks with either high-dose Peg-Intron plus RBV, Rebetron, or low-dose Peg-Intron plus RBV are shown. SVR was significantly higher with high-dose Peg-Intron plus RBV compared to the other two treatments.

HCV genotypes were the major determinants of rates of sustained virologic response to Pegasys plus ribavirin (Figure 9B). Patients with genotype 1 had sustained responses of 46 percent to Pegasys plus ribavirin, 37 percent to Rebetron, and 21 percent to Pegasys monotherapy. Patients with genotypes 2 and 3 had sustained responses of 76 percent to Pegasys plus ribavirin, 61 percent to Rebetron, and 45 percent to Pegasys monotherapy. Patients with genotypes 2 or 3 were more likely than patients with genotype 1 to experience a sustained response with any of the three treatment regimens. One can conclude that Pegasys plus ribavirin is preferred over both Pegasys monotherapy and Rebetron.

Side effects and rate of withdrawal from treatment with Pegasys plus ribavirin were similar to those observed with either Pegasys monotherapy or Rebetron. Patients reported a similar frequency of fatigue, headache, sleeplessness, nausea, and arthralgia (joint pains) in

Figure 9B1. Rates of Sustained Virologic Response: Pegasys Trial (Fried), Effect of Genotype

Figure 9B. Rates of sustained virologic response to the combination of pegylated interferon plus ribavirin (RBV) are given by genotype. Results in patients infected with HCV genotype 1 are shown as dark gray bars and results for patients infected with genotypes 2 or 3 are shown as light gray bars. Panel 1. The sustained virologic responses (%) after treatment for 48 weeks with either Pegasys plus ribavirin (RBV), Rebetron, or Pegasys monotherapy are shown by HCV genotype. SVR was significantly higher with Pegasys plus RBV (56%) compared to both Rebetron and Pegasys monotherapy for all genotypes. Patients infected with genotypes 2 or 3 have higher rates of SVR compared to patients with HCV genotype 1 infection.

all three treatment arms. Fever, muscle aching, and rigors (shaking, chills) were more common with Rebetron, compared to either Pegasys monotherapy or the combination of Pegasys plus ribavirin. Thirty percent of patients in the Rebetron arm experienced depression. In contrast, only 20 percent of patients on Pegasys monotherapy and 21 percent of patients on Pegasys plus ribavirin experienced depression.

Peg-Intron Plus Ribavirin. A multi-center international trial of 48 weeks evaluated the combination of Peg-Intron plus ribavirin (Manns). In this study 505 patients received Rebetron, 514 received low-dose Peg-Intron plus ribavirin, and 511 received high-dose Peg-Intron plus ribavirin. The low-dose Peg-Intron treatment consisted of Peg-Intron 1.5 micrograms per kilogram per week for four weeks followed by 0.5 micrograms per kilogram for 44 weeks plus ribavirin 1.0

Figure 9B. Panel 2. The sustained virologic responses (%) after treatment for 48 weeks with either high-dose Peg-Intron plus RBV, Rebetron, or low-dose Peg-Intron plus RBV are shown by genotype. SVR was significantly higher with high-dose Peg-Intron plus RBV compared to the other two treatments, but only in patients infected with HCV genotype 1. Once again, rates of SVR were higher in patients infected with HCV genotypes 2 or 3.

to 1.2 grams per day. The high-dose Peg-Intron regimen was Peg-Intron 1.5 micrograms per kilogram per week plus ribavirin 800 milligrams per day. Patients in the three groups were similar in age (mean of 43 to 44 years), gender distribution (mean of 63 percent to 67 percent were male), body weight (mean of 82 to 83 kilograms), genotype 1 (mean of 68 percent for all three groups), and percentage of patients with cirrhosis (mean of 10 percent for all three groups).

The sustained virologic responses at six months after discontinuation of treatment were 47 percent for Rebetron, 47 percent for low-dose Peg-Intron plus ribavirin, and 54 percent for high-dose Peg-Intron plus ribavirin. The improved sustained response with high-dose Peg-Intron plus ribavirin was significant (P =.012) when compared to either Rebetron or low-dose Peg-Intron plus ribavirin. High-dose Peg-Intron plus ribavirin had a 7 percent greater sustained response than Rebetron (Figure 9A).

The likelihood of sustained response with Peg-Intron plus ribavirin was clearly related to HCV genotype (Figure 9B). Patients with genotype 1 had sustained responses of 33 percent to Rebetron, 34 percent to low-dose Peg-Intron plus ribavirin, and 42 percent to high-dose Peg-Intron plus ribavirin. Patients with genotypes 2 or 3 had sustained responses of 79 percent to Rebetron, 80 percent to low-dose Peg-Intron plus ribavirin, and 82 percent to high-dose Peg-Intron plus ribavirin. Patients with genotypes 2 or 3 were more likely to experience sustained response with any of the three treatment regimens.

High-dose Peg-Intron plus ribavirin was superior to the other two treatments in patients with genotype 1. The 42 percent sustained response in genotype 1 patients was significantly better (P < .001) than the sustained response with either Rebetron (Figure 9B) or with low-dose Peg-Intron plus ribavirin. The 82 percent sustained response in genotype 2 and 3 patients was not significantly better than the sustained response achieved with either Rebetron or with low-dose Peg-Intron plus ribavirin. One can conclude that high-dose Peg-Intron plus ribavirin is preferred over both Rebetron and low-dose Peg-Intron plus ribavirin, especially for patients with genotype 1 HCV.

Side effects of high-dose Peg-Intron plus ribavirin were similar to those observed with either Rebetron or low-dose Peg-Intron plus ribavirin. Fever, nausea, and injection-site reactions were significantly more common with high-dose Peg-Intron plus ribavirin compared to Rebetron.

Dose of Ribavirin and Duration of Treatment. In a large multicenter international trial of Pegasys and ribavirin, Hadziyannis and colleagues examined the impact of dose of ribavirin and duration of treatment on sustained virologic response. The findings of this trial are the basis for most of our current general recommendations regarding therapy:

➤ Genotype 1 requires higher doses of ribavirin (1.0 to 1.2 g/d)
➤ Genotype 1 requires longer duration of treatment (48 weeks)
➤ Genotypes 2 and 3 can be treated at lower doses of ribavirin (800 mg/d)
➤ Genotypes 2 and 3 can be treated for shorter duration (24 weeks)

Early Treatment Effects that Predict Outcomes

Rapid Virologic Response. The term, Rapid Virologic Response, applies to the circumstance where HCV RNA is cleared from the blood within 4 weeks. Presence or absence of Rapid Virologic Response may modify some of the recommendations regarding duration of therapy. Patients with genotype 1 infection who experience Rapid Virologic Response may require only 24 weeks of treatment, and those infected with HCV genotypes 2 or 3 who experience Rapid Virologic Response may require as little as 12 weeks.

The 12-Week Guideline. In contrast to Rapid Virologic Response, which identifies the patients with most vigorous and effective virologic response, failure to achieve at least a 100-fold, or $2\log_{10}$, decline in HCV RNA by week 12 of treatment identifies patients who will not achieve viral clearance. Treatment is often stopped when the 12 week HCV RNA has failed to decline 100-fold from baseline (12-Week Guideline).

I will illustrate this point further with the following example. If your baseline HCV RNA level was 2,000,000 copies per ml prior to treatment, the HCV RNA level must drop below 20,000 copies per ml blood by week 12 in order for you to have a reasonable chance to clear HCV. If by week 12 your HCV RNA has not fallen 100-fold and remains above 20,000 copies per ml blood, your chance for sustained virologic response even if you continue treatment for a full 48 weeks is 0 to 2 percent. In this case the standard recommendation would be to discontinue treatment at week 12.

In conclusion, the combination of pegylated interferon with ribavirin represents the current standard-of-care in the treatment of patients with chronic hepatitis C. Two regimens, Pegasys plus ribavirin and Peg-Intron plus ribavirin, are currently used. Sustained response, side-effect profile, cost, ease of administration, compliance with treatment, and patient and physician preference may ultimately determine which regimen is used in a given patient.

The Patient's Experience: Treatment with Pegylated Interferon Plus Ribavirin

Note: Please refer to "The Patient's Experience" in chapter 8 for information about injections and the side effects of both interferon and ribavirin. Note also that each person reacts differently to treatment.

> With my first dose, I had the worst side effects ever. My teeth were chattering, and I had a fever. But by the next week, it wasn't as bad.
>
> Although I had a lot of the same side effects I had when I took Rebetron, everything started improving after I learned I was virus-free! My hair doesn't come out in handfuls anymore. Body aches are down, and the fatigue is a little better.

> The first dose was not as bad as regular interferon. I compare myself to others who are really sick, or so tired they can't do anything. It didn't make me feel like that.

> I take my shot on Monday night. On Tuesday or Wednesday, I get the reaction: a temperature, achy muscles. I take Tylenol®, and by the next morning I'm fine.
>
> When I took the first dose, I got chills and nausea. I went into work, and I started shaking. My teeth were chattering. I had the sweats. I missed three days of work, so I called the nurse and said I can't handle this. I can't miss work.
>
> The nurse was a big help. She encouraged me. After the second shot, my body got used to it. But I didn't like having dry, itchy skin, especially around the injection areas, and the tiredness and depression. I felt like a martyr.

> Why did I stick with it? I try to keep my word. If I tell someone I'm going to do something, I do it.
>
> And a year later, my blood tests show that the virus is still undetectable!

> I'd get tired if I carried groceries from the car to the house. The doctor thought that maybe I'd have to cut back on work, but I never did. Treatment did not interfere with my work, daily functions, or my family at all.

It's unbelievable to deal with your emotions. Every week they mutate, like the virus. Every week is different.

I have a blue-collar mentality. My dad always said a little hard work never killed anybody. So when I can't go out and do stuff, I feel bad.

The sprinkler broke. I got all my tools out. Where do you think they all are two months later? Still in the same place! I had to fix the pump or the lawn would die, but I had no energy, no will to put the tools back. It's a mental thing.

I call it "the day-after-the-shot day." It's pretty dramatic. That's when I have most of my body aches and pains. I can't function. I go to bed after work at 5 o'clock. I'm doing better now; I can stay up until 8.

I started at a high dose, but it was reduced because of my blood counts. The treatment wasn't agreeing with me, but I had no side effects, no fatigue, no weight loss. The only thing I can recall was the itching that started around six months. No rash—but I'd itch like crazy on the lower part of my ankles, legs, and the back of my neck.

The hardest part was trying to communicate what treatment is like to my family and friends. I had a hard time with that—with getting them to understand that I can't go out, that I'm exhausted and it wouldn't be any fun.

I've had hepatitis C for 30 years, and I think their attitude is, "What's new? Why are you whining?"

I responded. That was the wonderful part. I didn't expect it after other courses of therapy and a diagnosis of cirrhosis. Then I got a rash so bad, I had to quit taking ribavirin. It was all over my body—even in my mouth—and so painful I couldn't sleep.

I thought that without ribavirin, pegylated interferon alone wouldn't clear the virus. But it did!

I'd have a red spot where I injected the needle for a few days after the injection. Then it would go away. Over the year, the red spots turned black. I'd have black marks on my thighs. I refused to wear shorts. Two to three months after I was done with treatment, they totally went away.

I didn't go to church for six months. I just slept. It's a miracle I didn't lose my business. God had His hand in it.

Pegylated? It was Greek to me when I started. You get an education as you go. I was very optimistic, glad to have hope.

I felt blessed. That's as good a word as any. I never felt I was particularly deserving of anything special. Why was I picked to be someone who responded?

I'm the head of a national sales force. A lot of people were depending on me to keep them from being laid off when the company went through a period of turmoil while I was on treatment. I felt like a shepherd with a flock. I couldn't let them down. Maybe that's why I got the extra strength.

I didn't clear the virus, but a recent biopsy showed that the inflammation and fibrosis improved. My liver went from stage II back to stage I.

Myalgia kept me awake. I had this gnawing, irritating grinding in my muscles. The doctor put me on sleep medicine. I was so desperate for sleep.

It worked, and with no hangover, too. It just shut my mind off so I only took it at home. I had no problem getting off it after treatment.

I said, "Well, okay, I did not respond to the medicine. But it's not over yet because the Great Physician—God—is still at work, and I am not giving up." I refuse to believe that I will have to live the rest of my life with this virus inside me.

I didn't think regular interferon was a big deal. I wouldn't say that about pegylated interferon and ribavirin, but I've never gotten to the point where I can't function.

I filled out this form that asked me if I felt good or bad. I don't feel either. My sexual desire is gone. I feel like a machine. I do things because I have to do them.

The first test showed I was responding. Anybody who is going to take this treatment has to be committed. I've thought about quitting, but giving up would be worse. I've had hepatitis C since 1988, and I want to get rid of it.

Treatment made me more compassionate. I used to avoid people who were suffering from other diseases because I didn't know what to say. Now I go right up to them, and I ask them how they're REALLY doing.

Treatment Tips from Patients on Pegylated Interferon Plus Ribavirin

Note: See "Treatment Tips" in chapter 8 for additional suggestions.

I call it my bath therapy—soaking in a tub with mineral salts. It really helps me relax.

I try not to think about the side effects. I look at the end result and keep my eyes on the prize.

I had to rearrange my thinking around an emotional, mental wall. I hadn't talked to anyone until I confided in a friend who had cancer and chemotherapy. I'm lucky I picked him because he knows exactly what I'm going through.

Once I found out I was in remission, there was hope. So I finally told my dad.

If I walk up a flight of stairs, I'm huffing and puffing because ribavirin lowers your oxygen. I have to stop on the landing and take deep breaths to get more air into my system.

I try very hard to take a nap in my car at lunchtime. It helps me get through the workday.

I work full time. I was raised to think that when you quit, that's when you die. So you just keep going. When both my white and red blood counts dropped, I was doing what I had to do, but I was in a total fog. My boss said, "You're going to have to start writing things down."

The doctors reduced my doses of both interferon and ribavirin and I went on an antidepressant. That helped.

I took baths in an Aveeno bath treatment with oatmeal powder for the itching, and I used their anti-itch cream, too.

Baking soda and water worked as well as anything for the itching.

I'm exhausted all the time. I go to bed at 7 o'clock at night and get up at 7 o'clock in the morning. I'm rarely up to see the sunset.

Exercise helps. At first I got tired, but now I'm doing better. I started with 9 holes of golf, and I've worked my way up to 18.

I run out of gas, and I feel spaced out. I enjoy a nap now and then.

I never missed a day of work. I took the meds with me when I had to travel, icing them down.

I'd also time my shots. I started on Friday, and I'd have 36 hours with aches, pains, and headaches. By the time Monday came, I was feeling alright to work. I could do routine stuff. By Wednesday I was feeling like myself again. I would plan complicated projects on Thursday and Friday when I was mentally sharper.

I was always cold. It felt like I stayed cold for the whole 48 weeks of treatment. I never put on shorts that year. Instead, I wore insulated jeans.

I drink a lot of water. I have water bottles everywhere, at home, at work. I never drink pop. I only drink filtered water.

I don't concentrate as well on this interferon so I use a hand-held computer. I set it to buzz me when it's time to take the ribavirin. Then on the screen it asks me if I took it, and I have to insert "yes." I've never missed any ribavirin or injections.

I'd get redness at the site of the injection, but I learned to rotate the injection sites, move the needle around. The redness went away after a couple of months.

My faith and spirituality help me through it. I have wonderful church support with people praying for my healing.

One day at a time. I never understood that saying until the doctor told me I only had five years left. Okay, I thought. I'd better take that cruise now. When I think of something I always wanted to do and I can afford it, I do it now. I even went parasailing last May!

I look at it this way. The rash is ugly, but the fact that I have it means that at least my body knows something is going on!

I'm very conscious of what I eat. I cut back on sweets, junk food, and I eat a lot of fruit with fiber. I also drink lots of water and apple, cranberry, and orange juice. I even juice my own apples and veggies.

Special Considerations

Nonresponders and Relapsers. Nonresponse is defined by lack of viral clearance throughout treatment and followup. Relapse is defined by undetectable HCV RNA while on treatment but return of HCV RNA in your blood after treatment was discontinued. Nonresponse or relapse occurs for five main reasons:

1. The therapy used was ineffective.
2. The patient did not comply with prescribed treatment.
3. Treatment doses had to be reduced due to low levels of white cells, red cells, or platelets.
4. Length of treatment or dose was reduced due to side effects or poor quality of life.
5. The type of hepatitis C infection was relatively or absolutely resistant to the prior course of interferon-based treatment.

Recommendations regarding retreatment depend upon the type of your prior treatment and virologic response to your prior therapy. Also, you should realize that studies focusing on treatment of nonresponders and relapsers typically are enriched in patients infected with HCV geno-type 1. Patients infected with genotypes 2 or 3 may experience better outcomes with retreatment compared to patients infected with HCV genotype 1. Your prior therapy could have included interferon or pegylated interferon monotherapy, interferon plus ribavirin, or pegylated interferon plus ribavirin.

Retreatment with pegylated interferon plus ribavirin is most effective for patients whose prior therapy was either interferon or pegylated interferon monotherapy. In the HALT C trial, the sustained virologic response rate after retreatment of nonresponders to monotherapy with pegylated interferon plus ribavirin was 28 percent.

In contrast, retreatment of nonresponders to interferon plus ribavirin with pegylated interferon plus ribavirin is less effective. In the HALT C Trial, the sustained virologic response rate was only 12 percent. Higher response rates, up to ~40 percent, have been reported in small series using daily high-dose interferon (9 to 15 ug/d) plus ribavirin, but these results require confirmation in larger trials.

Effectiveness of retreatment of patients who have had nonresponse or relapse to pegylated interferon plus ribavirin with a second course of pegylated interferon plus ribavirin is under investigation. Early results indicate modest, if any, beneficial effect. Higher response rates, 20 to 25 percent, have been reported in small series using daily high-dose interferon alfacon-1 plus ribavirin. As noted above, these early encouraging reports with interferon alfacon-1 will require confirmation in larger trials. Also, this daily, high-dose regimen is associated with significant side effects and requires a highly motivated patient and careful medical supervision.

If you received prior therapy, you may ask the question, "Does it make any sense to be re-treated?" In my view, any patient who failed to clear hepatitis C on any previous treatment regimen is potentially a candidate for re-treatment with ribavirin in combination with either pegylated interferon or daily interferon alfacon-1. The decision to re-treat must be made only after careful consideration of all variables by your treating physician.

My first treatment was just interferon, not the cocktail. It was a piece of cake. I seemed to adjust in a month-and-a-half, but I lost my response. I relapsed. And then I went into denial. I thought maybe my symptoms were a weird residual thing left over from the malaria I had in the army.

After several years of depression and putting hepatitis C on the back burner, I started to get a dull ache in my liver area. I decided that I needed to get proactive and understand the disease. When my doctor told me I might qualify for a study of pegylated interferon, I went for it because I don't have any health insurance.

Actually, the first time I took interferon was not a piece of cake, but the pegylated interferon with ribavirin was much harder. It got my attention. But I trained myself to be very positive.

At the end of the month, I told my nurse that my blood tests were going to be normal. She said that would be unusual. A few days later, she called with the results. They were normal!

Tom

African Americans. In nearly every study of interferon, pegylated interferon, and combination therapies the rate of sustained virologic response has been lower in African Americans compared to other study populations. However, the number of African Americans was much lower than the number of other participants in these trials making statistical comparison less valid. In addition, a higher proportion of African Americans was infected with HCV genotype 1.

The results of the recently completed NIH study of treatment of African Americans, VIRAHEP-C, were presented at the American Association for the Study of Liver Diseases meeting in 2005. In this study, all patients were infected with HCV genotype 1 and an equal number of African Americans and Caucasian patients with chronic hepatitis C were compared. On-treatment and sustained virologic responses were consistently and significantly lower in African Americans. Sustained virologic responses were 28 percent versus 50 percent for African Americans and Caucasians, respectively. These differences were not attributable to differences in doses of medications, and the mechanisms responsible for the reduced response are under study.

Cirrhosis. As a general principle, if your liver disease is more severe you will have less chance for sustained virologic response. In the large trials of pegylated interferon plus ribavirin, sustained virologic response rates were approximately 10 percent lower in patients with advanced fibrosis or cirrhosis (fibrosis stage 3 or 4 out of 4). In these trials, all the patients with cirrhosis were very well compensated. None had experienced clinical complications of liver failure (ascites, varices, encephalopathy, infections, jaundice) and nearly all had stable and nearly normal laboratory tests.

We treated sicker patients who had experienced complications of liver disease, many of whom were ultimately listed and underwent transplantation. The regimen we used, LADR, started at low doses and gradually increased both interferon and ribavirin. Only 24 percent of all these patients and 13 percent of patients infected with HCV genotype 1 achieved sustained virologic response.

In the HALT C Trial of retreatment of nonresponders to prior interferon or interferon plus ribavirin with pegylated interferon plus ribavirin, sustained virologic response in those with fibrosis and least severe disease was 23 percent but only 9 percent in those with cirrhosis and most severe disease.

Treatment of patients with cirrhosis requires close supervision and frequent monitoring of laboratory tests. Complications, such as infection, bleeding, worsening ascites, and encephalopathy, may arise either due to underlying severity of disease or the effects of treatment, and early intervention is warranted. For these reasons, treating patients with cirrhosis who have had clinical decompensation should only be done in liver centers or by physicians with extensive experience in the treatment of patients with chronic hepatitis C and management of advanced liver disease. Some considerations prior to treating patients with cirrhosis include evaluation and eradication of varices by endoscopic ligation therapy, prophylactic antibiotics to prevent spontaneous bacterial peritonitis, and use of pre-emptive lactulose, neomycin, or rifaximine to reduce risk of encephalopathy.

Renal Failure. Patients with renal failure, especially those on dialysis have an increased prevalence of infection with chronic hepatitis C. Generally, patients with renal failure respond well to interferon and have a sustained virologic response to interferon or pegylated interferon monotherapy that is equivalent or even superior to patients with chronic hepatitis C without renal failure. In contrast, kidney dysfunction impairs the excretion of ribavirin, leading to its accumulation in blood and tissue increasing hemolysis, bone marrow suppression, and mucosal and skin injury. It has been my practice to limit use of ribavirin and use primarily pegylated interferon monotherapy in patients with renal disease. If ribavirin is used it is typically administered at very low doses under careful supervision by an experienced physician.

Acute Hepatitis C. Acute hepatitis C is diagnosed by conversion from negative to positive HCV antibody in a patient with acute hepatitis and positive HCV RNA. In some cases, HCV antibody has already developed at time of initial presentation so seroconversion of antibody cannot be documented. The diagnosis of acute hepatitis C is then defined by absence of underlying chronic liver disease, clinically acute hepatitis, and positive HCV RNA.

In more than 50 percent of cases, acute hepatitis C resolves spontaneously. This has prompted some to suggest that treatment be delayed for three to six months and only be administered to the group of patients who fail to clear spontaneously. The problem with this strategy is that waiting for three to six months may diminish the ability of treatment to clear infection. We know that fully-established chronic hepatitis C has only a 50 to 60 percent chance for sustained virologic response. In contrast, early initiation of therapy after diagnosis of acute hepatitis C yields a sustained virologic response of ~ 95 percent. For these reasons, I have generally recommended 6 months of treatment with pegylated interferon monotherapy for patients immediately after documentation of acute hepatitis C. Ribavirin does not seem to add to the efficacy of interferon or pegylated interferon in the treatment of acute hepatitis C and is not currently recommended.

Maintenance Therapy

Maintenance therapy has been investigated in three large clinical trials, HALT-C, COPILOT, and EPIC. The results of HALT-C have been published in the *New England Journal of Medicine* (2008) and results from both COPILOT and EPIC have been presented at national and international meetings.

Definition and Goals. Maintenance therapy is defined as indefinite long-term treatment to suppress disease activity, stabilize injury, and halt disease or clinical progression. In the case of chronic hepatitis C, pegylated interferon given at half of the usual therapeutic optimum is the leading candidate for maintenance treatment. In maintenance regimens pegylated interferon is given as monotherapy. The typical maintenance dose of Pegasys is 90 µg weekly, and the dose for Peg-Intron is 0.5 µg per kg per week. Goals of maintenance therapy of chronic hepatitis C include stabilization or reduction in hepatic fibrosis, reduction in risk of hepatoma, and prevention of clinical complications or deterioration.

Criteria for Selection of Patients. The two main criteria for selection of potential patients for maintenance therapy were:

> ➤ Failure of prior therapy to clear hepatitis C (HCV RNA positive)
> ➤ Significant fibrosis
>> • Stage 3 or 4 by Metavir Fibrosis Score
>> • Stage 4, 5, or 6 by Ishak Fibrosis Score

Outcomes. The National Institutes of Health–sponsored HALT C (Hepatitis C Antiviral Long-Term treatment to prevent Cirrhosis) trial was an ongoing multicenter U.S. trial of maintenance pegylated interferon to prevent fibrosis progression and clinical decompensation. Patients were first treated with 24 weeks of pegylated interferon alfa-2a 180 ug/wk plus ribavirin 1.0–1.2 g/d. The results of this Lead-In phase of treatment in HALT C patients with cirrhosis are described above. Virologic nonresponders at week 20 were randomized to either no further therapy (N=533) or 90 ug/wk of pegylated interferon alfa-2a (N=517) for an additional three and a half years. Study end points included histologic progression, and development of clinical decompensation, liver cancer, need for liver transplantation, or death.

The HALT-C Trial failed to demonstrate any benefit of maintenance therapy. The combined rate of clinical and histological outcomes were 33.8% in the control group and 34.1% in the treated group. Based upon the results of HALT-C, maintenance therapy with low-dose peginterferon to prevent disease progression in chronic hepatitis C is not currently recommended.

A subsequent study of the HALT-C data, examining the relationship of virologic response to peginterferon and outcomes, suggested that patients with more that 10,000-fold decrease in HCV RNA had lowest rates for clinical outcomes. This finding was not statistically significant, however, due to the few numbers of patients who achieved this level of viral suppression.

COPILOT (Colchicine versus Peg-Intron Long-term Trial) is another large, U.S. multicenter study of maintenance peginterferon therapy. In this study, prior nonresponders with fibrosis or cirrhosis (80 percent of cases) are randomized to receive either peginterferon alfa-2b (0.5 ug/kg/wk) or colchicine for four years. Preliminary data after one year indicate a trend toward lower viral load and a lower frequency of clinical events in patients treated with peginterferon. A followup report of two-year data, indicated an annual event rate (included death, transplant, hepatoma, 2 point or more progression in CTP (Child-Turcotte-Pugh) score, and variceal hemorrhage) of 7 percent in the colchicine-treated arm versus 3.5 percent in the peginterferon maintenance arm (P=.003).

The results of a third maintenance trial, EPIC (Efficacy of Peg Interferon in Hepatitis C), compare peginterferon alfa-2b to no treatment, and were just presented at EASL, 2009. Similar to the results in HALT-C, EPIC failed to demonstrate benefit of maintenance therapy. A subgroup analysis suggested that patients with pre-existing portal hypertension may have had fewer clinical events with peginterferon maintenance.

The final results from COPILOT and EPIC have not yet been published. Nonetheless, it does not seem likely that low-dose peginterferon will emerge as an effective maintenance treatment to prevent disease progression in patients with chronic hepatitis C. The linkage of virologic response, a greater than 10,000-fold reduction in HCV RNA, with reduced outcomes suggest that future maintenance strategies must incorporate antiviral drugs that achieve near complete viral suppression.

In summary, I have been impressed by the current results of treatment using pegylated interferon with ribavirin. Today more than 50 percent of patients with hepatitis C may be cured of their infection. However, side effects of treatment remain problematic and we still must face the fact that nearly 50 percent of treated patients do not respond and fail to clear HCV. Certain populations are more resistant to treatment and reasons for this resistance must be defined to improve chances for better outcomes. Maintenance therapy using low dose peginterferon is probably ineffective, but future maintenance regimens with new anti-HCV drugs might be beneficial. Although the advances in treatment of HCV have been considerable, my hope is that future treatments will be even more successful in the upcoming years.

After Treatment, What Next?

If You Are a Sustained Responder. A sustained response is the most desirable outcome after antiviral treatment. Most patients with a sustained response have cleared the virus from their blood and have improvement in their liver biopsy (fewer inflammatory cells and less damage).

Long-term sustained responders (more than three years) may have halted the progression of their liver disease and are likely to have actually cleared hepatitis C completely. However, there is always the risk, albeit small (~1 percent), that hepatitis C may only be dormant and reactivate, flaring at a later date. Patients should continue to undergo periodic biochemical tests, measurement of HCV RNA annually for two years after SVR, and undergo physical examinations.

If you had advanced fibrosis or cirrhosis, you are at risk for liver cancer even if you are a sustained responder and no longer have hepatitis C. I recommend continued surveillance for liver cancer through your physician. Surveillance strategies vary and are of unproven benefit but a common one uses measurement of alpha fetoprotein every 6 months plus ultrasonography every 6 to 12 months (see Chapter 11).

If You Are a Relapser or Nonresponder. You still harbor HCV infection and are at risk for disease progression, development of cirrhosis and its complications, and liver cancer. Greatest risk for these outcomes and complications is in patients who have had extensive fibrosis or cirrhosis on liver biopsy. Routine blood testing and clinical followup through your physician is recommended.

If you had advanced fibrosis or cirrhosis, you are at risk for liver cancer even if you are a sustained responder and no longer have hepatitis C. I recommend continued surveillance for liver cancer through your physician. Surveillance strategies vary and are of unproven benefit but a common one uses measurement of alpha fetoprotein every six months plus ultrasonography every six to 12 months (see Chapter 11).

You should understand that the continued use of alcohol can cause early progression to cirrhosis and liver failure. Smoking may increase your risk of liver cancer and active alcoholism is a contraindication to liver transplantation. Avoid cigarettes and alcohol.

Vaccinations. The National Institutes of Health (NIH) guidelines indicate that hepatitis C patients should undergo vaccination against both hepatitis A and B. Both vaccines are safe and highly effective in preventing infection; and, the two vaccines may now be co-administered (TWINRIX®). Check with your physician about vaccination.

No physician, insofar as he is a physician, considers his own good in what he prescribes, but the good of his patient.

Plato

Reference

1. The Hepatitis C Antiviral Long-Term Treatment Against Cirrhosis (HALT C) is the NIH-sponsored clinical trial of the use of Pegasys plus ribavirin in the treatment of nonresponders to prior therapy.★

★In the NIH-sponsored Hepatitis C Antiviral Long-Term Treatment Against Cirrhosis (HALT-C Pegasys plus ribavirin was used to treat nonresponders to prior therapy. Patients who remained RNA positive after 20 to 24 weeks of treatment were then randomized to maintenance therapy wit dose peginterferon or no treatment for another 3.5 years. Followup, after the end of the mainte treatment period, was extended for a total of 6 years.

10

LIVER TRANSPLANTS
A Miracle of Modern Medicine

I was on the liver transplant waiting list for—oh, gosh—nine months. Finally, they gave me a pager because it was getting close. The second day, early in the morning, I was sleeping in that ozone where you're just starting to wake up, when I heard the pager go off. I bolted out of bed. I hadn't moved like that for months because I'd been so sick.

I reached for my pager, but it wasn't blinking. My heart was just pounding! Then I heard the garbage truck in the alley; it was the warning beep as the truck backed up.

The real call came three weeks later at 4:30 A.M. The doctors kept asking me if I was afraid, if I was sure I wanted to do this. "My God, yes!" I said. "Let's get this show on the road."

Tom

SOME PEOPLE with hepatitis C develop cirrhosis, liver failure, and need a liver transplant to survive. Liver transplantation is the most complicated therapy for people with end-stage hepatitis C, but it can produce seemingly miraculous results.

Pre-transplant patients go through a difficult time. They suffer from a variety of symptoms, including jaundice, sleeplessness, itching, fluid buildup, mental confusion, and hemorrhaging. A successful transplant cures these symptoms, and the patient can lead a full, productive life.

This chapter covers the following topics:

- Liver Transplantation: A Brief History
- Who Gets a Liver Transplant?
  The Most Common Diagnosis: Hepatitis C
  Signs That You Need a Transplant
  MELD Score
  Denial of Transplants
  Paying for Transplants
- The Transplant Team
- Waiting for a Liver
  The Evaluation Process
  The Waiting List
  Transplant Support Groups
- Types of Donors
  Deceased Donor
  Extended Criteria Donor
  Living Donor
  Our First Case of Adult-to-Adult, Living-Donor
    Liver Transplantation in Colorado
- How is it Done? The Operations
  Donor Surgery
    Deceased Donor
    Liver Donation from "Non-Heart-Beating Donor"
    Living Donor
  Recipient Surgery
   General Principles
   Unique Aspects of Surgery for Recipients of Right Lobes
    From Living Donor
- How long am I in the Hospital?
  The Hospital Stay
- Living with a New Liver
  Medications to Prevent Rejection
- Managing Complications
  Rejection
  Recurrence of Hepatitis C
  Psychological Transformation
- What are my Chances? The Outcomes.

- How Organs Are Allocated in the US
  UNOS and UNOS Regions
  MELD Score
  PELD Score
- Center-Specific Results

Liver Transplantation: A Brief History

The first liver transplant was performed by Dr. Thomas Starzl in 1963 at the University of Colorado in Denver. Twenty years later, in 1983, a National Institutes of Health (NIH) consensus conference on the therapeutic role of liver transplantation concluded, "After extensive review and consideration…liver transplantation is a therapeutic modality for end-stage liver disease that deserves broader application."

At that time, only six centers in North America and four in Europe performed liver transplantation. Since then there has been a dramatic increase in the number of liver transplants performed. On June 30, 2005, there were 126 programs in liver transplantation and 17,661 patients were on the recipient waiting list in the United States. From July 1, 2004 to June 30, 2005, 6082 deceased donor and 307 living donor liver transplantations were performed, and 10.1 percent patients died on the waitlist without transplant within one year of listing. The first adult-to-pediatric, living-donor, liver transplant in the US was performed in 1989. The first adult-to-adult, living-donor liver transplant in the US was performed in 1997. Adult-to-adult, living-donor, liver transplantation, has been increasingly utilized to meet the rising recipient need for donor livers.

I suggest three websites for you to visit regarding most current information and statistics on liver transplantation in the United States:

www.unos.org
www.ustransplant.org
www.a-s-t.org

Who Gets a Liver Transplant?

The Most Common Diagnosis: Hepatitis C. Liver transplantation is the most successful therapy for patients with a wide array of diseases that ultimately result in liver failure. Currently, the most common diagnosis for transplant is cirrhosis due to chronic hepatitis C. Laennec's cirrhosis, caused by alcohol, ranks second, but co-infection with hepatitis C is common in these patients—illustrating once again that the combination of alcohol and hepatitis C speeds the progression of liver disease.

Signs That You Need a Transplant. Obvious clinical signs and symptoms usually accompany advanced liver disease, including:

- ascites (accumulation of fluid in the abdomen)
- encephalopathy (alteration of mental function)
- variceal hemorrhage (bleeding from veins in the esophagus or stomach)
- worsening nutritional status
- diminishing quality of life

Patients who have a spontaneous infection in the ascites fluid, low serum albumin (< 2.8 grams/deciliter), clotting problems (prothrombin time > 5 seconds prolonged), and severe sustained jaundice should be given urgent consideration for transplantation. All of the above findings indicate severe liver dysfunction and are late signs of end-stage liver disease.

> *I found out I had hepatitis C when I came to the hospital a year ago. I had a lot of fluid in my stomach. They drained me and sent me home. I couldn't sleep. I'd lay down, stand up. The only way I could get some sleep was to fill the bathtub up so I could get some buoyancy, which relieved the pain in my stomach.*
>
> *The second time I had to go to the hospital, they did an ultrasound. That's how I found out I needed a transplant.*
>
> *Chris*

Many people with cirrhosis have few or no findings of liver disease. Doctors say that these patients have "compensated" cirrhosis, and that it may be too early to consider liver transplantation. However, the waiting list for liver transplants is expanding, while the pool of donors is staying about the same. Patients often wait on the list for one, two, or more years before they get a liver.

Once you have cirrhosis, your doctor must monitor your blood tests closely and watch for any physical signs of decompensation in order to time the referral for liver transplantation. Unfortunately, not all patients with compensated cirrhosis are the same; some will remain stable for several years, but others may deteriorate relatively rapidly.

The course of hepatitis C varies greatly, so your physician must make an imperfect estimate of your chances of having a life-threatening complication over a one- to two-year followup period. If your doctor estimates that you have more than a 10 percent chance of sustaining a complication within one year, you should be evaluated for transplantation.

MELD Score. Generally, the standard liver blood tests will deteriorate prior to any clinical event. That is why your physician draws blood and runs tests. Early markers of cirrhosis are low platelet count, elevated bilirubin, and elevated alkaline phosphatase. Severity of liver disease and prognosis can be determined from a combination of laboratory tests and clinical features. Today the most commonly used clinical score of severity of liver disease is the Model for End-stage Liver Disease (MELD) Score. MELD Score is calculated from bilirubin, INR, and creatinine (see chapter 4 for discussion of liver blood tests). The score ranges from 6, which indicates least severe disease, to 40, which is the most severe disease. For patients with chronic hepatitis C and cirrhosis, we currently recommend that patients with MELD scores 10 or greater be referred to a liver center for consideration for liver transplantation.

Priority for liver transplantation is assigned on the basis of MELD Score; patients with the highest scores have highest priority for allocation of a deceased donor organ for liver transplantation. In the absence of other critieria for listing, such as liver cancer, patients with chronic hepatitis C are not listed for transplantation until they have achieved a MELD Score of 12 or higher. The average MELD score at which deceased donor livers are transplanted in the United States is approximately 26.

Denial of Transplants. You may be denied a liver transplant if you have active HIV infection or AIDS, incurable cancer, active infection in the blood, active alcohol abuse, or severe underlying heart, lung, or multi-organ disease. If you are elderly, morbidly obese, or have had prior extensive abdominal surgery, a clotted portal vein, extensive liver cancer, an isolated liver cancer larger than five centimeters, or cancer of the bile ducts, you might be excluded from transplantation.

Paying for Transplants. See chapter 7, "Taking Care of Yourself Financially."

The Transplant Team

Liver transplantation is a complex procedure requiring many specialists to care for you. Usually, your transplant team consists of a hepatologist, a hepatology nurse, a transplant surgeon, a transplant anesthesiologist, a transplant nurse coordinator (who keeps you informed and tells you when a liver becomes available), a social worker (who provides you and your family with emotional support), a psychiatrist (who meets with you and your family to evaluate your strengths and weaknesses and make recommendations to help you through the transplant experience), a nutritionist (who deals with pre-transplant issues, such as overweight problems or nutritional wasting, and helps with recommendations for your post-transplant nutritional needs), and a financial coordinator. Your outcome is improved if your liver transplant program has a "team" approach and performs more than 20 transplants a year.

Waiting for a Liver

The Evaluation Process. You will be asked to take many diagnostic tests and meet with a psychiatrist and social worker. Usually, you meet with each person on the transplant team. The process can take a couple of days. When all the tests and interviews are completed, the team meets to approve or deny your candidacy for transplantation and may suggest additional evaluations or consultations.

I had two days of evaluation, from early morning until 5 o'clock in the evening. The tests were tough, but I got a lot of kindness and attention. I met everybody—the psychiatrist, the surgical team. I had to bring my whole family to the social worker. Oh boy, I've never had such tests. At my first stop, they took 21 vials of blood!

They were very frank with me. They wouldn't waste a liver if other things were wrong with me. My previous doctor had told me I was too old to get a liver. I'm 61. The transplant team said I checked out to be in pretty good health for my age, and now I'm on the waiting list.

Carla

At my evaluation, the psychiatrist must have asked me ten times if I was a closet drinker. I know they have to find out if you're an active alcoholic, but I found it offensive. Everyone assumes that you're an alcoholic if you need a liver transplant. That's the first thing you have to overcome.

Bea

When they asked me why I thought I should get a transplant, I said, "I have seven grandchildren. I have much to teach and share. When I get my liver, as soon as I'm able, I intend to educate people and speak to people about becoming donors."

Leonora

In trying to evaluate your ability to tolerate transplant surgery, the transplant team will give you some diagnostic tests. Depending on your condition, the tests may include blood tests, colonoscopy (view of the entire colon through a colonoscope), CT scan (a radiologic test that lets doctors see the anatomy and size of your liver), ECG (an electrocardiogram), endoscopy (a procedure that allows doctors to look for ulcers, masses, varices, or bleeding in the esophagus or stomach), ERCP (a procedure performed when there is concern about blockage or narrowing in the bile ducts), flexible sigmoidoscopy (a procedure that lets the physician look at the lower colon for polyps, hemorrhoids, ulcers, and colon or rectal cancer), pulmonary function tests (a breathing test that measures the function of your lungs), and ultrasound (a test that gives information about the size and shape of your liver through sound waves). If you have conditions that require additional tests, you may be asked to meet with a consultant, such as a cardiologist.

The Waiting List. As previously noted, the number of patients on the waiting list continues to expand (Figure 10A). Current patients placed on the list can wait for more than two years for a donor liver. This is an incredibly difficult and apprehensive period. While waiting, you may have to deal with life changes, physical symptoms, and financial changes. If you're the major breadwinner who can't go to work, you may lose the social network from your job.

Life is on hold. I haven't had too many problems, except mentally— I worry a lot. The toxins make your mind goofy. I can't remember things or make good judgments.

And it's hard on my wife. This mental problem has been developing over years, and we didn't know why, so we've had a lot of marital problems. We go to counseling, and we've learned to fight fair, but she's scared of the hepatitis C. She doesn't have any desire to be intimate with me at all. It's pretty hard.

It's hard for me to accept knowing that I'm dying. I only have 10 to 15 percent usage of my liver. I've been in and out of the hospital five times. Sometimes I wonder if I'll die before I get a liver.

Thomas

I've been on the waiting list for seven months. It's like an out-of-body experience—as if it's happening to someone else, not to me. Sometimes I realize I have lots to get in order, because a percentage of people don't make it. You want a liver to come, and yet you don't.

Normally, I can battle the depression, but last night I couldn't sleep. I tossed and turned. When that happens, I start cooking. I love to cook.

Johanna

I waited 515 days for my liver—and each day was a little more painful and difficult than the day before.

I think the secret of my success during surgery was maintaining a positive attitude. I packed my suitcase in August with a red flannel robe and a Santa Claus hat. It was hot, and I felt lousy, so why did I pack for Christmas?

I was baking Christmas cookies with my grandchildren when the phone rang. Laughing and covered from head to toe in flour, I asked my husband to tell whoever it was that I was too busy for a transplant. It was the call from the hospital. I got my liver that night.

Deanne

Increasingly, transplants are performed in sicker patients who are hospitalized or in intensive care. As noted previously, the average MELD Score at time of liver transplantation in the United States is approximately 26. Patients with this level of severity of liver disease are typically jaundiced with mild to moderate renal failure and poor clotting ability. Often fluid retention with ascites and encephalopathy complicate the clinical picture.

It's critical at this stage to talk about your struggles with a good friend or therapist. Keeping a personal journal is helpful. You are going

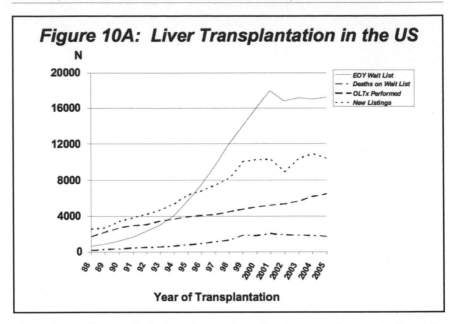

Figure 10A: This graph displays the number of patients on the waiting list at the end of the year (EOY) (solid line), new listings (dotted line), liver transplants performed (dashed line), and deaths (dashed-dotted line) by year of liver transplantation. At the end of 2005 there were 17,234 patients on the waiting list. During 2005 there were 10,435 new listings, 6444 transplants, and 1696 deaths of patients on the waiting list. There are currently nearly twice as many new listings each year as there are transplants performed. The number of deaths on the waiting list has stabilized since institution of MELD score for organ allocation in 2002.

through a fundamental shift in how you think of yourself and preparing for the psychological changes of the transplant.

Transplant Support Groups. Transplant support groups can be a source of strength and encouragement for pre- and post-transplant patients. The long waiting period, difficult symptoms, the trauma of surgery, the psychological shift of accepting another person's organ—all of these issues are unique to transplant patients. No one else can truly understand what it's like.

I feel a lot more comfortable in the support group now than I did six months ago. Getting to know the people, being involved with their lives, and caring for each other have helped.

When people get their transplants, it's like day and night. I look at myself as night, and they're day. Sam, he just got his. I watched him go through his struggle, and he looked really bad. It's amazing what a new liver can do for a person. It's a shot in the arm. Their facial expressions change. They glow.

I feel happier, less depressed. I don't participate a lot in the group, but I'm learning. When I get my transplant, I'll go to the group because it seems to be a help to new people who come in.

The tiredness, not sleeping, itching—no one else can know how bad you feel. They wouldn't believe it if you told them. You need to talk, to vent. If I talked to my family, I'd cry and they'd cry. You don't need that. How you feel is how you feel.

It helped me to see others waiting. I was a basket case, but I began to accept that it was going to happen. I'd get my liver.

I cried at the group the first time I went. To see all those people—it was overwhelming. For the first time, my husband felt positive about the transplant. He had been reluctant to have me go through it, but he saw so many people looking so good and doing so well.

I think everyone should be required to go to a transplant support group. At first I dug my heels in and refused to go. I had the feeling I was assisting Mother Nature and wondered whether I had the right to do that. When I saw others in the support group, I decided if I could have that quality of life back, I'd go for it.

Your transplant team can refer you to a support group, or you can check the resources listed at the end of this chapter. In addition to support groups, many people tell me they find it helpful to read about other liver transplant patients' experiences and about the procedure itself. Here are some books my patients recommend:

Resources:

Green, Reg. *The Nicholas Effect: A Boy's Gift to the World*. Sepastopol: O'Reilly, 1999.

Maier, Frank with Ginny Maier. *Sweet Reprieve*. New York: Crown, 1991.

McCartney, Scott. *Defying the Gods*. New York: Macmillan, 1994.

Schomaker, Mary Zimmeth. *Life Line, How One Night Changed Five Lives*. Far Hills: New Horizon, 1996.

Starzl, Thomas E. *The Puzzle People*. Pittsburgh: University of Pittsburgh, 1992.

Types of Donor Livers

Deceased Donor. Liver transplantation is made possible only through the act of organ donation. In most states, you can sign an organ donor permission statement on your driver's license; a witnessed signature is a legal form of consent. Most organ procurement organizations, however, request additional consent from the closest living relative. These organizations identify potential donors by interacting with emergency rooms and intensive care units.

Organ donation is one of the highest forms of giving and caring, and the vast majority of religious denominations endorse it. The generosity of organ donation makes possible the miracle of transplantation. Here is Judy Ferrin's story:

> At the hospital, the doctors diagnosed my daughter, Allison, with toxic shock syndrome. She went from laughing and joking with me to sleeping, a coma, and dying within 24 hours. She was 19 years old.
>
> Just three weeks before, the two of us were watching a little boy on TV who needed a new heart. We decided to donate our organs if something happened to us—so I knew what her wishes were, and I told her nurse.
>
> The night before the funeral, I tossed and turned. I felt a need to speak at the service, but I was so afraid. We got a call from the doctor that morning. They had successfully transplanted her kidneys. Other organs were also transplanted, but that was the first, the turning point. A wave of relief went over me. And I was able to speak about Allison to the hundreds of people who came to mourn with our family.
>
> When we give to other people, it helps us through our grief. It helps us as much as the people we give to.

Did you know that the liver donor usually donates as many as seven organs for seven different patients? Standard liver donors are patients under age 65 who are brain-dead but whose hearts are beating. They have no underlying malignancy, and they test negative for AIDS and active hepatitis B. The donors must have stable heart function with acceptable liver tests, serum sodium less than 170, and preferably been hospitalized for fewer than seven days. Donors and recipients must have compatible blood types and approximately similar body size but not identical gender.

Extended Criteria Donor. As noted above, there is a tremendous shortage of organ donors in the U.S. (Figure 10A). For this reason, transplant surgeons have begun to use grafts that fall outside the criteria for ideal grafts; these grafts are called extended criteria donor grafts. Features of an extended critieria donor or graft could include older donor age, fat accumulation in liver cells of the graft, grafts from donors who have either hepatitis C or hepatitis B, injured grafts, and grafts with damaged vessels. Recently there have been several transplants using grafts from non-heart-beating donors (described in more detail below).

Once recovered, the donated organs are flushed with a special solution that preserves them for up to 48 hours. Extended criteria donor livers are more susceptible to injury and damage prior to transplantation. Although most of the latter grafts function very well, there is slightly greater risk of poor graft function, bile duct complications, and need for retransplantation.

Patients frequently ask whether organs from donors who test positive for hepatitis C can be used for transplantation. Yes, but the recipient will acquire hepatitis C. One study followed 29 recipients of organs from 13 donors who tested positive for hepatitis C. Twenty-eight of the 29 recipients tested positive for hepatitis C after the transplant. For this reason, we restrict the use of these donor livers primarily to recipients who already have hepatitis C.

Despite efforts to use all potential donor organs, we currently face a crisis in supply and availability of donor organs. We encourage all readers of this book to work with their local organ procurement organizations to increase public awareness of the critical need and value of organ donation. It's important for all family members to discuss organ and tissue donation. Everyone should consider signing a Uniform Donor Card.

Resource: For more information on organ donation, contact the Coalition on Donation, an alliance of national organizations and local coalitions that educates the public about organ donation at 804-782-4920; email: coalition@donatelife.net; website: www.shareyourlife.org.

How can physicians attempt to deal with the crisis in availability of donor organs? The cadaveric supply of donor livers has remained relatively constant at about 5,500 to 6,000 donor livers each year for the past three years. The current U.S. waiting list is nearly 18,000.

We need to increase the donor pool in innovative ways in order to meet the expanding need for donor organs. Use of older donors, livers with increased amounts of fat, and hepatitis C antibody-positive livers has failed to substantially expand the donor pool. **Splitting of deceased donor livers** for use in two recipients works well for a pediatric (left lateral segment) and adult recipient (right lobe + left medial segment); splits for two adult recipients works less well. For this reason, our center and many others have embarked upon the use of adult living donors (right lobe donation) for adults.

Living Donors. You may be thinking, "By the time I need a transplant, there will be too many people on the waiting list, and I won't ever get one!" A partial solution for the shortage of donors is living-donor liver transplantation, where a portion of a living donor's liver is removed and then transplanted. The Japanese, for example, still debate the concept of brain death so nearly all liver donations in Japan are from live donors. In the United States, from 1989 until 1997 virtually all live donor transplant operations were performed in pediatric recipients. Typically a parent would donate a part of their left liver lobe, the left lateral segment, to son or daughter. In 1997 the first adult-to-adult right liver lobe donation and transplantation was reported from the United States and since that time there are nearly five times as many adult-to-adult transplants as compared to adult-to-pediatric transplants (Figure 10B).

At the time of this writing, the University of Colorado had performed 112 adult-to-adult live-donor liver transplantations with the vast majority between relatives, although close friends and personal relationships may be considered. All donors are alive and tolerated the liver resection. Their livers regenerated back to normal size within 16 weeks. In 2001, we published a paper describing the impact of right lobe donation on the quality of life of the first 30 living donors in our program:

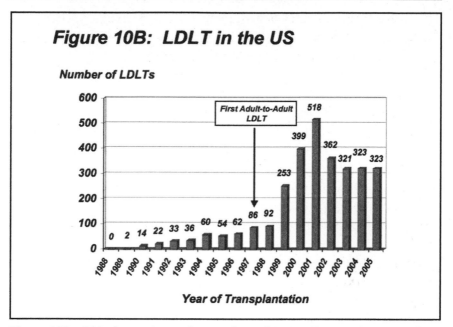

Figure 10B: LDLT in the US

Figure 10B: This figure shows the number of Living Donor Liver Transplants (LDLTs) performed in the United States between 1988 and 2005. The first US case was adult-to-pediatric and occurred in 1989. The first adult-to-adult LDLT in the U.S. occurred in 1997. Prior to 1999, most LDLTs were performed in pediatric recipients using adult donors. Since 1999 the LDLT activity in the U.S. has been dominated by adult-to-adult LDLT. Over 500 cases of LDLT were performed in 2001, but in that year there was a donor death from a transplant program in New York and most U.S. programs subsequently cutback activity while re-examining their own processes and procedures.

- 75 percent of donors recovered completely and returned to normal life within an average of 3.4 months after surgery.
- 96 percent returned to work at an average of 2.4 months.
- 42 percent described a change in body image related to the scar from the incision.
- 71 percent had mild ongoing abdominal discomfort.

Personal relationships between donor and recipient were the same or better in 96 percent of cases. The relationship of the donor to his or her life partner was the same or better in 88 percent of cases. Most donors reported out-of-pocket expenses not covered by insurance plans; the mean out-of-pocket expenses were $3,660. All patients reported that under the same circumstances they would donate again, and 96 percent of the donors felt that they benefited from the experience. A multi-center study of donor quality of life is currently being conducted by centers participating in the NIH-sponsored A2ALL Study.

In our program, we have developed selection criteria for both donor and recipient. Our current criteria for selection of recipients center around two concepts. First, we feel that recipients should have an excellent chance for favorable post-transplant outcome. Second, the recipient should be in urgent need of a transplant for survival and might die while waiting for standard cadaveric transplantation.

Donors for living-donor liver transplantation must be relatively young (less than 50 years old), normal body size, healthy without medical problems, and they cannot have a history of prior abdominal surgery. Donors and recipients should have compatible blood types and an emotional bond. Unlike other transplants, livers do not need to be matched by tissue type. The donor liver, however, must be of sufficient size that a lobe will be large enough for the recipient.

Our First Case of Adult-to-Adult, Living-Donor, Liver Transplantation in Colorado. In 1997 Karen Frederick had been fighting for her life for 14 long months on the liver transplant waiting list. Her older sister, Christine Larsen, was a little taller, bigger, and had the same blood type:

> *Karen's skin was gray. Her mind was gone. She couldn't walk or make a sentence. She didn't know who people were. She knew me on occasion, but she'd fade in and out.*
>
> *Christine*

> *I had to have a transplant, so I came to terms with it. But if anything happened to my sister, I don't know if I could live with it. My doctor said I had to accept that it was her decision.*
>
> *Karen*

> *After the operation, we lived in the same hospital room for seven days. Later we learned the doctors felt the sibling rivalry would make us*

get better quicker. They were right. We got into who could blowcomb their hair sooner, faster, better.

Christine

We prepared for our hospital stay by buying matching T-shirts with funny faces and boxer shorts.

Karen

I was surprised. Even the first day after the operation, she was making more sense. She lost that gray color.

Christine

I got her right lobe. They told us it would take six weeks for both of our livers to grow back to normal size. Ten days after the operation, Christine was leaving to go home. On our way to the airport, we stopped at the hospital for CT scans. And we both had full-sized livers!

Karen

I love coffee ice cream, and Karen never did until after the transplant. "Look what you've done," she tells me.

I love cilantro. She hates it. When she starts to eat cilantro, I'll know that the livers are in perfect shape!

Christine

At the airport, when Christine was going home, I was tearful. "I can never thank you enough," I said. Then I gave her a quick hug and zoom, we were off. Neither of us is big on mushy stuff. But she knows how I feel.

Karen

The living donor undergoes careful medical, psychological, and social evaluation. Potential donors may be rejected because their livers are unsuitable or they have underlying medical conditions that increase the risk of complications from surgery.

Risks to a Living Donor. Risk to the living donor are real and not inconsequential. The current estimate of the risk of death is 1 death in 300 to 500 liver donations. Other complications can occur, however, including development of clots in legs or lungs, bleeding internally, from the wound, or into the gut, bile duct injury, bile leak, bowel obstruction, and infection. The overall rate of significant complications in donors is approximately 2 to 16 percent. In our study of the quality of life after right lobe donation, 71 percent of donors reported mild ongoing symptoms (mainly abdominal discomfort) that they related to the surgery.

The liver is the only internal human organ that regenerates. Within 12 weeks of surgery the overall size of both the right lobe that was implanted into the recipient and the left lobe remaining in the donor have returned to approximately 80% of the size of the total liver prior to donation. When the liver regenerates in the donor the remaining left lobe enlarges and occupies the center to left side of the upper abdomen. In the recipient the right lobe enlarges and occupies the right side of the upper abdomen.

How Is It Done? The Operations.

The human body has two kidneys, two lungs—but only one liver. Scientists have created artificial kidneys (kidney dialysis) and even artificial hearts, and there have been gains in development of a bioartificial liver. However, no one has yet been able to duplicate the hundreds of functions of the liver in an effective liver dialysis machine or bioartificial liver. Liver transplant surgery, therefore, has no fall-back position, no margin for error.

Donor Surgery

Deceased Donor. After declaration and confirmation of brain death by the patient's care providers, the potential donor remains on life support to maintain blood flow through organs that are to be used later for transplantation. The organ procurement team is not involved with the management of the patient prior to the donation, declaration of brain death, or the consent of the donor or donor's family. Once consent for donation has been obtained, the potential donor's blood is checked for HIV infection, active hepatitis, and other medical conditions, including malignancy, that could compromise outcome of the graft or recipient. The donor is then taken to the operating room where teams work to procure the organs and tissues for subsequent transplantation. After organ procurement, the donor is taken off life support.

Liver Donation from "Non-Heart-Beating Donor." Patients who may become non-heart-beating donors (NHBD) are managed according to Organ Procurement Organization (OPO) protocols which are consistent with recommendations of the Institute of Medicine. Although these patients lack the strict criteria for brain death, they have experienced catastrophic brain injury, require machines for ventilation (cannot breathe on their own), and their health care team has determined that further resuscitation efforts are futile. The decision to withdraw life support, which usually means stopping mechanical ventilation, is made by the health care team and family. No member of the organ procurement or transplantation teams is involved with the decision to withdraw life support. After the family and health care team have decided to withdraw life support, the OPO coordinator approaches the family and fully explains the NHBD procedures. Informed consent from the family is required prior to proceeding with the operation for procurement of organs.

Upon completion of the process for consent, the patient is then a potential NHBD donor and is taken to the operating room. The organ procurement team prepares the potential donor for the surgery by cleansing and sterilizing the skin, and draping the body. After this and prior to any incision, the organ procurement team exits the operating room and does not participate in withdrawal of life support or declaration of death. The potential donor is managed by the donor's care team up until the time of the surgical procedures to procure the organs. Life support is discontinued by the donor's care team which then monitors the patient and waits for the heartbeat to cease and the absence of blood pressure (cardiopulmonary arrest). If arrest does not occur within one hour of stopping life support, the donation process ceases and the patient is returned to the intensive care unit without the procurement of any organs. This potential outcome of the donation process is explained to the family during the process of obtaining informed consent. If arrest occurs, a period of at least five minutes of cardiopulmonary arrest, lack of any heartbeat or blood pressure, is required prior to declaration of death. Five minutes of cardiopulmonary arrest results in irreversible brain injury and brain death. The donor's care team, not involved with organ procurement or transplantation, declares and confirms the donor death.

Rapid recovery techniques are used to procure the organs and perfuse them with preservation solution to minimize the damage done by lack of any oxygen delivery that occurred during the five minutes of cardiopulmonary arrest required for declaration of donor death. Damage done to organs due to lack of blood flow and oxygen delivery is called ischemic injury. There is greater risk of ischemic injury in donor livers obtained from NHBD donors compared to standard deceased donors or living donors. Ischemic injury in these grafts translates into greater risk of bile duct complications in recipients. Strategies to minimize ischemic damage to NHBD organs are being evaluated. Despite the increased risk of bile duct complications, the shortage of standard deceased donor livers relative to the large number of waiting list candidates continues to push the activity in NHBD liver transplantation.

Living Donor. In living donor liver transplantation, recipient surgery and donor surgery are tightly coordinated and occurring simultaneously (Figure 10C). Anatomic matching of living donors and recipients is made possible by current imaging techniques such as MRI and CT angiography which provide detailed visualization of both donor and recipient vascular anatomy. The donor surgery begins first and recipient surgery begins midway through the donor operation. Rarely, the donor's surgery might be halted if unsuspected vascular or biliary anomalies are found or other problems are encountered that would preclude proceeding with the operation and donation.

Surgery to remove the right lobe from a living donor for use in transplantation is far more complicated that the standard surgical resection of a right lobe containing disease or a mass. In standard resections for a diseased lobe or liver mass, the blood flow to the right lobe is first eliminated by clamping the vessel. Bile ducts are tied and the resection follows, removing a right lobe that is completely devoid of blood supply. This resected lobe is dead tissue that cannot be used for transplantation.

In right lobe donation the surgeon performing the operation must maintain blood supply to the right lobe while he is cutting across the liver to remove the right lobe for transplantation into the recipient. The transection of the liver, cutting it into right and left lobes, is accomplished while maintaining blood supply to both lobes. After transection

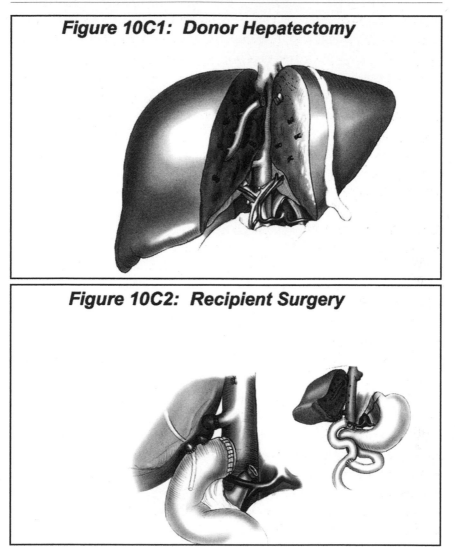

Figure 10C1: Donor Hepatectomy

Figure 10C2: Recipient Surgery

Figure 10C: Panel 1: This figure depicts the splitting of the donor liver into right and left lobes. The surgery is technically demanding since blood flow is maintained to both lobes of the liver throughout the transection (splitting) of the liver. Several major vessels, including portal vein, hepatic artery, vena cava, and hepatic veins must be identified and branches ligated and cut. The biliary tree exiting the right liver lobe must be carefully assessed, ligated, and cut. Panel 2: This figure shows the implantation of the living donor's right lobe into the recipient. Bile ducts from the right lobe are usually sewed to a loop of intestine (roux-en-Y) and the graft's vessels are connected to recipient vessels, similar to the way the connections are made in deceased donor liver transplantation.

of the liver, the vessels and bile ducts are clamped, the right lobe is removed and flushed with perfusion solution, and the graft is implanted immediately into the recipient.

Recipient Surgery

General Principles. Although the original method pioneered by Dr. Starzl has been modified, the basic technique remains essentially unchanged. The operation has three phases:

1. dissection to access the patient's liver
2. removal of the patient's liver
3. connection of the donated liver

First, the surgeon meticulously dissects tissues and promptly controls bleeding vessels to expose the patient's liver. This process takes about one to two hours. Blood loss ranges from zero to five pints of red blood cells.

In the next phase, the surgeon clamps the blood vessels supplying your liver and removes the liver. Then the surgeon and anesthesiologist work together to maintain adequate blood clotting factors. The anesthesiologist carefully monitors your blood and blood pressure to give you the proper fluids and blood products. In the last phase, the surgeon positions the donor liver in your abdomen and sews the blood vessels together. This procedure takes from one and a half to three hours; blood loss ranges from zero to five pints.

Once all the vessels are connected, the surgeon must unclamp the main vessels. After unclamping, one of the more critical periods of the procedure begins—especially if your blood clotting is poor. After you stabilize, your surgeon connects your bile duct to the donor bile duct and removes the donor gallbladder.

Livers typically begin to function immediately after their blood supply is established. Clotting improves, and the liver makes bile on the operating table!

"The most critical moment in the operation," says University of Colorado's Chief of Transplantation, Dr. Igal Kam, "is when we release the clamps holding the vessels going to the new liver, and the new liver changes in color from pale or dark brown to a more pink-brown, because new blood is flowing to the liver. When we see the yellow-brown bile start to appear from the bile duct, we can relax because we know the liver is going to work. There's no room for mistakes in this procedure.

"About 40 to 50 percent of patients go off the respirator in the operating room and we can talk to them. After six to eight hours of surgery, it's great to talk to the patient. We deal with very sick people who sometimes have only hours to live. After the transplant, then we see the miracle."

Unique Aspects of Surgery for Recipients of Right Lobes from Living Donors. Although the general scheme of surgery for recipients of right lobes from living donors is very similar to that of recipients of whole livers from deceased donors, the operation is technically challenging and requires considerable surgical expertise. In most cases the bile ducts from the right lobe grafts are sewed into a loop of small intestine (roux-en-Y), and not directly sewed to the recipient's bile ducts (Figure 10C). Also, because the right hepatic artery and right portal vein are shorter than the main portal vein available in whole liver grafts, a greater length of recipient hepatic artery and portal vein or vascular grafts are required.

How Long Am I in the Hospital?

The Hospital Stay. After the operation you may be monitored in an intensive care unit (ICU), especially if you had complex medical problems, or complicated surgery. In contrast, you may have had an uncomplicated surgery and few medical concerns, in which case you might bypass the ICU and transfer from recovery room directly to the transplant inpatient floor. If you are transferred to the ICU and have no complications, you'll spend 24 to 48 hours in the ICU and then transfer to the inpatient transplant unit.

In intensive care I was in la-la land from the prednisone IV. For two days I thought I was in an alien spaceship. Other patients were in the ship, and that's how they were making us well. My vision was foggy. Everything sounded as if it came from a long metal tube, echoing, distorted. But I was happy, fine with that.

When I went to a regular room, I was still foggy and doped up. It was uncomfortable, not painful. I was cranky, though—had some major mood swings. After four days, they got me moving again. On my first walk, the IV stand got away from me, and I almost fell on my face. Then

I progressed to day passes—went out for a few hours and came back. I was there two and a half weeks.

Harry

My legs were like tree trunks, they were so swollen with fluid. You couldn't tell I had five toes; it looked like one big toe. A week after the surgery, I had lost 60 pounds. The doctors would come in and tickle my toes, just for fun.

Janet

Usually, patients stay in the hospital from five to 20 days depending on their condition. The average length of initial hospital stay is about 11 to 12 days. Some people require extensive rehabilitation, such as physical therapy or nursing, due to their weakened situation before or after the transplant.

After discharge you'll be monitored in transplant outpatient clinics for a few weeks to a few months, and then you'll return to the care of your referring primary care physician or gastroenterologist. The transplant center continues to guide patient management through close cooperation with referring physicians.

Living with a New Liver

Although recovery is highly variable from patient to patient, most people require from three to six months to physically recover from surgery and adjust to new medications. An inspiration to transplant recipients, Chris Klug, a 28-year-old American snowboarder, took the gold in the World Cup parallel giant slalom on January 17, 2001—less than nine months after his liver transplant for primary sclerosing cholangitis! Almost unbelievably, Chris later accomplished a seemingly impossible feat, the bronze medal in snowboarding at the Winter Olympics in Salt Lake City, Utah in 2002. Chris has never forgotten what organ donation meant to him and his success. He founded the Chris Klug Foundation for Organ Donation and travels throughout the United States to support donors and donor families.

Liver transplantation is a profound event that affects every part of a patient's life—the mind as well as the body. Patients must learn to live with lifelong medications, deal with the fear of rejection of the organ, and come to terms with a profound physical and psychological transformation.

Medications to Prevent Rejection. After the transplant, you need to take medications for the rest of your life to prevent your immune system from rejecting your new liver. The medications are called immunosuppressants and include the following: cyclosporine (Sandimmune®, Neoral®, Gengraf®), tacrolimus (Prograf®), sirolimus (Rapamune®), everolimus (Certican®), azathioprine (Imuran®), steroids (Prednisone®, Solumedrol®), and mycophenolate mofetil (Cellcept®, Myfortic®).

Most patients take either cyclosporine or tacrolimus as primary therapy, and use the other agents to strengthen the anti-rejection effect. In the first six to 12 months it's common to take two or three anti-rejection medications. After that period most patients remain on cyclosporine or tacrolimus either alone or in combination with azathioprine, mycophenolate mofetil, sirolimus, everolimus, or steroids.

> So many pills! I had eight of one kind. Taking my medication was like eating a snack. When I went to the pharmacy to pick up my first prescription, they gave it to me in a shopping bag—and then another little bag.
>
> The bill was $1,668 the first month. Ten months later, it's down to about $300.
>
> *Al*

Although the medications have side effects, most of them are dose-related and respond to either lowering the dose of the specific immunosuppressant or changing to another medication.

Never change doses by yourself. All dose adjustments of immunosuppressants require the supervision of your doctor. If you take too little immunosuppression, you run the risk of rejecting your liver transplant. If you take too much immunosuppression, you risk infection, renal (kidney) failure, hypertension, hyperlipidemia (excess blood cholesterol and fat), and diabetes mellitus.

Managing Complications

It's essential that your transplant team supervise you closely during your post-transplant outpatient care. The most serious problems are rejection and recurrence of hepatitis C.

Rejection. If rejection occurs, it typically does so within the first six months of the transplant and is indicated by a rise in liver enzymes. Elevations of liver enzymes and bilirubin occur, although the first change noted is usually an increase in AST. In some cases, rejection is very mild and does not require additional immunosuppressive treatment. If you experience more severe rejection, you might note fever (up to 102°F), poor appetite, fatigue, and malaise.

> *When my wife had a transplant, I was more scared than she was. I still have fear. If she gets sick, even a common cold or the flu, I still get scared. This is our second chance; there has to be a reason.*
>
> *Roger*

Nearly all rejections occur within six months of transplantation, but occasionally rejection happens later. "Late rejection" usually results from low levels of immunosuppressive therapy due to improper dosing, addition of a new medication, or development of a simultaneous illness such as diarrhea or liver dysfunction. Rejection usually responds to intravenous steroids or other strategies (intravenous antibody treatments such as OKT3®, or Thymoglobulin®).

Recurrent episodes of hepatitis C in post-transplant cases are often mistaken for rejection. Recurrent hepatitis C must be carefully considered before one embarks on a course to treat rejection.

Recurrence of Hepatitis C. How do patients with hepatitis C fare after liver transplantation? Many, perhaps the majority, do extremely well with little evidence of significant damage over years of follow-up. However, analysis of the five-year survival after liver transplant suggests that graft and patient survival is lower even as early as one year post-transplant compared to the survival of patients transplanted for other reasons (Figure 10D). Some patients have aggressive recurrence of hepatitis C and may progress rapidly to significant fibrosis or even cirrhosis. Current estimates indicate that 10 to 25 percent of patients will develop cirrhosis in the liver graft due to recurrence of hepatitis C within three to five years of the transplant. For this reason, most transplant hepatologists have advocated aggressive antiviral therapy for hepatitis C in either the pre- or post-transplant setting in liver transplant candidates or recipients.

If you have active hepatitis C with positive HCV RNA in your blood prior to liver transplantation, you should expect hepatitis C to

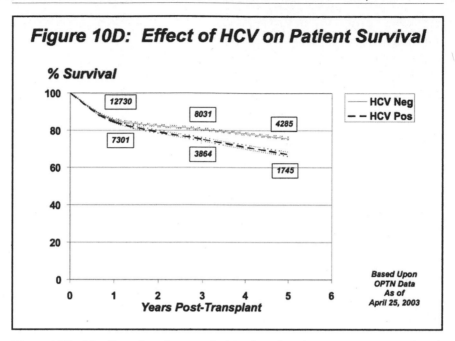

Figure 10D: Effect of HCV on Patient Survival

Figure 10D: Unadjusted patient survival is plotted against years post-transplantation and is based on data from the OPTN at www.unos.org. The solid line depicts survival for patients without hepatitis C and the dashed line depicts the survival for patients with hepatitis C. The dotted lines around the solid and dashed lines are the 95% confidence limits for each plot. Patient survival is lower for patients transplanted for chronic hepatitis C after one year post-transplant, compared to patients transplanted for other reasons. Two causes of the dropoff in survival in patients transplanted for chronic hepatitis C are recurrent disease and rapid progression to cirrhosis and liver failure and recurrence of hepatoma.

infect your liver graft. We don't yet know how to prevent reinfection of your liver graft. In contrast to hepatitis B, where immunoglobulin (HBIG) and antiviral treatments (lamivudine, adefovir, entecavir) are effective, HCV-specific immunoglobulin has not been effective and there are no available antivirals (see chapter 14, "Research Trends" and chapter 15, "Advances in Treatment").

We, in Colorado, have used pre-transplant treatment with a low-dose regimen of interferon and ribavirin (LADR) and have been able to prevent recurrence of HCV infection and graft hepatitis in some patients. However, treatment with interferon and ribavirin is often not practical because pre-transplant patients are typically quite ill, have low white blood cell counts, low platelets, and a liver that's in poor condition. Most patients with MELD score 18 or less might be candidates as their disease and overall condition is less severe. Carefully selected patients with MELD from 18 to 25 might also be candidates. However, this treatment has to be monitored very carefully and should only be administered through liver centers or by physicians with extensive experience in the treatment of hepatitis C and patients with advanced liver disease. In our experience, complications attributed or associated with treatment were more likely in patients with more advanced disease. There is currently an ongoing NIH-sponsored clinical trial of pre-transplant peginterferon/ribavirin, conducted by the Adult-to-Adult Living Donor Liver Transplantation study. Results will be presented at AASLD, November 2009.

Although pre-emptive treatment, prior to development of hepatitis C in the liver graft, has been used it is not widely accepted or practiced. Most transplant hepatologists currently initiate antiviral treatment only in patients with documented recurrent hepatitis C. Recurrence is defined by positive HCV RNA, elevated ALT, and chronic active hepatitis C on liver biopsy. When hepatitis C recurs, you usually don't have symptoms and doctors detect it as an increase in blood levels of liver enzymes as early as one week after the transplant. Recurrent hepatitis C is often confused with rejection since the histologic features of rejection and hepatitis C on liver biopsies overlap considerably. Often, transplant hepatologists treat selected patients based upon clinical impression and experience.

Post-transplant treatment is very similar to regimens of antiviral therapy for chronic hepatitis C used in nontransplant populations. The preferred regimen is peginterferon plus ribavirin but some unique features of therapy of transplant recipients deserve mention.

First, immunosuppressive medications, especially cyclosporine and tacrolimus, lower your kidney function. Ribavirin, one of the key hepatitis C drugs, is cleared through the kidney. For this reason, liver recipients on cyclosporine or tacrolimus experience greater toxicity from ribavirin when used in standard doses. This toxicity includes anemia, rashes, mouth sores, sore throat, and cough. As a consequence most liver recipients can only tolerate a low dose of ribavirin, which may compromise their chance to respond and be cleared of hepatitis C with treatment.

Second, liver recipients may be more susceptible to low cell counts and infections associated with interferon-based treatment. Many centers initiate therapy with low doses of peginterferon and ribavirin and increase doses as tolerate (similar to LADR regimen used in patients with advanced liver disease).In the author's experience, the liver recipient with hepatitis C treated with interferon and ribavirin also seems more resistant to use of growth factors (erythropoeitin or G-CSF) to stimulate the bone marrow to raise the low cell counts. Also, immunosuppressive medications increase the risk that a liver recipient will experience infection and addition of interferon may further increase this risk.

Third, interferon treatment may increase the risk of rejection. In liver recipients, most patients tolerate interferon well and there is no apparent risk of rejection related to interferon per se. However, we have observed severe rejection in a few liver recipients who cleared HCV RNA from their blood. This means that liver recipients on interferon therapy must be monitored very carefully, especially during a period of viral clearance and that immunosuppressive medications may need to be modified to insure adequant immunosuppressive drug levels.

Psychological Transformation. Post-transplant patients go through a period of accepting the "gift of life." The feelings are common to everyone and include curiosity about the donor, feelings of guilt that someone had to die so they could live, and a sense of indebtedness—of feeling overwhelmed and struggling with how to repay an enormous gift.

Michael Talamantes, transplant social worker at the University of Colorado Health Sciences Center, says that patients often write a letter of thanks to the donor's family. The donor's identity is kept confidential, so the letter is sent through official channels. If the donor's family members wish to reply, they will. And if not, it's important to respect their privacy.

Feelings of guilt over the donor's death take time to work through. Although it seems obvious that the donor's death is independent of your need for a liver, the feelings are almost universal.

> *I'm small, so I got a liver from a young boy. It blew my mind. What happened to that young man that he passed away? He was only 16 years old, still a baby. It makes me feel bad because I've been through it all.*

At first I got depressed. Then I thought maybe that's why I'm doing so well—because I've got a young, healthy liver. Finally, I said, the Lord must have wanted it this way. When I get better, I'll write to his parents …

Tomas

The sense of indebtedness is often overwhelming. Some people do community service or visit patients in the hospital who are awaiting transplants. Every patient is touched in some way.

When I got the call for my liver, my heart went down to my toes. I was really scared. I went into the hospital restroom and confessed all my sins, restored my soul.

Afterwards, when I recovered, I thought how beautiful the trees looked and how beautiful even the weeds looked. I went back to that restroom and thanked the Lord.

Tomas

As in every new experience, you may have contradictory feelings. It's important to pay attention to them.

Everyone talks about the "gift of life." I don't feel that way. To me, $300,000 doesn't qualify as a gift!

Sonya

It's a gift. It's unfortunate that the donor had to die, but I'm not the cause of it. Before I knew I would need a transplant, I put on my license I was a donor. I made the same decision, and I honor my donor's decision.

Sandy

Whatever normal, contradictory feelings you have, you need to sort through them to adjust to your new sense of yourself. To complicate matters, you may get mixed messages from others. Are you a hero, a biotechnological miracle, or does your boss see you as damaged goods, a drain on the company's health insurance? Whatever your experiences, they are profound indeed. You are not alone in wrestling with these issues.

People who haven't had a transplant don't understand. All they see is machinery and medicines. It's really important to talk. If someone calls me, it cheers me up to just listen, to say I was there. It can't get any bet-ter than that—to talk to someone who's been there, done that.

Evie

What Are My Chances? Outcomes.

The success of transplantation has increased steadily over the last two decades. In the United States prior to 1979, results were poor, with one-year patient survival of 32 percent. In Europe prior to 1985, the one-year patient survival was only 34 percent. But, current one-year survival exceeds 85 percent in the United States and 83 percent in Europe. These statistics reflect the average results in all centers in the United States and Europe; individual transplant centers have achieved one-year patient survivals approaching 95 percent (see Center-Specific data at www.us transplant.org). In addition, long-term results are steadily improving. In the United States, current one- and three-year patient survival rates are 88 percent and 78 percent, for deceased donor transplantation and 90 percent and 83 percent for living donor liver transplantation, respectively (Figure 10E). As noted above, the survival of patients transplanted for chronic hepatitis C is slightly worse than the survival of patients trans-planted for other indications. However, patient survival is still excellent and will undoubtedly improve as more effective antiviral therapies for hepatitis C are developed over the next several years.

The reality is, however, that not all patients survive. Deaths occurring within the first six months are due to nonfunction of the donor's liver, clotting of the main artery to the liver, infection, multi-organ failure, or rejection. When deaths occur later, more than one year after the transplant, they are more commonly due to malignancy or complications of athero-sclerosis and less often due to rejection or infection. A major concern in the long-term outcome after liver transplantation is the development of kidney disease from immunosuppressive therapies and chronic hepatitis C. Liver recipients, having weathered all the medical and surgical issues surrounding liver transplantation, may yet face another challenge, the prospect of chronic dialysis or kidney transplantation.

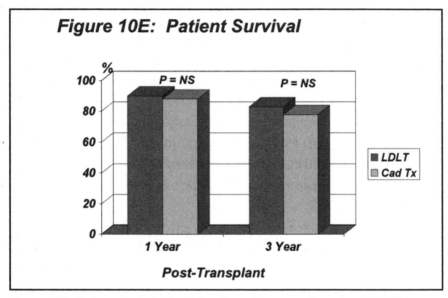

Figure 10E: Patient survival after living donor liver transplantation (LDLT) is compared to patient survival after deceased donor liver transplantation (Cad Tx). There were no differences in survival of patients undergoing LDLT compared to patients undergoing Cad Tx at 1, 3, and 5 years post-transplantation.

Despite these complexities, the outlook for transplant recipients is very hopeful. We anticipate that future immunosuppressive protocols will reduce adverse metabolic effects and continue to improve the long-term outlook for transplant recipients. New drugs and strategies may increase the chance that the goal of tolerance to the liver graft, allowing removal of all immunosuppressive medications, may be achieved. Advances in immunosuppression and new drugs to control or eliminate HCV may reduce or eliminate many of the late metabolic complications, including kidney failure. Our ultimate goal, of course, is to restore you to your normal health and life.

How Organs Are Allocated

UNOS and UNOS Regions. In the United States, the United Network for Organ-Sharing (UNOS) regulates the distribution or allocation of donor organs. Here's how it works.

The United States is divided into 11 regions for organ procurement and allocation. Several local organ procurement organizations (OPOs) exist within each region. When a patient is approved for transplantation, he or she is placed on local, regional, and national waiting lists. Typically, more than 80 percent of recipients receive organs from local donors.

MELD Score. In the United States, since February, 2002, prioritization has been based primarily on MELD score which is calculated from bilirubin, INR, and creatinine (see chapter 4 for discussion of these laboratory tests). UNOS status 1, the most urgent priority, was retained in the current system for patients with fulminant hepatic failure. In Europe, the system of prioritization of recipients and allocation of donor organs has varied widely between countries. The Eurotransplant network implemented MELD at least in some countries in 2006.

Prior to the introduction of MELD score in February 2002, the UNOS system of status 1, 2A, 2B, and 3 was used in the United States. UNOS status relied heavily on Child-Turcotte-Pugh (CTP) score to grade severity of illness and determine priority. But, two components of the CTP score, encephalopathy and ascites, were not readily verifiable. Furthermore, within these medical urgency categories, waiting patients were given priority for transplant based upon time on the UNOS list. Subsequent studies had shown that waiting time did not correlate with death on the waiting list.

The MELD score is superior to the old UNOS status system because it lacks subjectivity and eliminates waiting time as a major determinant of prioritization for liver transplantation. MELD score is highly predictive of three-month mortality in cirrhotics; mortality rate is 10 percent to 60 percent over the range of MELD scores of 20 to 35 and more than 80 percent for MELD scores over 35. After its first year of implementation, the allocation system based on MELD has been associated with reduced registrations and improved transplantation rates, and has not altered waiting list or post-transplant mortality. As noted in previous discussion, MELD 12 is the threshhold for listing patients with hepatitis C, because that is the MELD score where survival with transplantation exceeds survival without transplantation. If you have cirrhosis and are interested in calculating your own MELD score, visit http://www.unos. org/resources/MeldPeldCalculator.asp.

PELD Score. The Pediatric End-stage Liver Disease (PELD) score is a similar model developed for the allocation of liver transplants in the pediatric population. The variables included in this model are age younger than one year, serum albumin level, serum bilirubin, INR and growth failure (<2 SD below the age-based mean) (Table 2). Similar to MELD score, PELD accurately predicts the three-month probability of waiting list death for children with chronic liver disease.

Center-Specific Results

Statistics regarding performance of liver transplantation in the United States are displayed on the website of the Scientific Registry of Transplant Recipients at www.ustransplant.org. Overall results for the United States as a whole and individual center statistics are available. If you are considering transplantation at a given center you can check on their overall activity and results at this website. The statistics are periodically updated, with the most recent analyses completed for transplants up to December 2005. Patient and graft survivals for one- and three-year outcomes are given in combined totals and for each individual center. Results are also adjusted for differences in patient populations according to variables known to influence outcome after liver transplantation: UNOS listing status, diagnosis of fulminant hepatic failure, age, renal failure, presence of hepatitis B, and presence of primary liver cancer. Using this stratification method, results from each center can be compared to the expected outcome. Centers of excellence could be defined as those centers whose actual outcomes for patient and graft survival exceed the expected outcomes.

Many people have suggested that the current number of 126 transplant programs is far in excess of what the donor organ pool can provide. More than half the programs in the United States perform fewer than 20 liver transplants per year; 75 percent of all liver transplants are performed by only 25 percent of the programs.

A recent study examined the impact of transplant program activity on recipient outcome and found that transplant teams that perform more than 20 transplants per year achieved optimal patient and graft survival. According to this analysis, the chance to die after liver transplantation was almost twice as great when the transplant was done by a program performing fewer than 20 transplants per year. Because more than half the programs in the United States perform fewer than 20 transplants a year, one must question the wisdom of encouraging the proliferation of transplant centers.

Some states have invoked the concept of "certification of need" to ensure a balance between the regional need for transplantation and the number of transplant centers. Further increases in the number of transplant centers should be discouraged unless dictated by regional need.

Resource: Call the toll-free UNOS patient information hotline at 1-888-TXINFO1 (888-894-6361); website: www.unos.org.

Resource: Regional organ recovery organizations are a good source of information. To locate your region's organization, call the UNOS patient information number listed above.

Resource: For information on national organizations and local coalitions that educate the public about organ donation, call the Coalition on Donation: 804-782-4920; email: coalition@donatelife.net; website: www.shareyourlife.org. You may also request a free brochure on organ donation from the coalition by calling 800-355-SHARE.

Resource: For information about transplants and organ donation, call a nationwide support group for transplant patients and their families, Transplant Recipients International Organization (TRIO): 800-TRIO-386.

Resource: A uniform donor card is enclosed in this book. Discuss organ and tissue donation with family members. After completing and signing the Uniform Donor Card, be sure to have your signature witnessed by two people.

> *To every thing there is a season, and a time to every purpose under the heaven...*
>
> *A time to weep, and a time to laugh; a time to mourn, and a time to dance...*
>
> *Ecclesiastes*

11

LIVER CANCER
Are You at Risk?

Just the word "cancer" scares me. I thought I'd die. I have four kids, and I was just terrified.

Six years after I was diagnosed with hepatitis C, I weighed 89 pounds. I had no appetite. My liver enzymes went sky high. The doctors sent me for a CT scan and found liver cancer. Thank God they put me on the transplant waiting list because it gave me hope.

After ten months I got my new liver. My weight's back; I'm 120 pounds. The cancer blood tests are good. "How's the hepatitis C?" I ask my nurse. "Very quiet," she says.

See this bulge here? My new liver is too large for me. But I just wear big shirts—and I'm still alive!

Carolyn

MOST OF MY PATIENTS DON'T realize that hepatitis C can cause liver cancer (hepatoma). But before you panic or worry unnecessarily, consider the following:

1. Only a minority of patients with hepatitis C will ever develop liver cancer.
2. Effective therapies exist for tumors detected early.

3. Liver cancer is almost entirely restricted to those with advanced liver disease who have extensive fibrosis (stage III) or cirrhosis.

Of course, you're wondering if *you* are in danger. This chapter provides you with information regarding risk factors, warning signs, screening and diagnostic tests for liver cancer, and results of current treatment. Here are the topics I'll cover:

- Overview: What Is Liver Cancer?
  Primary Liver Cancer (Hepatoma)
  Secondary Liver Cancer
  Is Primary Liver Cancer on the Rise?
- Common Risk Factors
  Stage of Hepatitis C
  Duration of Infection
  Other Liver Diseases
  Viral Genotype, Viral RNA Level, Quasispecies
- Interferon: Does It Reduce the Risk of Primary Liver Cancer?
- Warning Signs
  No Symptoms but with Underlying Cirrhosis
  Deterioration in Liver Function
  Pain
  Sudden Development of Portal Hypertension
  Other Symptoms
- Testing
  Early Screening Guidelines
        Blood Tests (Serial Measurement of Alpha-fetoprotein)
        Radiologic Imaging
  Diagnostic Tests
- Treatment
  Cancer Staging
        Early Stage
        Advanced Stage
        Metastic Liver Cancer
  Hepatic Resection
  Transplantation
  Chemoembolization
  High-Frequency Radio Waves (Radiofrequency Tumor Ablation)
  Alcohol Injection, Cryosurgery
  Chemotherapy
- Summary

Overview: What Is Liver Cancer?

Primary Liver Cancer (Hepatoma). Primary liver cancer, also known as hepatoma or hepatocellular carcinoma, is a malignant tumor that originates within the liver. Nearly all hepatomas originate from cells composed of the main tissue of the liver (hepatocytes), rather than from cells of the biliary tract, fibrous tissue, blood vessels, or fat.

Secondary Liver Cancer. In the United States, primary liver cancer is relatively rare. Most cancers migrate to the liver, are called secondary cancers, and have their primary site in other organs of the body, such as the colon, breast, or lung. Secondary liver cancers frequently appear as multiple liver masses, while primary liver cancers commonly appear as a solitary mass.

Physicians distinguish secondary from primary liver cancers by imaging the liver (ultrasonography, CT, MRT) and biopsing the tissue. The finding of secondary liver cancer means that tumor cells have traveled far from their primary site, typically indicating a poor chance of survival. Liver transplantation is not indicated for secondary liver cancers.

Is Primary Liver Cancer on the Rise? In the past, primary liver cancers were so rare that doctors often selected these cases for presentation at medical Grand Rounds lectures. Today, we diagnose primary liver cancer with increasing frequency, especially in patients with chronic hepatitis C. The Centers for Disease Control and Prevention report that the incidence of hepatoma increased from 1.4 to 2.4 per 100,000 people between 1979 and 1995. More recent statistics continue to demonstrate an increase in the incidence of hepatoma—in fact, liver cancer is currently the cancer with the greatest increase in mortality rate in the United States. Hepatitis C is the underlying cause of liver disease in the majority of the increased numbers of cases of liver cancer.

Common Risk Factors

Stage of Hepatitis C. The most important predictor of liver cancer is the condition of the liver tissue (histologic stage). Noncirrhotic patients with low fibrosis scores (fibrosis stages 0 to 2) have a low risk (less than 0.1%/yr). In contrast, patients with extensive fibrosis (stage 3) run an intermediate risk (0.8%/yr), and those with cirrhosis are at greatest risk (>1.4%/yr). In the HALT-C Trial, patients with compensated cirrhosis had an annual risk of developing hepatoma of 1.4%. Studies of patients with decompensated cirrhosis, like patients on waiting lists for liver transplantation have a much higher annual risk, >4%/yr.

Various studies have yielded similar results. In five other studies, the risk of developing liver cancer in patients with established cirrhosis ranged from 1.2 percent per year to 9.5 percent per year. Patients with early compensated cirrhosis, like those enrolled in HALT-C, had the lowest risk, ~1%/yr, but those with advanced cirrhosis had a much higher risk, ranging from 5 to 10 percent per year.

Patients without significant fibrosis are at low risk for hepatoma and do not require screening. In contrast, patients with advanced fibrosis or cirrhosis run a considerable lifetime risk of developing hepatoma and should undergo screening—current screening is with a minimum of alpha-fetoprotein every 6 months and radiologic imaging of the liver, usually by ultrasonography, every 6 to 12 months.

One clinical note: the development of liver cancer may present as sudden deterioration in an otherwise stable compensated patient with cirrhosis. Patients who suddenly deteriorate (see Chapter 4) should undergo diagnostic studies to rule out liver cancer.

Duration of Infection. Most data suggest that the median time period for developing hepatoma is approximately 30 years from the date of infection and 10 years after the onset of cirrhosis. If you don't have cirrhosis but have had hepatitis C for 30 years, you may still be at risk for liver cancer—screening for liver cancer may be warranted and you should discuss this with your physician. However, this issue has not been adequately studied and the exact risk is unknown.

Other Liver Diseases. Any liver disease that hastens the development of cirrhosis may also increase the likelihood of developing hepatoma. The three most common concurrent hepatic diseases in hepatitis C patients that accelerate disease progression are chronic alcohol use, hepatitis B, and genetic hemochromatosis.

Multiple studies have now conclusively demonstrated that patients with hepatitis C who drink alcohol add fuel to the hepatitis C fire. Chronic daily consumption of alcohol is associated with acceleration to cirrhosis, increased risk for liver failure, increased risk for needing liver transplantation, and increased risk for development of liver cancer. Similar risks have been observed in patients with hepatitis C who are co-infected with hepatitis B. In addition, hemochromatosis, the most common genetic liver disease, causes excessive accumulation of iron in the liver, which also accelerates liver disease due to hepatitis C and, therefore, potentially increases the risk of liver cancer.

Viral Genotype, Viral RNA Level, Quasispecies. Genotype 1b has been associated with longer duration of disease, more aggressive disease activity, increased likelihood for progression to cirrhosis, and increased need for liver transplantation. Therefore, it's not surprising that this genotype has also been linked to hepatoma, though it is not known whether genotype 1b is an independent predictor of liver cancer. Levels of HCV RNA in the blood and the diversity of the hepatitis C virus RNAs (quasispecies) have not been proven to correlate with the risk of developing hepatoma.

Interferon Does Not Reduce the Risk of Primary Liver Cancer

It is well-established that clearing HCV with antiviral therapy reduces the future risk of liver cancer—risk of cancer is not eliminated, but dramatically reduced.

Past studies suggested that interferon or peginterferon therapy could reduce risk of liver cancer. However, the studies were retrospective and uncontrolled.

In the HALT-C Trial, over 1000 patients were randomized to either peginterferon alfa-2a, 90 μg/wk, for 3.5 years, or no treatment, and followed for more than 5 years. The incidence of liver cancer was compared between patients who were treated and those who were not treated—the incidence of liver cancer was identical. In HALT-C, a carefully controlled, randomized prospective trial, maintenance with peginterferon mono-therapy had no impact on incidence of liver cancer.

Warning Signs of Liver Cancer

No Symptoms but with Underlying Cirrhosis. Many patients develop hepatoma without any changes in symptoms or obvious progression of their disease. That's why I recommend screening tests, such as alpha-fetoprotein and ultrasonography for all patients with bridging fibrosis (stage III) or cirrhosis. Detection of early stage hepatoma with screening tests may result in more effective treatment and better outcomes.

Deterioration in Liver Function. A stable cirrhotic patient may be fully employed, have normal levels of energy, conduct normal social activities, and have stable liver tests. When such a patient develops hepatoma, liver function may deteriorate for no other apparent reason. Signs of deterioration are increasing fatigue, mental confusion (encephalopathy), fluid retention (ascites, edema), or gastrointestinal bleeding. Alternatively, the patient's liver tests may suddenly deteriorate with rising bilirubin, diminishing clotting factors, increase in liver enzymes, and drop in serum albumin. Some patients experience only a loss of appetite, fever, and unexplained weight loss.

In March my husband was starting to feel tired. A checkup showed his blood work was fine, and the liver scan came back great.

In mid-April he ran twice around the track and was exhausted. He said he hurt his back and took muscle relaxers. A week later, he vomited blood all over the bathroom floor. He told me it was just juice mixed with the medicine—but I saw blood clots.

At the hospital they found out his stomach was bleeding. A CT scan showed liver cancer. Since his first test, the thing had grown to over 20 centimeters. They couldn't operate on the cancer because it was the size of his liver.

"No go," said the doctor. "It's too big."

Claudine

Pain. A tumor can grow rapidly, causing the liver capsule to expand, and tumor cells can invade adjacent nerve roots, blood vessels, and lymphatics. As the hepatoma enlarges and impinges on adjacent structures, it can create significant pain and discomfort. Development of persistent moderate to severe pain in the right upper quadrant of the abdomen in a patient with cirrhosis may point to the diagnosis of hepatoma.

Sudden Development of Portal Hypertension. Hepatoma is a vascular tumor and often invades vascular structures, such as blood or fluid-bearing vessels or ducts. If the tumor enters the portal vein, it may plug the vessel or cause blood clotting that blocks the vein. An acute rise in portal pressure related to this blockage may result in an upper gastrointestinal bleed (variceal hemorrhage), swelling of the abdomen (ascites) or ankles, worsening of existing ascites, development of diuretic-resistant ascites, mental confusion (encephalopathy), or worsening of existing encephalopathy.

My husband's final request was to see the ocean one more time. He wanted to say goodbye to his sisters in California. The night before our flight, I heard him yell. Vomiting blood, he collapsed at the bottom of the stairs.

At the hospital I freaked out, and I was crying, crying. The pain was like a monster in his stomach. "No, no," he said, "I want to go see my sisters!" That whole last week he talked about God. He knew he'd be with the Lord when he died.

His sisters flew in. He was still awake and able to recognize them. The next morning he got very confused. He died that night.

Annie

Other Symptoms. Patients may attribute certain nonspecific symptoms (fatigue, loss of appetite, poor energy) to their ongoing hepatitis C when the symptoms may be related to emergence of hepatoma. These patients often delay notifying their physicians for several months. Such a delay may convert a potentially treatable tumor to one that has spread beyond the confines of the liver and may no longer be treatable.

Testing

Early Screening Guidelines. Doctors have not yet established guidelines for screening for hepatoma in patients with hepatitis C. However, recent clinical trials have indicated that screening with both alpha-fetoprotein and ultrasonography detects early tumors and results in improved patient survival. Nonetheless, many of my comments on screening come from my own experience and represent my bias regarding the most cost-effective and sensitive approach to this problem.

Again, I want to emphasize that most patients with hepatitis C will not develop primary liver cancer. Noncirrhotic patients appear to be at an exceedingly low risk, and only those with advanced fibrosis or cirrhosis who have had the disease for more than 20 years are at excess risk. Therefore, all comments regarding screening apply only to patients with bridging fibrosis (stage III) or cirrhosis.

The two screening tests doctors use to detect liver cancer are (1) blood tests (serial measurement of alpha-fetoprotein, AFP-L3, DCP) and (2) radiologic imaging.

1. Blood Tests (Serial Measurement of Alpha-fetoprotein). Hepatoma cells synthesize a protein called alpha-fetoprotein and release the protein into the bloodstream. A very high alpha-fetoprotein [>500 nanograms (ng) per milliliter (ml)] or a sustained rise in alpha-fetoprotein on serial measurements (with the last value > 150 ng/ml) may predict the development of hepatoma. A subtype of alpha-fetoprotein (L3) may be more specific for cancer. Other blood tests, such as AFP-L3 or DCP, are under investigation.

The accuracy of alpha-fetoprotein, used alone, in predicting hepatoma is poor. Therefore, doctors may order supplemental radiologic tests, biopsies, or even a surgical incision (laparotomy). In addition, 20 to 50 percent of the hepatomas that occur in patients with hepatitis C may lack the ability to produce alpha-fetoprotein. In such cases, the tumors progress undetected by the serial alpha-fetoprotein measurements. Radiologic imaging of the liver is required to screen for these tumors.

2. **Radiologic Imaging.** Although CT scans and magnetic resonance imaging (MRI) with enhancing agents may be slightly more sensitive than ultrasonography, they are prohibitively expensive for use in screening. Ultrasonography, on the other hand, which can detect the majority of early hepatomas, is much less costly and is the radiologic screening choice.

I currently advise my cirrhotic patients and those with extensive fibrosis to have alpha-fetoprotein measurements and ultrasonography, alternating with CT or MRI, of the liver every six months.

Diagnostic Tests. If screening tests detect a lesion that might be cancerous, doctors may biopsy the mass with the guidance of ultrasonography or CT. Other imaging studies (CT, MRI, or angiography) can detect early hepatoma in the patient with rising alpha-fetoprotein or worsening of symptoms when ultrasonography fails to reveal a definite lesion. The type of imaging study is ordered at your physician's discretion.

Treatment

Cancer Staging. In order to select proper treatment, the physician must determine the stage of the hepatoma. This is usually done with radiologic imaging, laparoscopy, or abdominal exploratory surgery.

1. **Early Stage (T1 or T2).** Patients with a solitary tumor less than five centimeters in diameter or patients with up to three tumors, all less than three centimeters in diameter, may be candidates for surgery to remove the tumor (hepatic resection) or liver transplantation. Recurrence of the tumor is common if resection is performed. Cure and excellent long-term survival are the rule with liver transplantation.

2. **Advanced Stage (T3, T4, Metastases).** More advanced stages of hepatoma usually represent multiple tumor nodules involving one or both liver lobes. The tumor may have invaded the main liver vessels. Advanced stage tumors have a poorer prognosis, and typically doctors do not advise resection or transplantation.

   Most patients cannot undergo resection due to the extensive nature of the disease and the risk of precipitating liver failure because of underlying cirrhosis. Only a small subgroup is considered for transplantation. However, the outcome after liver transplantation is poor for patients with advanced stage hepatomas because of recurrence of cancer. Patients with advanced stage cancer are considered for palliative treatment with either chemoembolization, cryosurgery, or radiofrequency thermal ablation. A new drug, sorafenib, has recently been FDA approved for treatment of advanced hepatoma—it slows tumor growth and prolongs survival by several months.

3. **Metastatic Liver Cancer.** Patients with widespread tumor that has metastasized (spread) beyond the confines of the liver are not candidates for surgery, transplantation, cryotherapy, or chemoembolization. They are evaluated only for standard chemotherapy.

   Hepatic Resection. Surgeons achieve the best results in the treatment of hepatoma when they perform a liver resection to surgically remove a solitary tumor (less than five centimeters) in a patient with a noncirrhotic liver. These patients may be cured of their cancer and usually enjoy long-term survival.

   However, this represents an uncommon clinical scenario when it comes to hepatoma in patients with hepatitis C. As I have already mentioned, the patient with hepatitis C who develops a liver cancer usually has cirrhosis and a disease duration of hepatitis C for greater than 30 years.

   My wife was prepped for surgery. First, the doctors did a biopsy. "The other side of her liver is all cirrhosed," they told me. "You have 30 days before she gets real sick." They said to wind up her affairs—wills and such—and see to our family.

   When we got home, she only had energy to go to the post office and the bank. And that was it for the day.

   Owen

Unfortunately, cirrhosis precludes a successful resection because resections for hepatoma usually require removing 25 to 75 percent of the liver tissue. A normal liver can tolerate a massive resection since regeneration is rapid (usually within 12 weeks) and the remaining liver cells are functioning normally. That's not the case when a person has cirrhosis and hepatitis C. The remaining liver cannot effectively regenerate, and its function is severely impaired. When a surgeon performs a large resection on a cirrhotic patient, the operation may lead to liver failure. For these reasons liver resections are usually restricted to patients without cirrhosis or to those cirrhotic patients who have no evidence of clinical or biochemical deterioration in liver function or portal hypertension.

Transplantation. Results from a number of centers agree: Cirrhotic patients with solitary liver cancers, small in size (less than five centimeters in diameter) or up to three tumors (all less than three centimeters in diameter), should be considered for transplantation.

Patients with advanced stages of hepatoma or metastatic disease almost uniformly experience early post-transplant recurrence of tumor and death from metastatic disease. Transplantation is not indicated for the latter patients.

Even for hepatomas in favorable stages, time can run out—tumors can increase in size and number, invade blood vessels, and metastasize. The U.S. waiting list for liver transplantation remains at approximately 15,000, but only about 6,000 liver transplants are performed annually. Under MELD, patients with hepatoma are given priority, 22 MELD points initially, and then 10% increases in MELD score every 3 months. Solitary tumors below 2 cm are not eligible for MELD upgrade—only patients with solitary tumors >2 cm or with multiple tumors, less than 3 in total, are eligible for MELD upgrade.

The average MELD score at the time of liver transplantation in the U.S. is currently (in the year 2009) around 26. The average doubling time of a liver cancer is between 3 and 6 months. If the tumor exceeds 5 cm in diameter, MELD upgrade is denied. So, if you have a 2 cm tumor that doubles every 6 months, you will likely get transplanted—initial MELD is 22, 3 months later MELD is 24, and after another 3 months MELD will have increased to 27. You have reached priority for transplant, and your tumor has only doubled from 2 to 4 cm—success! In contrast, if you have a 2 cm tumor that is more aggressive and doubles every 3 months, you may not get transplanted. Why? Your MELD increase would be the same, from 22 to 27 over 6 months; but, after 3 months the tumor has doubled to 4 cm, and over the next 3 months it doubled again, to 8 cm. Now, your tumor is too large and you are denied the MELD upgrade! The only option for transplant becomes living donor liver transplantation.

> *Four years ago, the doctor thought my liver was bruised from all the biopsies I had. He said it could be a hepatoma, but I didn't know that meant cancer. When the doctor told me the biopsy was positive, all the blood ran out of my face; my knees gave out. Three months later, I got my liver transplant.*
>
> *I remember hallucinating about dying when I was in the hospital. I saw the place where I go fishing—a nice, peaceful place with green grass and a stream running through. I wanted to lie down, go to sleep, give up.*
>
> *But I had just rebuilt my Harley-Davidson. In my fantasy I got on my cycle and rode it for two days down this highway with a white dotted line in the middle of the road. I heard the roar of the exhaust and smelled the pine trees.*
>
> *It was the turning point. I didn't quit fighting—and the cancer is gone. That dang Harley-Davidson saved my life. I feel like I won the lotto!*
>
> *Jack*

Chemoembolization. Chemoembolization is commonly used prior to liver transplantation to destroy at least part of the tumor and prevent growth. This procedure does not cure cancer. However, it can help destroy local tumors, reduce the tumor mass, provide significant relief, or in the case of a solitary tumor, keep the tumor from spreading outside the liver until a donor liver becomes available.

> *My family was 100 percent for the transplant, but my husband got so worried and scared for me, he lost 30 pounds. He was nothing but skin and bones.*
>
> *They put me in the hospital and gave me chemoembolization twice. I lost all my hair. It was scary, but I made it to my transplant. I have a lot of faith in God. That's what got me through—that and my family.*
>
> *Krista*

The technique, transarterial chemoembolization (TACE), involves placing a catheter through a vessel in the groin (the femoral artery) and advancing it into the liver's main artery (the hepatic artery). Then special types of chemotherapy or radioactive beads are infused through the catheter into the artery feeding the tumor. Because cancer cells retain the chemotherapy for a prolonged time, they are destroyed.

In the absence of resection or transplantation, chemoembolization is not curative, and the patient should understand that the tumor will probably recur. Nonetheless, chemoembolization of the tumor has been associated with prolonged survival and reduced symptoms of pain and weight loss. In transplant candidates, chemoembolization may sustain the patient until successful transplantation can take place.

High-Frequency Radio Waves (Radiofrequency Tumor Ablation). This treatment of hepatoma remains under study. The technique involves CT-guided puncture of the hepatoma and positioning the prongs of a special instrument within the tumor mass. High-frequency radio waves (near the microwave limit) generated within the tumor mass destroy the tumor. Overall effectiveness and clinical outcome of this treatment for hepatoma is similar to TACE.

Alcohol Injection, Cryosurgery. These two approaches are also limited to hepatomas that cannot be resected or transplanted. The goal of these treatments is to reduce tumor size and relieve painful symptoms.

Alcohol injection is done with the guidance of a CT scan to ensure proper placement of the treatment catheter within the tumor. Absolute alcohol dehydrates the tissues, causing the immediate death of cells, and starts a clotting process within the tumor that destroys it.

Cryosurgery involves the use of a flexible fiberoptic instrument (laparoscopy) with the guidance of an ultrasound probe to properly position the cryosurgical instrument within the tumor. When the probe is positioned, the tumor cells are destroyed by freezing.

Chemotherapy. Hepatoma is one of the most resistant tumors to both radiation and chemotherapy. Early experience with external beam radiation suggested that doses of radiation required for effective anti-tumor activity exceeded safety standards. In addition, clinical experience with radiation therapy of hepatomas was uniformly dismal and disappointing. For this reason, radiation is employed only rarely in the treatment of these tumors. Some evidence suggests that chemotherapy can be partially effective in reducing tumor burden and relieving symptoms.

As stated previously, new therapies such as sorafenib, targeting specific tumor pathways, have yielded better results but remain palliative.

Summary

Primary liver cancer is an extremely serious, life-threatening complication of chronic hepatitis C, but it occurs mainly in patients with advanced disease and cirrhosis. Hepatitis C patients with bridging fibrosis or cirrhosis should be aware of the danger of liver cancer, undergo screening by their physician, and know the warning signs.

Early hepatoma is treatable, but most patients with large tumors or multiple tumors cannot be treated by liver resection or transplantation. Cirrhotic patients with solitary and small hepatomas should be considered for early liver transplantation and possibly living-donor transplantation. A number of new approaches can reduce but not cure inoperable tumors: chemoembolization, radiofrequency thermal ablation, alcohol ablation, cryosurgery, and systemic chemotherapy.

Liver cancer is an increasingly important issue for hepatitis C patients, families, physicians, surgeons, transplant programs, and the health care system in general. We in the medical community know that we sorely need new ideas and new treatments.

The first wealth is health.

Emerson

12

Co-Infection with HIV/AIDS or Hepatitis B

Triple Trouble

In 1996 the doctors took me off AZT and put me on triple combination drug therapy. My T-cells went up, and my viral load went down. The nurse said they could probably keep me alive for a long time if I stayed off drugs and cocaine.

Meanwhile, two friends with AIDS killed themselves. The loneliness, deaths, and suicides were too much. Then I found out I had hepatitis C in August. I was tired all the time, so they tested me—and the tests came back reactive for hepatitis B and C.

I cried. I started reading about hepatitis C, and none of it looked good. Another virus. Now I have three viruses in my body.

Jay

THIS CHAPTER DISCUSSES two types of viral co-infections: HCV with either HIV or hepatitis B. If you are battling hepatitis C, it can be devastating to discover that you have another viral infection—HIV or hepatitis B. In the case of HIV co-infection it is more likely that you were first diagnosed with HIV, only to discover later, when liver tests became abnormal, that you were also infected with hepatitis C or hepatitis C plus hepatitis B. Co-infection is not uncommon due to the shared routes of transmission of HCV, HBV, and HIV.

You know from personal experience what it means to live with one dangerous virus, and now you have to face co-infection. Nothing can prepare you for the shock. Once again, you go through the cycle of fear, anger, and denial.

Until a few years ago, doctors did not focus on treating hepatitis C in patients with HIV infection because patients with HIV often had AIDS and limited years to live. Also, the only available treatment, interferon monotherapy, was only modestly effective in patients with HCV mono-infection, and it was not likely to be effective in HIV patients with AIDS who had severely impaired immune responses. Now, however, introduction of new highly active HIV drugs (HAART therapy) has produced a growing number of HIV-infected patients with strengthened immune systems who are enjoying longer life spans. At the same time, the treatment of hepatitis C was vastly improved by the introduction of combination therapy with ribavirin and development of pegylated interferons. With these hopeful and encouraging developments, treatment of hepatitis C in patients with HIV infection becomes a greater concern. The U.S. Public Health Service declared hepatitis an "official" opportunistic infection in patients with HIV.

When you have hepatitis C, co-infection with hepatitis B alters your prognosis and raises treatment issues. Patients co-infected with hepatitis B tend to have more aggressive liver disease with a greater likelihood of progression to cirrhosis and the need for a liver transplant. Also, the risk of cancer increases. When dealing with hepatitis B and C co-infection, your doctor must assess and determine which of many potential treatment strategies is most appropriate for you.

In this chapter, I will discuss the following topics:

- Overview of HIV Co-Infection
  What Is HIV/AIDS?
  Are You at Risk for Co-Infection?
  Testing Problems
  Population Trends
- Current Treatment of HIV Infection (HAART)
  What is HIV?

Highly Active Anti-Retroviral Therapies (HAART)
- Impact of Infection with Hepatitis C Virus (HCV) in HIV-Infected Persons
  Effect of Hepatitis C (HCV) Infection on HIV
  Effect of HIV Infection on HCV Infection
- Does HIV Co-Infection Affect the Rate of Progression of Liver Disease?
- Antiviral Therapy of Hepatitis C in Patients Co-Infected with HIV
  Pegylated Interferon Plus Ribavirin, The Current Standard
  Are New Treatments on the Horizon for Co-Infected Patients?
- Co-Infection with Hepatitis B
- Liver Transplantation
  Transplantation before HAART
  Transplantation after HAART
- Summary

Overview of HIV Co-Infection

What Is HIV/AIDS? The human immunodeficiency virus (HIV) destroys the immune system that helps the body fight illness and infection. HIV infects lymphocytes, the main immune cells in the body, and causes acquired immunodeficiency syndrome (AIDS). Severe damage to the immune system results in susceptibility to a wide array of infections and malignancy (cancer). These latter complications are collectively called AIDS-defining illness.

According to the Centers for Disease Control and Prevention (CDC) 2003 figures, an estimated 1,039,000 to 1,185,000 people were living with HIV in the United States. The cumulative estimated number of persons diagnosed with AIDS through 2003 was 929,985.

Are You at Risk for Co-Infection? Approximately 25% of patients with HIV infection living in the Western World are also infected with the hepatitis C virus (HCV). In the United States, up to 8% of patients with chronic hepatitis C may be co-infected with HIV. Behaviors that transmit HIV also transmit hepatitis C (such as sharing intravenous drug needles or receiving blood transfusions, organ transplants, or hemophilia treatment before tests screened the nation's blood supply). When HIV patients are infected with both HIV and HCV, it is called an HIV/HCV co-infection. Approximately 60 to 80 percent of patients who acquired HIV from intravenous drug use and 16 to 25 percent of patients who acquired HIV from sexual contact are co-infected with HCV.

In my experience, HIV treatment clinics diagnose most cases of hepatitis C and HIV co-infection because symptoms relating to HIV usually show up before those of hepatitis C. In fact, I have diagnosed unsuspected HIV in only a handful of patients with chronic hepatitis C (despite routine HIV testing of our hepatitis C population) during my years directing our hepatology clinics.

> *I'm a vet. In 1996 I had outpatient treatment, and my blood came back positive for HIV. The diagnosis threw me. I just gave up.*
>
> *It was an avalanche. Where am I going? What am I going to do? Then this year rolled around. My doctor wanted me to take a hepatitis B shot. That's when I found out I had hepatitis C.*
>
> *Joel*

Testing Problems. Researchers have documented that antibody tests for hepatitis C in patients with HIV may fluctuate; spontaneous conversion of hepatitis C from positive to negative antibodies may occur—up to 6% of patients with active HIV/HCV co-infection will test negative to HCV Ab.

For these reasons, if you have HIV infection I recommend that you be screened for HCV using tests that detect HCV RNA (see chapter 2 on HCV RNA testing), such as polymerase chain reaction (PCR) assay for HCV RNA. Despite the shortcomings of detection of HCV by use of antibody tests in patients with HIV, the data from the following studies described below are still useful in identifying trends.

Population Trends. Risk of co-infection with hepatitis C relates to how HIV was acquired. Patients who acquired HIV from blood-borne routes, as opposed to sexual routes, are more likely to be co-infected with hepatitis C. Patients who acquired HIV from intravenous drug use have a 60 to 80 percent chance of also harboring hepatitis C. Hemophiliacs who acquired HIV from transfusion with unpasteurized plasma-derived factor VIII concentrates have rates of co-infection of hepatitis C greater than 70 percent. These co-infection statistics are strikingly elevated when one compares them to the hepatitis C prevalence of 16 to 25 percent among male homosexuals with HIV without history of either transfusions or intravenous drug use.

When they told me I had HIV and they could keep me alive for five years tops, I was terrified. I thought I'd be dead very soon. I fell off the wagon after six months of sobriety. Figuring it didn't make any difference, I drank, I did drugs—anything to numb myself.

I suppose that's how I got hepatitis C in the first place.

Carl

Resource: For information on co-infection with HIV and hepatitis, access this website: www.hivandhepatitis.com.

Current Treatment of HIV Infection (HAART)

What is HIV? HIV is an RNA virus acquired by blood-borne routes or sexual activity. The virus, first identified in 1983 as the cause of AIDS, was given the name human T-cell lymphotropic virus type III (HTLV-III) in the United States because of its known association with lymphocytes. HIV infects the body's immune cells (lymphocytes), which then become dysfunctional or nonfunctional, or die, thus severely impairing the body's immune system. Before current effective anti–HIV therapy, most patients succumbed to either the ravages of infectious disease or malignancy (AIDS).

I've known 35 people who died from AIDS since 1985. When they put me on AZT, I figured I had two years left. That's what I had seen. The only thing that kept me going was taking care of my friend Jonathon, who went blind a month before he died. It was very hard.

Bill

Highly Active Anti-Retroviral Therapies (HAART). Certain classes of drugs, reverse transcriptase inhibitors, polymerase inhibitors, and protease inhibitors, dramatically altered the course of HIV infection. Today, most patients with HIV are treated with a combination of three to four drugs, and they experience significant improvement. HAART has improved patients' survival in HIV/AIDS from less than 5 years to over 20 years.

Seven years after my HIV diagnosis, the nurses called me at work. My T-cells were 160. I had AIDS! Confused, depressed, I flunked the memory tests and a CT scan showed I had a shrinkage of the brain. They put me on AZT.

Four years later, I went on HAART. My T-cells went up. Now I'm more scared of hepatitis C than HIV. After 14 years of being HIV-positive, you learn to deal with it, but this hepatitis thing is new. I'm dealing with all that uncertainty all over again.

John

How effective are these highly active anti-retroviral therapies (HAART)? Steven C. Johnson, M.D., Associate Professor of Medicine and Director of the University Hospital HIV/AIDS Clinical Program, University of Colorado Health Sciences Center, recently reviewed outcomes over a three-year period.[1] From 1995 through 1997 the percentage of HIV/AIDS patients treated with HAART increased from less than 10 percent to over 80 percent. The rate of hospitalization fell from 6.4 to 1.1 inpatient days per patient-year. Decreases in days of hospitalization resulted in significant cost reductions. The incidence of the three major opportunistic infections (infections that develop only because of the patient's immune deficiency)—pneumocystis pneumonia, mycobacterium avium complex disease, and cytomegalovirus retinitis (CMV)—decreased dramatically. Death from opportunistic infection or advanced HIV declined markedly from 15 percent of the clinic population in 1994 to 2 percent in 1998.

Hepatitis and end-stage liver disease, however, emerged as an important cause of sickness and death in this population. In 1995 hepatitis and liver disease accounted for only 4 percent of deaths, but two years later the number rose to 14 percent! Now, in the year 2005, cirrhosis due to chronic hepatitis C is a leading cause of both morbidity and mortality in patients with HIV infection on HAART therapy.

Resources: For more information about HIV/AIDS and sexually transmitted diseases, contact the CDC Info Hotline: 1-800-342-2437 or 1-800-227-8922, or the CDC website: www.cdc.gov.

Impact of HCV in HIV-Infected Persons

Effect of Hepatitis C (HCV) Infection on HIV. Some studies have suggested that HCV infection may increase the rate of progression of HIV infection to AIDS and AIDS-defining illness. Other studies have not observed this effect. Although there is no consistent evidence for a direct effect of hepatitis C on HIV, the major clinical issue is clear: hepatitis C can complicate therapy of HIV. Currently, the Federal Drug Administration has licensed more than 20 drugs for treatment of HIV in the United States. Nearly all of these medications, but in particular the protease inhibitors, are metabolized by the liver.

As liver disease due to hepatitis C progresses from hepatitis to cirrhosis, the liver is less able to metabolize these compounds. Changes in liver function may make it necessary to change either the drugs used or the doses of individual drugs. In addition, the anti-HIV drugs may be toxic to the liver. Instances of liver enzyme elevations, jaundice, and even fatal cases of severe liver toxicity from anti-HIV medications are well documented. Certain anti-HIV drugs, particularly the nucleoside reverse transcriptase inhibitors DDI, DDC, or D4T, may interact with ribavirin and increase risk of lactic acidosis, pancreatitis, and liver failure. Careful monitoring of electrolytes, kidney function, liver tests, blood counts, amylase, and lipase is necessary in patients on a combination of anti-HIV and anti-HCV treatments.

I had never heard of hepatitis C before. I figured I already had HIV-AIDS, so what difference did hepatitis C make? My doctors pulled me off all my AIDS meds twice because my liver enzymes went crazy. My whole body went crazy. I was nauseous and had vomiting.

Turned out I had a fungus in my esophagus from not being on the medications. I'm sick if I take the medicine and sick if I don't.

Anna

Effect of HIV Infection on HCV Infection. As described in preceding chapters, a chronic hepatitis C patient's own immune system can injure the liver as the immune system tries to destroy infected liver cells (immune-mediated injury). In contrast, after a transplant the viral levels are very high due to the use of immunosuppressive medications, and the virus itself destroys liver cells. Thus, HIV infection, which destroys components of the immune response, may either slow or accelerate liver disease due to hepatitis C.

Because HIV infection affects the immune system, it might impair a patient's immune response to hepatitis C and result in higher levels of the hepatitis C virus. One French study compared 75 patients with hepatitis C to 75 patients co-infected with hepatitis C and HIV.

Co-infected patients were more likely to have positive HCV RNA in their blood, and their HCV RNA levels were significantly higher. However, the level of HCV RNA did not correlate with CD4 count (a measure of the degree of immune deficiency), p24 antigen levels (a specific HIV protein), or HIV RNA level.

In contrast, a German study of 21 co-infected hemophiliacs and 22 hemophiliacs with isolated hepatitis C failed to show a difference in HCV RNA viral levels between these two groups. Another study retrospectively examined stored serum for HCV RNA levels in groups of hemophiliacs infected with hepatitis C. Those who subsequently developed HIV experienced a significant increase in HCV RNA level, which correlated with the reduction in CD4 count.

One fear is that HAART medications may actually accelerate the progression of hepatitis C to cirrhosis and therefore compromise the effectiveness of therapy against HIV. Researchers examined this issue in a study of HAART therapy in 51 patients with "HCV-related chronic liver disease." HAART therapy was associated with an increase in HCV RNA viral load and elevations in liver enzymes (AST/ALT) within one to three months of starting treatment. Liver biopsies revealed liver cell injury and inflammation. Seven patients were taken off HAART due to signs of liver failure. This effect was mainly due to HAART because a much smaller number of patients not on HAART (four out of 148) experienced symptoms of liver failure. However, the worsened liver inflammation noted early in HAART therapy had largely subsided by nine months on HAART. Additional research is needed in this area.

A recent study examined the development of abnormal liver tests after 394 HIV patients began HAART treatment. Seven percent were co-infected with hepatitis B and 14 percent had hepatitis C. The risk of developing abnormal liver tests was greater in HIV patients who had chronic hepatitis (37 percent in co-infected patients vs. 12 percent in HIV patients without either HBV or HCV). Although inconclusive, these data suggest that the immune deficiency caused by HIV may promote hepatitis C viral replication and potentially hasten the progression of liver disease.

Does HIV Co-Infection Affect the Rate of Progression of Liver Disease?

The CDC has reported that the percentage of HIV patients with death due to liver disease steadily increased from 1987 to 1997. According to data from the U.S. National Vital Statistics System, the percent of death certificates listing "sequelae (consequences) of chronic liver disease" increased from 1.3 percent in 1987, to 2.2 percent in 1995, to 3.5 percent in 1997.

Further analysis of death certificates indicated that liver disease caused, contributed, or was secondarily involved in approximately 10 percent of all deaths in 1997. Patients dying with a diagnosis of chronic hepatitis C increased from 0.9 percent in 1995 to 2.3 percent in 1997 (tests for hepatitis C were not available until 1990). Patients dying with a diagnosis of chronic hepatitis B increased from 0.5 percent in 1987, to 0.8 percent in 1995, to 1.3 percent in 1997.

The observed increase in deaths related to "sequelae of chronic liver disease" exceeded the expected frequency by 46 percent. It is not known whether the increase in mortality rate was due to use of HAART medications, increased activity of hepatitis viruses, or reflected the natural progression of hepatitis B and C occurring in HIV patients who now live longer.

Only a few studies have examined the association between HIV infection and acceleration in liver disease related to hepatitis C. One large retrospective series from Spain examined 547 patients who acquired hepatitis C by blood-borne routes and found that 116 of these patients were co-infected with HIV. The researchers observed that co-infected people took less time to develop cirrhosis. At ten years of HCV infection, 14.9 percent of co-infected patients had cirrhosis, compared to only 2.6 percent of those infected only with hepatitis C.

A French series of 210 patients with hepatitis C, 60 of whom were co-infected with HIV, suggested that the incidence of cirrhosis was 3.5 times higher in co-infected patients. Another study from Spain examined liver histology and found that co-infected patients had more severe liver inflammation and later stages of fibrosis.

Although data are limited, these studies do suggest that hepatitis C-related liver disease may accelerate in HIV/HCV co-infection.

Antiviral Therapy of Hepatitis C in Patients Co-Infected with HIV

Pegylated Interferon Plus Ribavirin, the Current Standard. Older studies and reports indicated that rates of sustained virologic response with interferon monotherapy and the combination of interferon plus ribavirin were approximately 50 percent lower in co-infected patients compared to patients with HCV mono-infection. Four randomized controlled trials have established pegylated interferon plus ribavirin as the current treatment standard: ACTG 5071, APRICOT, RIBAVIC, and Barcelona. The remainder of this section describes the results from these trials and highlights the promises and pitfalls of the current standard-of-treatment, pegylated interferon plus ribavirin.

The study by the AIDS Clinical Trials Group, ACTG 5071, randomized 133 patients with co-infection to treatment with either interferon plus ribavirin versus pegylated interferon (Pegasys) plus ribavirin. Seventy-eight percent were infected with HCV genotype 1, 33 percent were Black, and 82 percent had high levels of HCV RNA (greater than 1 million IU HCV RNA/ml). Rates of sustained virologic response were significantly higher with pegylated interferon plus ribavirin (27 percent versus 12 percent for all patients; 14 percent versus 6 percent for patients infected with HCV genotype 1) (Figure 12A).

In the APRICOT study 860 patients were assigned to either pegylated interferon (Pegasys) plus ribavirin, interferon plus ribavirin, or pegylated interferon monotherapy. Only 61 percent were infected with HCV genotype 1, 11 percent were Black, and 72 percent had high level HCV RNA (greater than 800,000 IU HCV RNA/ml). Rates of sustained virologic response were highest in patients treated with pegylated interferon plus ribavirin (40, 20, and 12 percent, respectively) (Figure 12A). The sustained virologic response for patients with HCV genotype 1 was nearly 30 percent.

In RIBAVIC, 412 patients were randomized to either pegylated interferon (Peg-Intron) plus ribavirin or interferon plus ribavirin. Fifty-eight percent of patients were infected with either HCV genotype 1 or 4. Rates of sustained virologic response were 26 percent for pegylated interferon plus ribavirin and 18 percent for interferon plus ribavirin (Figure 12A). Interpretation of the results from RIBAVIC is compromised by a 42 percent dropout rate for patients in the trial.

In the Barcelona trial (N=95), SVR in HCV genotype 1 was 38%. The slightly improved results with HCV genotype 1 in this trial may have been due to use of higher doses of ribavirin, and better suppression of HIV RNA with HAART.

The range of rates of sustained virologic response in patients with HIV/HCV co-infection, 26 to 40 percent, observed in these three trials is far below the reported rate of approximately 55 percent for patients with HCV mono-infection. In APRICOT, sustained virologic response

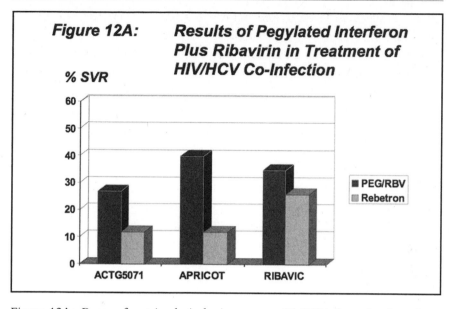

Figure 12A: Rates of sustained virologic response (% SVR) from the three large trials of pegylated interferon plus ribavirin for treatment of patients with HIV/HCV co-infection are shown. Results are displayed against the comparator therapy, Rebetron, which was the combination of standard nonpegylated interferon plus ribavirin. Characteristics of the three trials, ACTG5071, APRICOT, and RIB-AVIC, are discussed in the text.

for patients with HCV genotype 1 was only 30 percent. This is far below the reported rate of approximately 40 to 45 percent observed in patients with HCV mono-infection. Thus, although current treatment with pegylated interferon plus ribavirin has improved outcomes, it is still effective in only a minority of patients and is not as effective in HIV/HCV co-infection as it is in HCV mono-infection.

Safety is another factor when using pegylated interferon and ribavirin in HCV/HIV co-infected patients. Ribavirin-associated anemia is more common and more severe, particularly in patients taking AZT. Severe reactions, even death, have occurred in patients taking ribavirin and ddI—this combination is to be avoided. Since pegylated interferon may predispose to infection and SVR from treatment may require immune mechanisms, it is recommended that CD4 counts exceed 200/mm3 prior to therapy.

Are New Treatments on the Horizon for Co-Infected Patients? We are on the brink of a new era in the treatment of hepatitis C (see chapters 14 and 15). Several new drugs and therapeutic approaches are under development, but primarily in HCV mono-infected patients. The treatments which seem to offer the most promise include viramidine as a ribavirin substitute, HCV-specific protease inhibitors, and HCV-specific polymerase inhibitors, and others (see chapter 14). The new anti-HCV drugs will need to be cautiously and carefully evaluated in co-infected patients on HAART therapy due to the possibility of adverse interactions between HIV and HCV drugs. In the absence of cure, long-term, low-dose treatment pegylated interferon monotherapy to halt disease progression is currently being evaluated in SLAM-C, an ACTG trial. Your doctor may be able to tell you if you are a candidate for participating in trials of any of these therapies.

Resources: For more information about treatment and trials, call the following hotlines and information services:
AIDS Info: 800-448-0440 or 1-800-TRIALS-A
Project Inform: 800-822-7422

Co-Infection with Hepatitis B

The worst thing for me is the fatigue. Although everyone with hepatitis seems to suffer to some degree, my experience has been extreme. My doctor thinks that maybe because I have two viruses, B and C, my body fights twice as hard and causes me to be increasingly more tired.

Mel

How Common is HBV/HCV Co-infection? Ten to fifteen percent of persons with chronic hepatitis B have active HCV infection. Stated from the perspective of HCV, less that 5 percent of persons with chronic hepatitis C are actively infected and have chronic hepatitis B. However, serologic studies of patients with chronic hepatitis C indicate that a much higher proportion, up to one-third, may have been exposed to HBV. At least a proportion of these patients harbor HBV in a quiescent or dormant state; HBV can be activated when the patient's immune system is altered by disease or treatments such as steroids, anti-cancer drugs, or immunosuppressive medications. Given the current estimates of a minimum of 1.25 million persons in the United States with chronic hepatitis B, I calculate that there are at least 125,000 to 187,500 US residents actively co-infected with both HCV and HBV.

Increased Risks of Co-infection. Co-infection with hepatitis B and C results in greater liver damage, more rapid progression to cirrhosis, and increased risk for liver cancer. The risk for more aggressive disease with co-infection is not related to high viral levels or replication rates; in fact, the opposite has been found. Co-infected patients typically have lower HCV RNA and HBV DNA levels compared to mono-infected controls. Despite the lower levels of HCV and HBV, co-infected patients were more likely to have either moderate to severe chronic hepatitis or cirrhosis.

The effect of co-infection on risk of liver cancer is particularly striking. One study followed 290 patients with cirrhosis for 8 to 96 months and observed the following:

HBV Blood Test	HCV Blood Test	Incidence of Liver Cancer
HBsAg +	HCV Ab +	40%
HBsAg+	Negative	19.6%
Negative	HCV Ab +	12.2%
Negative	Negative	9.1%

(For more on the risk of developing liver cancer see chapter 11.)

Treatment for HBV/HCV Co-infection. In general, therapy is recommended for co-infected patients. Treatment strategies for co-infected patients have been simplified by recent results of studies of pegylated interferon therapy for HCV and HBV. First, as noted in chapter 9, pegylated interferon plus ribavirin is the current standard-of-treatment for chronic hepatitis C. Second, pegylated interferon alfa-2a (Pegasys), 180 ug/wk for 48 weeks, was approved by the FDA for treatment of chronic hepatitis B. Third, pegylated interferon and standard interferon stimulate the immune response against hepatitis B and induce a "flare" of active hepatitis. Generally this "flare" is well tolerated, asymptomatic, and is an indicator of effective response that could lead to clearance of HBV. However, flares in patients with compensated cirrhosis can lead to deterioration in liver function and clinical decompensation. For these reasons, pegylated interferon is relatively contraindicated in patients with chronic hepatitis B and cirrhosis. Nucleoside analogues (lamivudine, adefovir, tenofovir, entecavir, emtricitabine) are preferred in the treatment of chronic hepatitis B in patients with cirrhosis. Fourth, and finally, treatment of HBV is typically only warranted for patients with active replication, those with positive HBV DNA in blood. No specific treatment for HBV is warranted in co-infected patients with negative HBV DNA.

Given the above considerations, here are the treatment regimens that I currently recommend in my patients who are co-infected with HBV and HCV and have positive HCV RNA and HBV DNA:

	HCV Treatment	HBV Treatment
Patients without Cirrhosis		
Genotype 1, 4, 5, 6	PEG/RBV[1], 48 wks	No additional
Genotype 1 with RVR[2]	PEG/RBV, 24 wks	PEG for extra 24 wks
Genotype 2, 3	PEG/RBV, 24 wks	PEG for extra 24 wks
Genotype 2, 3 with RVR	PEG/RBV, 12–16 wks	PEG for extra 36 wks

[1]PEG/RBV, pegylated interferon (180 ug/wk for Pegays or 1.5 ug/kg/wk for Peg-Intron) plus ribavirin (1.0–1.2 g/d for genotypes 1, 4, 5, 6 or 800 mg/d for genotypes 2 and 3) combination therapy. [2] RVR, rapid virologic response defined as HCV RNA negative after 4 weeks of treatment.

Patients with Compensated Cirrhosis

Same regimens for HCV treatment as noted above, but pegylated interferon is relatively contraindicated in patients with chronic hepatitis B and cirrhosis. In this setting, I have used nucleoside analogues to suppress HBV replication while attempting to treat and eradicate HCV with pegylated interferon plus ribavirin. However, efficacy is limited and patients require close monitoring, frequent blood testing, and management by either hepatologists practicing in liver centers or physicians with considerable experience in treating chronic hepatitis C, chronic hepatitis B, and patients with cirrhosis.

With me, the C is the active virus and the B is apparently rather inert. I was so tired and irritable, I had to quit night school—and my goal was to finish college before my kids. When I tried to go back, there was no brain left. I had migraines, joint pain, arthritis.

I read that if you have B as well, the hepatitis is worse, so I decided to try treatment. I made my husband promise not to leave me if I went on interferon. The first night, my husband and I sat on the couch and waited for the side effects. We both fell asleep.

When I woke up, I had no joint pain. It's been eight months, and I feel better on interferon. My labs are good. The C is undetectable.

Ina

My son, a hemophiliac, is co-infected. He got non-A, non-B hepatitis at age 1. Later they diagnosed it as hepatitis C. He got it from the clotting factor they gave him to stop the bleeds. Today they heat the clotting factor to kill viruses.

He's 19 now and more concerned about being contagious with the hepatitis B in regard to his social life. His doctor started him on six months of combo therapy for the C but with daily doses of interferon to hit the B hard. In July he tested negative for the first time ever for hepatitis B surface antigens. And he tested less than 200 for a hepatitis C viral load after a six-month treatment of daily interferon and ribavirin!

Sophie

In clinical practice, a liver biopsy does not help to determine the dominance of one infection over the other, because the histologic (cell) changes with hepatitis B and C are similar. I use the liver biopsy to detect underlying cirrhosis—if cirrhosis is detected the management and treatment becomes more complicated!

I didn't have a clue I was sick until I had a bleed. I was in the hospital eight or nine days. When the tests came back, they were positive for hepatitis B and C. My biopsy showed I only had 25 percent liver function. I had cirrhosis so bad, the doctor said I was a candidate for a transplant. I had active hepatitis C and inactive hepatitis B. The fear was that after the transplant, because of the immunosuppressive drugs and the surgery, the B could flare up.

Juliet

Resource: For more information on hepatitis B, contact the organizations listed in the Resources section at the end of this book and the Hepatitis B Foundation, 700 E. Butler Ave., Doylestown, PA 18901-2697; phone: 215-489-4900; email: info@hepb.org; website: www.hepb.org.

Resource: For an online hepatitis B support group, contact the Hepatitis B Information and Support List: http://www. geocities.com/ Heartland/Estates/9350/hblist. html. To subscribe, send a blank email to: hepatitis-b-on@mail-list.com.

Resource: For up-to-the-minute research reports, subscribe to the free Hepatitis B Research List by sending a blank email to: HBV_Research-on@mail-list.com. The research bulletins from 1998 to the current year are archived at http://dispatch.mail-list.com/archives/hbv_research and can be accessed by an easy search engine.

Resource: Everson, Gregory T., M.D., and Hedy Weinberg. *Living with Hepatitis B: A Survivor's Guide.* New York: Hatherleigh Press, 2001.

Liver Transplantation

Patients who are co-infected with hepatitis B and C are considered candidates for liver transplantation using the same criteria established for chronic hepatitis B and chronic hepatitis C. In the case of HCV/HBV co-infection, transplant hepatologists have several therapeutic options to control HBV, including effective immune globulin (HBIG), lamivudine, adefovir, entecavir, telbivudine, tenofovir, emtricitabine, interferon, and pegylated interferon.

In contrast, transplantation for patients co-infected with HIV and HCV is controversial. Prior to HAART, liver transplantation in patients with active HIV was associated with very poor outcomes. With the development of HAART, results for patients with HIV infection have improved considerably.

Transplantation before HAART. Before HAART physicians refused to consider HIV-infected patients for liver transplantation for the following reasons:

1. The immunosuppressive medications used after transplantation to prevent rejection of the donor liver would have further compromised the HIV-induced immune deficiency and increased the risk of serious life-threatening infection or malignancy.
2. HIV patients typically had ongoing infections, malignancies, or other illnesses that prohibited transplantation.

3. HIV patients would likely have died of HIV-related complications despite liver transplantation, thereby wasting a donor liver.

Anecdotal reports of liver transplantation in HIV-infected patients before the era of HAART therapy indicated that HIV patients continued to have HIV after the transplant. They experienced a predictable downhill course. Therefore, many transplant centers disqualified HIV patients from receiving liver transplants. Effective control of HIV with HAART may have changed the outlook, and many transplant centers are reconsidering HIV patients with cirrhosis for liver transplantation. Current Medicare and Medicaid guidelines regarding HIV are under review and modification.

I'm really worried. If I get cirrhosis, they won't give me a transplant because I have HIV. That will be it. The end. No options.

At my hepatitis C support group they told me to take it one step at a time. First, I need a liver biopsy and a PCR viral load test. But I can't stop my mind from racing ahead and obsessing.

The only thing that keeps me going is God.

Reuben

Transplantation after HAART. HAART therapy may make liver transplantation an option for HIV-infected patients. Current experience suggests overall improvement in post-transplant outcome with HAART. However, outcomes after liver transplantation for HIV/HCV co-infection may be worse than outcomes after liver transplantation for HCV mono-infection. Other problems in the post-transplant setting include adverse interactions of HIV and immunosuppressive drugs or medications, mitochondrial toxicity, and opportunistic infection.

Summary

We are just beginning to address the growing problem of co-infection of hepatitis C patients with either HIV or hepatitis B. As patients with HIV/AIDS live decades longer due to new antiviral treatments, many of them will have to deal with hepatitis C treatment decisions as well. These are complicated issues because HIV/AIDS therapies affect the liver, and hepatitis C therapies affect the immune system.

My hope is that new studies, advances in drug therapy, and controlled research projects will yield more information about all of these viruses. Then physicians and patients can work together to make thoughtful plans for treatment and to offer more options to patients affected by hepatitis C in combination with either HIV or hepatitis B.

A journey of a thousand miles must begin with a single step.

Lao-tzu

Reference

1. Johnson, S. A. Hageman, H. Wing, M. Grodesky, N. Bathurst, P. Romfh, W. Williams. Effect of Antiretroviral Therapy on Clinical Outcomes and Cost in a University-Based HIV/AIDS Program: 1995–1997. Abstract 42211, 12th World AIDS Conference, Geneva, Switzerland, June 23–July 3, 1998.

13

CHILDREN WITH HEPATITIS C

A Growing Problem

Five years ago I donated blood. I got a letter with a box checked off: hepatitis C. I never had any symptoms, and the doctors think I got infected from transfusions I had years ago.

I really wasn't alarmed until they tested my husband and my three kids. My youngest—my 3-year-old baby girl—was the only one with hepatitis C. She had slightly elevated enzymes and her biopsy showed a little bit of scarring. The doctors want to give her interferon.

What do I do? She's so little. If I have hepatitis C, it's my problem, and I did it to myself. I'll deal with whatever treatment I have to. But to make the decision for my child is much, much harder.

Betsy

WHEN CHILDREN HAVE a serious infection, like hepatitis C, it affects the whole family.

I'm a nurse, so I was stuck and splashed on for years. In 1995 I found out I had hepatitis C. Seven years before, I had given birth to my first baby—a little boy, Andy. He never had any symptoms or signs of hepatitis C, but I got scared and had both my kids tested—sure I was paranoid. Andy's test was positive.

I was devastated, guilty. I felt it was my fault. My husband never accused me but said, "You were not careful enough in the operating room." I felt terrible.

Shanna

Researchers are continuing to study the natural history and outcomes of treatment in children. And that adds to a parent's anxiety. As a parent, you feel concerned about your family—and you're concerned about yourself, too, if you're ill with hepatitis C.

I can't continue raising my kids and working. I lie in the bathtub and bawl. My kids are active, and I need downtime. It's hard when you have hepatitis C and one of your kids has it too.

Sometimes I plug in a movie for them so I can lie down. I can hardly move. I feel like a terrible mother. I always said I'd never park them in front of a TV.

Janice

How do children get hepatitis C? Today most children become infected when the mother passes the infection to her baby at birth (the vertical route). Some older adolescents acquired hepatitis C from exposure to blood or blood products (through treatment of conditions such as congenital heart disease, malignancies, leukemia, hemophilia, and other illnesses) before blood was screened for the virus.

Some older adolescents may acquire hepatitis C through intravenous drug use. This age group has its own problems with care and management of hepatitis C. However, issues regarding diagnosis, medical treatment, progression of liver disease, and transplantation are probably similar to the adult population, and I refer you to those topics in previous chapters.

Note: Discussions and recommendations in this chapter are meant as guidelines. Please consult your pediatrician, or your pediatric gastroenterologist or hepatologist regarding specific issues in treatment and management.

Here are the topics we'll cover:

• Overview
• Does Your Baby Have Hepatitis C?
    Antibody Testing
    HCV RNA Assays
    Can Infection Be Prevented?
• Should Women with Hepatitis C Avoid Pregnancy or Breastfeeding?
• Can Your Child Participate in Regular Activities?
    Disclosure: To Tell or Not to Tell
    Chronic Disease and Your Family
    Resources for Children
• The Course of the Infection in Children
• Monitoring Children with Hepatitis C
    Liver Biopsy
    Blood Draws and Biopsies/Practical Suggestions
• Treatment
    Interferon Plus Ribavirin
    Pegylated Interferon
    Giving Injections
    Future Therapy
    Post-Treatment Follow-Up

Overview

Hepatitis C in children is a growing problem. According to the American Liver Foundation, one of every 500 children (0.2 percent) between the ages of 6 and 11 is chronically infected by hepatitis C. In children between the ages of 12 and 19, one of every 250 (0.4 percent) is infected.

Most transmissions of hepatitis C to an infant occur during delivery when the infant may be exposed to the mother's blood. Prior to 1992 a common route of acquisition of hepatitis C, even in young children, was previous exposure to blood or blood products through transfusion. Screening with current tests has virtually eliminated this mode of transmission.

A mother with hepatitis C may transmit the virus to her infant at birth. The risk of this type of transmission correlates with the presence of HCV RNA viral load in the mother's blood at the time of delivery. Mothers co-infected with HIV and hepatitis C are even more likely to transmit hepatitis C to their newborn.

Several studies have found that when mothers have hepatitis C, the chance that the infant will acquire the virus is approximately 6 percent. In contrast, the likelihood of transmission increases to more than 15 percent when mothers are co-infected with hepatitis C and HIV. The increased risk of transmission in HIV-positive mothers may be related to the relatively higher concentration of HCV RNA in their blood. The U.S. Public Health Service and the American Academy of Pediatrics (AAP) recommend that all children born of hepatitis C-infected mothers be tested for the hepatitis C virus.

Does Your Baby Have Hepatitis C?

There is a low chance (only 6 percent) that you, a mother infected with hepatitis C, would transmit hepatitis C to your baby. In the event you do transmit hepatitis C to your baby, about half the time your baby will clear the infection without any treatment.

Antibody Testing. Hepatitis C antibodies in the mother's blood cross the placental barrier and are detected in the baby's blood. This movement of the mother's antibodies to the baby is called passive transfer and does not mean that the virus itself has transferred to the baby. Hepatitis C antibodies do not protect the baby, and the infant may or may not develop hepatitis C infection.

Passively acquired antibodies usually persist for 6 to 12 months and never beyond 15 months. If the baby undergoes antibody testing 15 months or more after delivery and the HCV antibody is positive, it is likely that the infant is or has been infected with hepatitis C.

HCV RNA Assays. Because of the problems with antibody testing, most hepatologists favor measuring viral load with an HCV RNA assay, such as a PCR assay (see chapter 2), to determine whether the infant is actively infected with hepatitis C. In most cases, truly infected infants will test positive for HCV RNA within two months of birth. HCV RNA will remain positive as long as the virus continues to replicate and persist in the child.

Can Infection Be Prevented? We don't have an effective antiviral strategy to prevent infection of the newborn. Immune serum globulin, even when it contains a high concentration of the antibody against hepatitis C, does not prevent transmission, and no one has studied preemptive use of antiviral therapy (interferon, etc). In addition, it probably makes little sense to expose all babies to the risks of gamma globulin therapy or interferon when the vast majority will not acquire hepatitis C.

For these reasons physicians recommend simply monitoring for hepatitis C. Minimum testing requirements include measurement of the hepatitis C antibody 12 to 15 months after delivery. Hepatitis C infection could be detected earlier by measuring HCV RNA viral load two or more months after birth. Umbilical cord blood should not be used for testing of either the hepatitis C antibody or the HCV RNA viral load because it may be contaminated with maternal blood. If infection is detected, it should be reassessed at about two years of age because of spontaneous clearance.

Should Women with Hepatitis C Avoid Pregnancy or Breastfeeding?

The decision to proceed with childbearing is personal and individual. Most experts in this field conclude that women should not avoid pregnancy simply because they have hepatitis C, even though there is the potential risk of transmitting the virus to their infant. In otherwise healthy mothers, 94 percent of offspring will not acquire hepatitis C; only 6 percent get the infection, and the course of hepatitis C in these infants has been clinically mild in the majority of cases. However, the long-term consequences of chronic HCV infection acquired vertically have not been well studied.

Nonetheless, parents must realize that there is a risk and that we don't completely understand the long-term consequences of hepatitis C in an infant who acquires the virus. Some infants may develop hepatitis, progress to cirrhosis over several years, and may even require liver transplantation in the future. In addition, all infants who become chronic carriers may be at some risk for developing liver cancer—although we don't have any data on this yet.

Studies have examined the risk of the newborn acquiring hepatitis C related to the type of delivery. Early studies showed that the risk was similar whether the baby was delivered vaginally or by Cesarian section (C-section), and the U.S. Public Health Service has not recommended Cesarian section as the routine method of delivery. However, a recent study showed that delivery by elective Cesarean section prior to membrane rupture was associated with a lower transmission risk than either vaginal or emergent Cesarean section delivery. Additional studies are needed before elective Cesarian section can be recommended.

In addition, there is little evidence that breastfeeding increases the risk of transmitting hepatitis C. In one study, the number of cases of hepatitis C in breastfed and bottle-fed infants born of mothers infected with hepatitis C was the same (4 percent). Epidemiological studies indicate that breastfeeding has not been definitely shown to transmit hepatitis C to infants. Given these data, the U. S. Public Health Service does not currently restrict breastfeeding for mothers with hepatitis C. Of course, women should discuss this decision with their physicians and pediatricians.

However, recent information suggests that infants who are breastfed and whose mothers have active symptoms of hepatitis C may be at increased risk. Mothers with active, aggressive hepatitis C (for example, jaundice) should avoid or abstain from breastfeeding if their nipples are cracked or bleeding. Always consult with your doctor.

Can Your Child Participate in Regular Activities?

Hepatitis C is not spread by casual contact, and children with the virus may participate in all regular activities, including school, play, day care, childcare, extracurricular activities, and sports. One exception would be the child who has active skin wounds and sores. The official American Academy of Pediatrics (AAP) recommendation is that the open wound be completely covered with a secure bandage or dressing before participation in the activity.

Tell your child that he or she cannot give hepatitis C to friends, classmates, family, or other acquaintances by sneezing, coughing, holding, hugging, or kissing; by sharing food, water, eating utensils or drinking glasses; or by any other casual contact. The Centers for Disease Control guidelines don't disqualify anyone from school unless they show aggressive behavior, such as biting or scratching.

Hepatitis C can be spread by blood exposure, so cuts or abrasions should be carefully cleaned and bandaged to avoid contact with other children. In addition, the child should be told to avoid putting his or her fingers in other children's mouths (in order to prevent possible biting), sharing toothbrushes or razor blades, and making other contact with open sores or wounds.

Parents will be pleased to know that in December 2000, the AAP announced that athletes with HIV, HBV, or HCV should be allowed to participate in all sports and that doctors should maintain patient confidentiality. The AAP policy statement states that there is a "very low probability" that these infections would be transmitted among young athletes. The AAP recommends that athletic programs use Occupational Safety and Health Administration (OSHA) Universal Precautions and inform students and parents that there is a "very small but finite risk" of a blood-borne infection.

Resource: To read the entire policy statement, go to the AAP website: www.aap.org/policy/re9821.html.

Disclosure: To Tell or Not to Tell. One of the major problems you face as a parent is disclosure. It's important to tell doctors and dentists about your child's condition, but do you tell the daycare facility, the school, caregivers, friends?

"There is a disparity between the ideal and the real situation," says Marjanne Claassen, R.N., M.S., C.N.S., clinical nurse specialist and pediatric liver center nurse coordinator in the Section of Pediatric Gastroenterology, Hepatology and Nutrition at the Children's Hospital in Denver, Colorado. "The approach in schools is to use standard precautions. The ideal is that every staff member will deal with every child's blood in the same protective way. The OSHA standards require that all blood is assumed to be contaminated. Therefore, the school worker must assume that there are germs in everybody's blood, and of course with any blood-borne illness most children have it well before anyone knows they have it.

"Protective Personal Equipment (PPE—disposable protective gloves) is usually all that's needed. Because of standard precautions, the family has no legal obligation to tell anyone a child's diagnosis. That's the ideal.

"The reality is that the parent usually chooses to tell the school. I recommend that families notify the professional registered nurse in charge of their child's school. A registered nurse understands the issues of confidentiality and will be prepared to handle questions as they come up."

"Be knowledgeable yourself," says Nancy Butler-Simon, M.S., R.N., C.N.S., C.P.N.P. "Be right up front with the school nurse. Have a script. Educate people. The school nurse can help you do that. Panic is the most contagious thing on this planet; deal with it by teaching others. Nip anxiety in the bud with knowledge."

Aside from school, parents and children must also decide what friends to inform and how. Parents must find the balance between secrecy and privacy. It's important to communicate that hepatitis C is not transmitted casually, but is a blood-borne infection.

My biggest fear is they'll label him and say, "Stay away from him. He's got that virus!" But as my mother says, "Things happen. The dear Lord doesn't give you any more than you can handle."

My husband and I always tell the parents of our children's friends in case something should happen. The parents say, "Oh, I'll keep an eye out." It's not like they don't invite her over. They say, "Don't worry about it."

My mom tells my friends' moms what to do if I cut myself. She tells them to put gloves on and not touch my blood because I have hepatitis C.

Everyone in the family knows. The daycare providers knew when she was little. Nothing has ever had to be done to treat her differently.

My daughter doesn't tell her friends. She doesn't want to feel like she has the plague. She does know she needs to be careful with her blood. From the beginning I talked to her. "Don't let them use your toothbrush or razor. Don't use theirs. Put a bandage on a cut yourself."

My brother, Tommy's uncle, got really angry at me when I decided to delay treatment for Tommy. He yelled at me and grabbed my arm— my own brother. "You're killing him!" he said.
Tommy had no symptoms, and it was a hard call, but the hardest thing of all was the lack of support in my own family.

It helps that I have hepatitis C too. I wouldn't know how to deal with my 7-year-old daughter otherwise. I know what she's feeling when she comes to me with a concern.

My husband has to use gloves to help us clean up if my daughter or I are bleeding. He felt bad. I said, "Just do it. Just put them on."

As children approach adolescence, parents should discuss decisions about future behaviors. Ideally, the topics of body piercing, tattooing, illegal drugs, and safe sex will be introduced in the context of family values when children are young. Pre-adolescence is an opportunity to make youngsters aware that you can not only give diseases such as hepatitis C and AIDS, you can also get these illnesses from these exposures.

In summary, says Claassen, "Think carefully before you share your child's diagnosis. Balance responsibility with caution and with making your child's life as normal as possible. You don't want a big red 'H' on your child's head."

Resource: Many organizations offer information to parents. Some also provide sample letters that can be given to schools. Contact Parents of Kids with Infectious Diseases (877-55-PKIDS) and other groups listed in the Resources section at the end of this book.

Resource: The *Pediatric Hepatitis Report,* co-funded by the CDC and Parents of Kids with Infectious Diseases (PKIDs), is available online at the PKIDs website: www.pkids.org. The report covers hepatitis A through E, the latest treatment options, liver tests, children's civil rights, how to tell others about your child's disease, how to tell your child, and more. You may obtain a hard copy for a fee by contacting the organization. See the Resources section at the end of this book.

Chronic Disease and Your Family. Hepatitis C affects everyone in the family—in positive as well as negative ways (see chapter 5). What family friends do you tell, and when do you tell them? How do you deal with brothers and sisters who worry about the sick sibling but may be jealous over the extra attention paid to the child with hepatitis C?

Another big issue is body image. Children don't like to feel different. Sometimes, even if they have no symptoms of hepatitis C, they may think they look different. Talk to your children. Let them tell you their fears and reassure them. Above all, your child needs to know that hepatitis C is a medical condition, not a reason to feel ashamed.

Worry? No, I don't. Not really. My mom doesn't have really bad hepatitis C.

When my sister or mom gets hurt, we have to wear gloves. But mostly I don't talk about it. Sometimes something comes up, and you have to explain what it is, like when kids are talking about other diseases.

I tell them it's a sickness, and it affects your liver sometimes. For my sister, it does. It can kill you, but it doesn't most often. And sometimes they ask me questions I can't answer.

Hannah, age 9

Chronic disease is a strain, emotionally and financially. Your pediatrician and local children's hospital have resources to help you: social workers, specialists in financial matters, nurses, and doctors who've dealt with the same problems you're facing.

Talking to others, either informally or in support groups, can help you keep your perspective.

Resource: Contact the PKIDs Support List for parents (kids are encouraged to participate). Also, access the PKIDs research archives: www.pkids.org.

Resources for Children. The organizations listed in "Resources" at the back of this book provide avenues to support groups, online chat groups, videotapes, research archives, and educational packets. Your local children's hospital library also is a good source of information.

On Healthy Eating. A balanced, healthy diet is appropriate for people with liver disease (see chapter 5). Note: Parents of children with cirrhosis should consult their doctors about dietary restrictions. Access the USDA Food Pyramid for children at www.usda.gov/cnpp/Kids Pyra.

On Hepatitis.

Aronson, Virginia. *Everything You Need to Know About Hepatitis.* New York: Rosen Publishing Group, 2000 (middle school, high school).

Silverstein, Alvin, Virginia and Robert. *Hepatitis.* Springfield: Enslow Publishers, 1994 (middle school, high school).

Weinberg, Hedy and Shira Shump with Gregory T. Everson, M.D. *My Mom Has Hepatitis C.* Long Island City: Hatherleigh Press, 2000 (preschool, elementary).

On Issues of Chronic Illness.

Band-aids and Blackboards. A colorful website about growing up with medical problems with areas for kids, teens, and adults; website: www.lehman.cuny.edu/faculty/jfleitas/bandaides.

Heegard, Marge. *When Someone Has a Very Serious Illness.* Minneapolis: Woodland Press, 1991 (workbook for preschool and elementary).

Huegel, Kelly. *Young People and Chronic Illness (True Stories, Help, and Hope).* Minneapolis: Free Spirit, 1998 (middle school, high school).

LeVert Suzanne. *Face to Face with Chronic Illness.* New York: Messner/Simon & Schuster, 1993 (high school).

Moe, Barbara. *Coping with Chronic Illness.* New York: Rosen Publishing Group, 1992 (middle school, high school).

On Children Facing Liver Transplants:

Murphy-Melas, Elizabeth. *Pennies, Nickels & Dimes.* Santa Fe: Health Press, 1999.

Ribal, Lizzy. *Lizzy Gets a New Liver/Lizzy Tiene un Higado Nuevo.* Louisville: Bridge Resources, 1997.

Shadow Buddies. A website that offers condition-specific dolls for your child, including one for liver transplant patients (complete with hospital gown, "Y" incision, and Hickman catheter), with a link to Shadow Buddies Foundation; website: www.shadowbuddies.com.

The Course of the Infection in Children

We don't yet know the natural history or course of hepatitis C in children who acquire the disease vertically from mother to infant at the time of delivery. The rate of development of long-term consequences, such as cirrhosis, liver failure, or liver cancer, is uncertain, but in general the course appears to at least be slower or milder in children. Fewer children go to end stage disease at 20 to 30 years after acquiring HCV. Persistent infection with hepatitis C may occur in greater than 50 to 60 percent of infected newborns. Most infants with hepatitis C have a benign course, even though the majority demonstrate mild elevations in liver enzymes. Few (less than 15 percent) exhibit more severe liver injury including clinical jaundice. Less than 3 percent of children will have more aggressive hepatitis and progressive fibrosis.

One recent study examined liver biopsies performed in 74 boys and 35 girls with chronic hepatitis C, ages 4 to 14. All were positive for HCV antibody or had HCV RNA in blood samples, and all had persistently elevated ALT (greater than 1.5 times normal) for at least six months prior to the biopsy. Results were compared to biopsies from 120 adults.

Most of these children had acquired hepatitis C by exposure to blood or blood products (85 percent) and only 11 percent were vertically transmitted from mother to infant. When researchers studied the liver biopsies under a microscope, they discovered that children had milder degrees of inflammation and lower histologic stages compared to adults. This finding implies a slower progression of disease in children. In fact, none of the biopsies in children demonstrated cirrhosis. However, additional controlled studies to define rates of progression of hepatitis C in children are needed.

NOTE: All patients with underlying liver disease, including hepatitis C, should receive the hepatitis A and hepatitis B vaccines. Please consult your pediatrician, pediatric gastroenterologist, or hepatologist. The hepatitis A vaccine is recommended for children over 1 year of age.

Resource: If you can't afford vaccination shots or don't know where to get them, contact your city, county, or state health department, or call the Centers for Disease Control's Immunization Information Hotline at 800-232-2522. For Spanish language inquiries, call 800-232-0233.

Monitoring Children with Hepatitis C

According to Michael R. Narkewicz, M.D., medical director of the Pediatric Liver Center and Liver Transplant Program at the Children's Hospital in Denver and associate professor in pediatrics at the University of Colorado Medical School, Hewit Andrews Chair in Pediatric Liver Disease, there are no standard recommendations. "Here at the Pediatric Liver Center, our recommendation is that the child should have liver blood tests performed once or twice a year (more frequently if the liver blood tests are abnormal), alpha-fetoprotein (tumor marker) every six-twelve months, and an ultrasound at a minimum of every three years or if the alpha-fetoprotein is rising.

Liver Biopsy.

I was kind of sore after my biopsy, but I watched lots of movies. The nurses moved the bed up and down. And I got spaghetti, pizza, chocolate pudding, and Jell-O!

Haley, age 6

"I think liver biopsy is mandatory before deciding on a course of treatment," says Dr. Narkewicz, "because it tells us how much scarring has occurred in the liver and makes sure that the abnormal blood tests are the result of hepatitis C and not some other unsuspected liver disease.

"We do all our liver biopsies using the needle biopsy technique under sedation or anesthesia to make it more comfortable for the child, less anxiety-provoking, and to minimize risks. It is either a day surgical procedure or involves a short overnight stay. The major risk is bleeding, so we always assess children's blood clotting before a liver biopsy. The risk of significant bleeding in pediatric liver biopsies is about 1 percent."

Blood Draws and Biopsies/Practical Suggestions.

My older daughter, Leigh, was in kindergarten and having a really hard time. She was so worried that something was wrong with her sister, Tammy, that she cried a lot and had nightmares.

I finally learned to schedule Tammy's blood tests when Leigh was somewhere else. The blood tests didn't bother Tammy that much, but Leigh couldn't stand watching the needles, the blood.

So now Tammy and I get our blood drawn together.

Mother of Leigh and Tammy

When I was little, I couldn't stand to have my sister hurt from the blood draws. So I would cry too. I couldn't watch. I'd put my face against the wall and cry and Tammy, who was only 2, would say, "That didn't hurt."

Tammy's sister, Leigh

When a child has hepatitis C, parents frequently have to prepare their child for painful procedures, such as blood draws and biopsies. According to Butler-Simon, emotional pain and physical pain are equally challenging and often inseparable. Doctors and nurses often underestimate pain, but parents know their children best and should be advocates on their behalf.

In 1996 Laura's enzymes shot up into the 70s. They did a hepatitis screen, and sure enough, she had it. It meant constant blood tests. She had one experience where they stuck her five times. She'd scream and carry on. It was traumatic.

Then a nurse told us about this topical anesthetic cream, EMLA® Cream. You put a pretty fair amount over the vein and put a clear dressing on it. You can even use that sticky wrap you cover food with. Keep the cream in place for an hour. It makes life easier for kids afraid of a needle.

Mary

Here are some of Butler-Simon's practical suggestions:

- Use EMLA® Cream to numb the area before a blood draw. Left on the skin for an hour, it will numb the area up to a half-inch deep.
- Give Tylenol® beforehand (size- and age-recommended dosage).
- Prepare the child beforehand, using language and concepts that are developmentally appropriate. Explain the procedure directly, honestly, and simply.
- Bring something distracting with you—anything your child likes to hold, listen to, or watch.
- Teach your child to help herself (Take an imaginary journey? Put on a "magic" sock?).
- Offer choices. Which arm? Sit up or lie down?
- Use a "hug hold" to provide emotional support for a blood draw. Hold the child on your lap. You hug the child, and the child hugs you. Let the health care staff do the rest.

For a biopsy, stronger medication is used to keep the child still and prevent pain. Stay close by and provide a familiar comfort item to help the child relax.[1]

Treatment

I feel mixed up about interferon. I'm going to have to do some serious investigating. What if the treatment could cause my daughter problems later in her life?

I sit here and think, "If I don't do it, this could happen. If I do it, this could happen." I make lists—and I pray a lot and ask for direction.

Patricia

I tried at first to keep it from him. I was devastated, and I needed time to think. Then I decided that at 10 years old he needs to be a part of this, to make decisions, just as I do about my treatment. I would never start treatment without his consent.

He can say, "I'm not ready. Can we think about this?" A positive attitude is powerful.

Irene

*I put off my treatment so my daughter and I could do it together—
so I could be a support to her. I did her shot, and she did mine. It helped
both of us.*

*We'd lie in bed together and watch "Animal Planet." I'd notice that
she would look pale and tired around her eyes. "Darn this hep C thing,"
she'd say.*

"I know," I'd answer, "but we're doing the right thing."

Dana

Criteria for selecting pediatric patients for antiviral therapy are still being defined. Many patients do not have symptoms, have normal or low ALT levels, and exhibit only mild liver injury and early stages of fibrosis on liver biopsy.

In addition, antiviral therapy is difficult to maintain with young people. Complying with the strict regimen of shots and dealing with side effects present challenges.

Despite these concerns, children with significant liver injury or fibrosis should be considered for treatment, even though the effects of this treatment on disease progression are unknown. Children should be referred to and evaluated by a pediatric gastroenterologist with experience in managing antiviral therapy in this unique population.

Pegylated Interferon Plus Ribavirin. Pegylated interferon alfa-2b plus ribavirin has recently been approved by the FDA for use in pediatric cases of chronic hepatitis C. Because the results are superior to interferon monotherapy, interferon plus ribavirin, or pegylated interferon monotherapy, the combination of pegylated interferon plus ribavirin is the new standard of care for treatment of chronic hepatitis C in children.

Weekly Injections of Pegylated Interferon. If a family chooses interferon therapy, it raises complex emotional issues. The parent must administer an injection and then deal with interferon's side effects. No parent likes to poke a child with needles. Often, the mother has gone through treatment herself and knows what side effects her child is facing.

"I do the first dose in the clinic," says Claassen, "and we watch the child for a couple of hours. I have the parents inject me with a saline solution so they get over the fear of entering someone's body with a needle. It's a sacred barrier."

Butler-Simon recommends that the parent allow the nurse to give her a saline injection so she can see how small the needle is and how much easier a subcutaneous (under the skin) injection is than an intra-muscular one. "Am I inflicting pain: No. And the parent can see and feel that I'm not. That's what parents freak out about—hurting the child."

"Many parents have given a shot before—to themselves if they have hepatitis B or to a pet," says Claassen. "But still, even with experience, giving a shot to one's own child is different. We go through the steps to help them gain confidence, and they give the first shot here."

Tools that help parents, such as EMLA® Cream or ice to numb the skin, are like "training wheels," until the parent gains confidence. But it's a trade-off. The cream must stay on the skin for an hour, and during that hour anticipation and dread increase.

"First and foremost," says Butler-Simon, "is setting the attitude of the parent. Kids will respond to the parent's attitude, which should be 'no big deal, and if it is, we'll work through it,' rather than 'I'm so sorry, dear, but we have to do it.'"

Most parents want guidance on the mechanics of administering the injection. "For really young children, infants to age 3 or 4, it's best to give the shot in the butt," says Butler-Simon. "You can lay them in your lap with your leg over their legs, hanging them over your other leg, or place them on their belly on a couch. Distraction helps. Give them a doll that they can give a 'shot' to at the same time to help them feel that they have some control. Praise and stickers are helpful, but then move on. Don't drag the ritual out to the nth degree because you have to do it so frequently.

"At ages 4 to 5, children may be able to be more cooperative. To elicit a sense of control, you can encourage them to do the alcohol swab, for example. For young school-age children, a 'hug-hold' is a good option. You hold the child on your lap. The child hugs you, you hug the child, and another adult gives the shot."

"Sometimes," says Claassen, "you have to come up with a good hold and get it over with. We've never had anyone fail therapy because it involves shots!"

Ribavirin Liquid and Pills. Generally the administration of rib-avirin has been well tolerated in pediatric cases—a liquid formulation of ribavirin is available for weight-based dosing. In addition, side effects of ribavirin, such as anemia, are better tolerated in pediatric cases.

Dose modifications of either pegylated interferon or ribavirin may be necessary in up to 31% of cases, and 7% may not be able to tolerate side effects and drop from treatment.

Rates of SVR with Pegylated Interferon Plus Ribavirin. Rates of SVR are similar or higher than rates of SVR achieved in adults. Regardless of genotype, treatment is administered for 48 weeks in pediatric cases, there is no truncation of treatment at week 24 for genotypes 2 or 3. The overall rates of SVR are:

	SVR
Overall	59%
Genotype 1	48%
Genotype 2/3	100%

Given these impressive response rates, an increasing number of pediatric cases of chronic hepatitis C will undoubtedly undergo treatment.

What About Triple Therapy for Pediatric Cases? At the time of this writing, triple therapy (pegylated interferon plus ribavirin plus protease inhibitor [or other inhibitor-) was just under investigation in adults. There were no pediatric trials. For current information regarding new and emerging treatments and clinical trials for pediatric cases, explore the following resources.

Resources: For news of clinical trials for hepatitis C in children, contact PKIDs at 360-695-0293, website: www.pkids.org. Other websites that track clinical trials include www.centerwatch.com and the National Institutes of Health website: www.cc.nih.gov.

The American Liver Foundation created a national "Pediatric Liver Research Agenda 2000: A Blueprint for the Future, Research Goals and Strategies to Treat, Prevent, and Conquer Childhood Liver Diseases" under the leadership of Ronald Sokol, M.D., Director of Denver's Children's Hospital Pediatric General Clinical Research Center, Associate Medical Director of The Pediatric Liver Center, and Professor of Pediatrics at the University of Colorado Medical School. For a copy of the research agenda, call the ALF at 1-800-GO-LIVER, Ext. 136; website: www.liverfoundation.org/html/advores.htm.

Post-Treatment Follow-Up. Children who respond to interferon should be monitored for complete resolution of markers of viral infection. Non-responders to therapy should be monitored for disease progression.

Cirrhotic patients need to be monitored for early signs of liver decompensation (see chapter 4). These patients are at greatest risk for development of liver cancer because they have both cirrhosis and active viral replication. Evidence of decompensation or development of isolated hepatoma (liver cancer) is an indication for referral for liver transplantation.

Despite these concerns and the need for monitoring, most children with chronic hepatitis C have a relatively benign course with few symptoms and slow progression of liver disease. Time is on their side as treatment options expand, and the likelihood of cure with medical therapy becomes increasingly possible.

> *A child is one who stands halfway*
> *between an adult and a TV set.*
>
> *Anonymous*

Reference

1. Liver Center and Liver Transplantation Program of the Children's Hospital (Denver). "Preparing Children for Painful Procedures," Connections, Fall/Winter 2000, Vol. 13, No. 4: 4–5.

14

RESEARCH
TRENDS

Hope for the Future

In the years since my diagnosis in 1993, I've seen many advances in hepatitis C treatments made possible by research: combination therapy, pegylated interferons, living-donor liver transplants, and now, protease and polymerase inhibitors. Even the once-held belief that cirrhosis is an irreversible death sentence is now being questioned by the HALT C trial.

With each revision of this book, we're able to move more topics from the research chapter to the treatment chapters as theories become reality. In the third edition of "Living with Hepatitis C: A Survivor's Guide," pegylated interferon was just emerging as a therapy. Now, it's the standard for treatment! These exciting developments replace despair with hope. The future looks promising if we continue to raise public awareness and demand more research dollars.

Here's where we can do something. Each of us can talk about hepatitis C and educate others about this viral epidemic. Each of us can contribute time and money to finding the cure.

It's scary to know that a virus is circulating in your body, and that you can't get rid of it. Interferon-based therapies work for some people, but not for everyone. All of us who have been affected by hepatitis C know that there's got to be something better coming down the pike. And we wait and hope.

Hedy

H EPATITIS C RESEARCH falls into two broad and some-what overlapping categories: clinical research and basic research. Clinical research primarily determines whether new drug therapies are effective in treating hepatitis C. Basic research encompasses a wide variety of studies of hepatitis C, including, but not limited to: molecular biology, cell biology, cryobiology and liver cell transplantation, pathophysiology, and pharmacology.

In this chapter, we'll cover the following topics:

- Clinical Research: Testing New Drugs
    Phases of Clinical Trials
    Should You Consider Participating in a Study?
- Current Clinical Research for Treatment of Hepatitis C
    New Interferons
        Albuferon
        Lambda Interferon
    Ribavirin Substitutes
        Viramidine (Taribavirin)
    Targeting the Life-cycle of HCV
        Viral Entry Inhibitors
        Protease Inhibitors
        Polymerase Inhibitors
- Additional Therapies and Strategies under Consideration
    HCV Specific Immunoglobulins
    Vaccine Development
    Therapeutic Vaccines
    Small Interfering RNAs (siRNAs)
    Ribozymes
    Toll-like Receptor Agonists
- Anti-Fibrotic Therapies
    IL-10
    Gamma interferon
    Caspase Inhibitors

• Basic Research
   Mechanisms of Clearance of HCV or Development of Chronic
      Infection
   Animal and Cell Culture Models
   Cell Biology
   Liver Cell Transplantation
   Pathophysiology
   Pharmacology
• Research Funding

Clinical Research: Testing New Drugs

In the United States, pharmaceutical companies, the National Institutes of Health, and some large universities test promising new drugs and submit their results to the Food and Drug Administration (FDA). It is the responsibility of the FDA to critically examine the results of the studies and determine whether the new treatment is safe and effective through a careful system of checks and balances. State review boards also monitor studies and adverse reactions to medications. Drugs approved by the FDA become available to practicing physicians to use in the treatment of hepatitis C.

A well-defined process evaluates all new drugs. First, the drug's safety must be established through animal testing. These studies may also help to define the expected effectiveness and dose ranges of the drug when it is used later in humans. After a drug has undergone animal testing and has been approved by the FDA for clinical research with humans, the drug testing enters three phases.

Phases of Clinical Trials. Studies in Phase I (human toxicity) typically involve small numbers of patients or healthy controls who are given single doses of the drug in varying amounts. Patients are monitored very closely (physical examinations and blood testing) to detect any adverse effect of the medication. Researchers examine the absorption of the drug, its distribution in the body, metabolism, and elimination. Sometimes the cumulative toxicity of multiple doses of drug are examined in Phase I studies.

Phase II (dose finding) studies evaluate the response of the disease to the drug in larger numbers of study subjects. Researchers determine the effectiveness of several different doses of the drug administered over prolonged periods of time to find the "optimal dose" for use in humans. Patients are also carefully monitored for evidence of toxicity.

Phase III (pre-clinical testing) typically treats hundreds to thousands of patients. Again, effectiveness and toxicity are carefully evaluated. Researchers often compare the drug under investigation to existing therapies and medications to obtain a measure of whether the new treatment represents an advance above current treatment strategies. These are the final studies done to obtain FDA approval and will determine how the drug is labeled. After this phase is completed, the results are submitted to the FDA for review. Some of the new drugs to treat chronic hepatitis C, such as protease or polymerase inhibitors, are on a fast track for FDA approval. However, it may still take approximately two years or more for approval and the FDA may reject the drug or request more studies.

Ongoing clinical testing (post-marketing surveillance for problems that might arise) occurs after the FDA has approved the drug, usually for several years, and determines optimal ways to use the drug or new indications for using the drug.

Should You Consider Participating in a Study? Obviously, before you enroll in a specific study, you should take time to review the patient informed consent document that you will have to sign. Be sure to ask how often you will see a doctor; doctor appointments vary at different study sites. You should also consider all the pros and cons of any study.

On the positive side:

1. You may get to try a new treatment that is not available through general clinical practice.
2. Typically, you would receive frequent examinations and careful followup.
3. Study coordinators will keep you informed about your status and progress.
4. Most studies are sponsored by either pharmaceutical companies or research grants, and typically your treatment is delivered without expense to you or your insurer. However, the degree of compensation can vary and you (or your insurer) may be responsible for some of the bill. Some studies also give extra compensation to you for

expenses related to travel to the study site or for the time you spent participating in the research.

5. Your participation is kept confidential. Representatives from the FDA or study sponsors, however, have the right to review your study record.

6. You reserve the right to stop treatment and withdraw from the study at any time.

On the negative side:

1. Testing programs are rigid. You must make the time commitment to follow the protocol exactly. For example, you'll have to show up at certain times for followup tests.

2. Clinical trials are usually blinded. That means that you won't know what you're getting in terms of dosage or placebo, for example. If you have been given a placebo, the pharmaceutical company may offer the active drug to you (free of charge) at the end of your participation in the trial if you have completed the study.

3. Sponsors can stop the trials at any time.

4. You may experience a new, previously unreported side effect.

5. You must be prepared to reveal all aspects of your physical and emotional health.

6. You won't know the results of the whole study, or your individual results, until every participant has completed the protocol. It may take more than a year from your point of enrollment.

You may have heard that it may be possible to be treated with investigational drugs through compassionate-use protocols. Typically, drugs available on a compassionate-use basis have demonstrated effectiveness in studies but "registration trials" have not been done or completed and the drug has not received formal FDA approval. Compassionate-use is generally limited to patients with rare diseases and does not apply to patients with chronic hepatitis C.

Current Clinical Research for Treatment of Hepatitis C

In 2009, the year of this 5th edition of *Living with Hepatitis C: A Survivor's Guide* we entered a new era of clinical research and changing concepts of the treatment of hepatitis C. More than 20 small molecules were being tested in human trials. Two, telaprevir and boceprevir, were in

Phase III trials, a new interferon, Albuferon, had just completed Phase III testing, and the VISER studies of viramidine were finalized. Most of these developments are discussed in detail in Chapter 15. Herein, I will highlight some of the research issues related to these treatments.

New Interferons.

Albuferon. Albuferon has completed its Phase III trials and is in the final steps of evaluation by the FDA. It is a synthetic protein made from the fusion of the gene for albumin with the gene for interferon. The hybrid protein is larger than either albumin or interferon and is eliminated slowly, like albumin, over weeks. Albuferon appears to be similar to pegylated interferons in effectiveness against both HCV genotype 1 (ACHIEVE1 trial) and HCV genotypes 2/3 (ACHIEVE2/3 trial). Overall, the side effects with Albuferon are similar to those of pegylated interferons—although some concern has been raised regarding potential pulmonary toxicity when using high doses (1200 μg/week or more). The main advantage of Albuferon is the ability to dose every other week, compared to the weekly dosing requirement for pegylated interferons. Despite the seeming convenience of twice monthly dosing, data regarding quality of life (presumably improved by less frequent dosing, but not verified yet in reports), compliance with the treatment regimen, or tolerance to the therapy have yet to be reported. The results from ACHIEVE1 and ACHIEVE2/3 were under review by FDA at the time of this writing.

Lambda Interferon. All of the interferons, standard or pegylated, which are FDA approved for treatment of chronic hepatitis C are alpha interferons. They interact with the same cell surface receptors, and induce similar changes in cells to exert antiviral effects against hepatitis C. Lambda interferons exert antiviral effects similar to the alpha interferons but they interact with distinctly different cell surface receptors and regulate different intra-cellular antiviral pathways. Recently it has been shown that lambda interferon has activity against hepatitis C, and in early experience in humans has few, if any, side effects. Lambda interferon is just beginning early Phase clinical trials for chronic hepatitis C.

Ribavirin Substitutes. Viramidine was developed as a substitute for ribavirin. Viramidin is taken orally, delivered to the liver via the portal circulation and converted to ribavirin within the liver. After viramidine is metabolized to ribavirin, ribavirin is concentrated in the liver, and relatively less is delivered to the rest of the body. Since ribavirin concentrations in the liver would be higher after viramidine compared to standard ribavirin, viramidine would theoretically be more effective than ribavirin in treating HCV. In addition, with viramidine less ribavirin is delivered to the rest of the body—so, theoretically, viramidine would have the additional advantage of less ribavirin-related toxicity, such as anemia. Two clinical trials, VISER-1 and VISER-2 (unpublished results), compared viramidine to standard ribavirin in combination with pegylated interferon alfa-2a or alfa-2b. Viramidine was associated with reduction in ribavirin-related toxicity and reduced rates of anemia. Unfortunately, the lowering of toxicity was not accompanied by superior, or even equivalent, effectiveness—rates of SVR were lower with viramidine. A recent dose-finding study reported that the combination of pegylated interferon alfa-2a with viramidine was associated with a rate of SVR (37%) equivalent to pegylated interferon alfa-2a with ribavirin (44%). Rates of significant anemia were significantly lower with viramidine (4% vs 27%). The future status of viramidine in the treatment of chronic hepatitis C is a bit unclear. Perhaps it will have a role in the treatment of patients with chronic hepatitis C who have co-morbid conditions, such as renal insufficiency or prior transplantation and need for calcineurin inhibitors, where ribavirin-induced anemia is particularly problematic.

Targeting the Life-cycle of HCV.

Viral Entry Inhibitors. The uptake of HCV into liver cells involves a very complicated set of interactions with a variety of proteins and factors residing on the surface of liver cells. Efforts are underway to fully characterize these pathways of viral entry and to develop compounds to block the pathways, preventing entry of HCV into the liver cell. Although this strategy would be ineffective for persons already infected, blocking viral entry into liver cells could be useful in management of transplant recipients to prevent reinfection of liver allografts, or as adjunctive therapy with other antiviral agents. Viral entry inhibitors based upon cyclic D,L-α-peptides are currently under investigation in the laboratory.

Protease Inhibitors. Drugs have now been developed that inhibit the HCV-specific serine protease. This enzyme activity of HCV is necessary for creation of all the individual proteins that assemble to form the virus and complete its life cyle or replication. The first HCV-specific protease inhibitor was BILN 2061, developed by Boehringer-Ingle-heim. In Phase I studies of patients with HCV genotype 1 infection, HCV RNA plummeted to nearly undetectable levels within 24 to 48 h of initiation of treatment with BILN 2061. Unfortunately, toxicity testing revealed potential cardiotoxicity and development of BILN 2061 for treatment of human infection was discontinued.

Despite the problems of toxicity with BILN 2061, several effective inhibitors of the HCV protease have emerged, and, at the time of this writing, telaprevir and boceprevir were in Phase III trials (see chapter 15). Other inhibitors are at earlier Phases of testing but also look promising as potential new therapies for chronic hepatitis C.

Two key issues surround the development of HCV protease inhibitors—viral resistance and toxicity. During treatment with an HCV protease inhibitor, forms of HCV emerge (resistant virions) that are resistant to the inhibitor—this is called viral resistance. How is this detected? The response of HCV RNA during treatment provides a clue to the emergence of resistant virions. Initially, with treatment with protease inhibitor, HCV RNA drops rapidly and may even become undetectable. But, with continued treatment HCV RNA increases—the resistant HCV virus is emerging in the face of the protease inhibitor!

What does this mean clinically? HCV protease inhibitors cannot be administered alone, as monotherapy.

Can resistant HCV be blocked or treated? Pegylated interferon plus ribavirin when co-administered with HCV protease inhibitors effectively inhibits the emergence of strains of HCV resistant to the protease inhibitor.

What does this mean clinically? The current HCV protease inhibitors under development for treatment of chronic hepatitis C are given as "triple therapy"—protease inhibitor plus pegylated interferon plus ribavirin.

Because "triple therapy" is the current paradigm for development of HCV protease inhibitor therapy, toxicity (not only of the HCV protease inhibitor but also the backbone of pegylated interferon and ribavirin) may limit future treatment regimens. In the telaprevir trials, special attention is directed towards specific strategies to manage skin rash, and anemia and in the boceprevir trials focus is placed on management of anemia and gastrointestinal symptoms. Optimal management of the side effects, adverse events, and toxicities of the new drugs will be a key to the overall success of "triple therapy".

Polymerase Inhibitors. Two very promising polymerase inhibitors, NM283 and R1626, progressed to Phase II clinical trials but lack of substantial efficacy and development of toxicity limited their development. NM283 exhibited dose-dependent gastrointestinal toxicity and R1626 showed dose-dependent bone marrow suppression. The current (as of 2009) most promising polymerase inhibitor is R7128, which is now entering later Phase II testing (see chapter 15).

As with protease inhibitors, the future of treatment of hepatitis C with polymerase inhibitors appears to be very bright. Undoubtedly it won't be long before treatment of chronic hepatitis C evolves to combinations of protease plus polymerase inhibitors, or other drug classes. In the not too distant future, we might even be using interferon-free or ribavirin-free treatment protocols and regimens (see chapter 15 for early results of the first study of the combination of an inhibitors of HCV protease with an inhibitor of HCV polymerase without co-administration of pegylated interferon or ribavirin).

Additional Therapies and Strategies under Consideration

HCV-Specific Immunoglobulins. Treatment with high-titer antibody against HCV could be one strategy for reducing risk of hepatitis C in the setting of liver transplantation, peri-natal exposure, or needle-stick accidents. The effectiveness of this approach has been clearly demonstrated by use of HBIG (hepatitis B immunoglobulin) in prevention of transmission of hepatitis B. Immunoglobulin preparations with high titers of antibody against HCV have been developed, but none have yet been proven effective in prevention of HCV transmission after liver transplantation.

Vaccine Development. To date, researchers have made only partial and slow progress toward the development of a vaccine against hepatitis C. When vaccines were developed for hepatitis B, researchers knew that antibodies against a specific hepatitis B antigen protected against subsequent infection with hepatitis B.

Unfortunately, no naturally occurring protective antibodies have been identified for hepatitis C; all of the antibodies that have been identified do not protect against subsequent infection with hepatitis C. In addition, hepatitis C is genetically diverse, which makes it difficult to develop a single vaccine effective against all forms of the virus. Nonetheless, some advances have been made, and work is in progress.

Therapeutic Vaccines. One of the central themes to explain the development of chronic hepatitis C is impairment of the T-cell immune response to HCV. Vaccines have now been developed that incorporate the proteins or peptides of HCV into other proteins, molecules, or complex mixtures. This HCV protein/peptide complex is selected to stimulate HCV-specific T-cell responses that would then ultimately lead to recognition of HCV by the immune system, enhancement of the immune response, and eradication of HCV. One therapeutic vaccine from GlobeImmune, Inc., in early Phases of testing, has demonstrated some ability to stimulate HCV-specific immune responses in patients with chronic hepatitis C. In addition, in combination with pegylated interferon alfa-2a and ribavirin, this vaccine has improved early on-treatment virologic responses. It is not known whether this vaccine when used with other antiviral strategies will enhance rates of SVR.

Small Interfering RNAs. Treatment of viral infections with RNA is particularly appealing because the therapeutic RNAs can be designed to bind specifically and exclusively to HCV. Early attempts with this treatment included RNAs that would bind to and destroy HCV RNA (Heptazyme—an HCV-specific ribozyme) or oligonucleotides that would bind to and inactivate HCV RNA. Unfortunately, these approaches have been ineffective in treatment of hepatitis C. A new approach uses small RNA fragments (small interfering RNAs, siRNAs) that bind specifically to HCV and inactivate the virus. SiRNA treatment has yet to enter into clinical trials.

Ribozymes. Ribozymes are RNA molecules that bind to specific regions of other RNAs and cleave the bound RNA (RNA RNAases). Recently, ribozymes have been synthesized that specifically bind to hepatitis C RNA and cleave the virus, inactivating it and preventing its replication. Although Phase I trials of the hepatitis C-specific ribozyme (HeptazymeTM) indicated no adverse reactions, during Phase II rashes were noted and in toxicology studies in primates one monkey developed blindness. Heptazyme was removed from further testing.

Toll–like Receptor Agonists. One mechanism of recognition and activation of the immune response against HCV is mediated through a group of proteins on the surface of immune cells. These proteins are called Toll-like receptors. One drug, isatoribine, selectively activates Toll-like Receptor 7, and may be useful in treatment of hepatitis C. Isatoribine, 800 mg daily, was administered for 7 days to 12 persons with chronic hepatitis C who had never been treated previously. HCV RNA decreased by an average of 0.76 log10, suggesting possible beneficial antiviral effects. Additional studies of Toll-like receptor agonists are underway.

Anti-Fibrotic Therapies

IL-10. Interleukin-10 (IL-10) has been evaluated mainly for its potential use as an anti-fibrotic agent. It is a naturally occurring compound in our bodies that regulates inflammatory reactions to infection or injury. In the liver, inflammation stimulates pathways of fibrosis. Studies of model systems suggested that IL-10 could suppress inflammation and limit or even reverse fibrosis. One pilot study of a small number of patients with hepatitis C suggested that IL-10 could potentially reverse fibrosis.

For this reason, IL-10 was examined in a large multi-center trial where biopsies were performed at the start and periodically throughout the trial. Treatment biopsies demonstrated reduction in inflammation but no consistent improvement in fibrosis. In addition, side effects included headaches and dizziness, and there has been concern over possible neurotoxicity. IL-10 has been withdrawn from further testing in clinical trials.

Gamma-Interferon. Gamma-interferon is another potential anti-fibrotic agent, and, like IL-10, is a natural compound in our bodies that regulates inflammatory reactions to infection or injury. Gamma-interferon also reduces the transformation of specific cells within the liver (stellate cells) to another form or cell type (myofiboblasts) that increase fibrosis. The group of hepatitis C patients targeted for this treatment is that of nonresponders to prior treatment with the combination of interferon-alfa plus ribavirin who have significant liver fibrosis. This group is at risk for clinical deterioration, need for liver transplantation, and development of liver cancer as the liver fibrosis progresses. The rationale for treatment is that inhibition or regression of fibrosis by gamma-interferon might reduce these risks. However, initial trials of gamma-interferon in patients with chronic hepatitis C have failed to demonstrated an anti-fibrotic effect and additional studies are not currently planned.

Caspase Inhibitors. The development of hepatic fibrosis is a complex process involving multiple metabolic pathways. A number of these pathways are current targets for drug development. Perhaps the one with greatest current promise is reduction in death rates of liver cells by inhibiting one of the key enzymes, caspase. Liver cell death may stimulate pathways that increase liver fibrosis and inhibition of liver cell death may reduce liver fibrosis. Caspase inhibitors are just now entering clinical trials but early results suggest potential beneficial effect on hepatic fibrosis.

Basic Research

Mechanisms of Clearance of HCV or Development of Chronic Infection. This is a very important and emerging area of current and future research. When HCV infects a liver cell, the proteins of the virus interact with the proteins and signals within the liver cell. By this interaction, HCV disrupts the natural processes within your liver cell to clear HCV—in other words, HCV sets up the house it wants to live in! With potent new antivirals, HCV replication might be lowered to such a low level, and your liver cell's mechanisms for clearing HCV could be restored. A key area of research is to understand the interaction of HCV with your liver cell's proteins, genes, and metabolism.

HCV constantly mutates to produce multiple variants. New antiviral medicines might work against some (but not all) forms of HCV, allowing for emergence of resistant strains. Mechanisms of action and development of viral variants with resistance to antiviral agents are currently under intense investigation. This research is critical to optimizing the best combinations of protease inhibitors, polymerase inhibitors, and other drugs in treatment regimens.

In addition to viral mechanisms of resistance, immune responses are key to clearance of HCV and prevention of relapse. After an acute infection with HCV, a person may clear the infection (15 to 45% of the time), or develop chronic infection and live with HCV for the rest of their life, unless cured by antiviral treatment. Why does one person clear HCV and another develop chronic infection? Differences in the immune response to HCV are likely at the core of the answer to this question. For this reason, several groups are now examining key immune responses in cohorts of patients who have experienced acute hepatitis C. The results may lead to more effective vaccine development or even new immune-based strategies to treat patients with chronic hepatitis C.

Animal and Cell Culture Models. Studies of hepatitis C have been hampered by lack of a convenient experimental model of the infection. The ideal model for studying hepatitis C would be one that mimics the infection in humans and is affordable, widely available, and allows for easily reproducible manipulation of experimental conditions.

Even though there have been significant recent advances, the ideal system for studying HCV remains elusive.

Primates have generally served as the main animal model. The chimpanzee is 98.5 percent genetically similar to humans and a wide array of information has been gained from the study of hepatitis C in chimpanzees: viral transmission, time course of viral infection, characterization of the virus, and testing of infectivity of HCV clones. However, studies of hepatitis C in chimpanzees are difficult due to lack of availability and expense. The chimpanzee is the only primate susceptible to infection with hepatitis C. Other primates, including cynomolgus monkey, rhesus monkey, green monkey, Japanese monkey, and doguera baboon, have been intravenously inoculated with hepatitis C and failed to develop infection. Results have been conflicting in transmission studies done with marmosets, tupaias, and tamarins.

Non-primates lack susceptibility to infection with hepatitis C. However, genetic manipulations have now yielded the "trimeric mouse" model. In the model, the mouse liver is populated by human hepatocytes which can now sustain and support HCV infection and replication. The hope is that this whole animal model will be useful not only in studying HCV infection and replication and response to antiviral therapy, but that it may also serve as a model for studying the development and progression of disease and fibrosis.

Within the last two years, scientists have had success in developing cell culture systems that express and maintain HCV replication. The hope is that these models will be very useful in studying HCV infection, replication, response to anti-viral therapy, and mechanisms of resistance to anti-viral medications. However, cell culture systems will still be inadequate for examining all aspects of hepatitis C infection and will give little or no information regarding mechanisms of progression of liver damage.

Cell Biology. Despite what we do know about the hepatitis C genes and many of the proteins produced, little is known about the interaction between the hepatitis C virus and the liver cell. Future studies in this area should yield fruitful information for designing therapies, but right now many questions remain unanswered, including the following:

- What attracts hepatitis C to the liver and not to other tissues?
- How does hepatitis C bind to the surface of a liver cell and get into it?
- Once hepatitis C enters the liver cell, how does it survive?

- Why doesn't the liver cell simply swallow it up and digest it?
- What cellular systems in the liver cell are required to aid the replication of the virus?
- What are the key determinants of assembly of the viral proteins and genes to form an active infectious particle?
- What processes within the liver cell control the secretion of the viral particle out of the cell?

An example of the interaction between proteins of HCV and key molecular pathways inside liver cells is the inhibition of interferon-responsive proteins. Interferon's mechanism of action inside cells is mediated first by binding of interferon to its receptor at the surface of the cell. Then, through complex signaling within the cell, proteins are produced by the cell that inhibit HCV. Interestingly, specific proteins produced by HCV block the production of these interferon-responsive proteins, thereby blocking or inhibiting the anti-viral action of interferon. HCV sets up defenses that make it difficult for interferon to work effectively—I mentioned earlier that HCV sets up its own "house," but perhaps a better analogy is that HCV sets up its own "castle".

Liver Cell Transplantation. Early experience with liver cell transplantation was hampered by lack of adequate supply of viable liver cells and inability to isolate and expand stem cells that could repopulate a diseased liver. Now, with the advent of methods for isolation, storage, and subsequent use of human stem cells, this research may once again emerge and have relevance for the treatment of end-stage liver disease.

Pathophysiology. One interesting feature of hepatitis C (and viral hepatitis in general) is that the hepatitis C infection probably is not sufficient to destroy or damage liver cells by itself. We don't fully understand the complex process of liver cell injury and the formation of fibrous tissue in the liver. Finally, repair mechanisms, such as liver regeneration, are poorly defined.

Many different laboratories are studying the effects of cofactors that may contribute to liver cell injury, fibrosis, regeneration, and progression to cirrhosis. These cofactors include processes such as excessive iron accumulation, oxidative stress, abnormal bile salts, and inflammatory mediators released by immune cells.

In the absence of effective therapies to eradicate hepatitis C, therapies that can modify basic mechanisms of cell injury and fibrosis may reduce the rate of progression to cirrhosis and the need for liver transplantation, slow the progression to liver failure, and reduce the rate of death from liver disease.

Pharmacology. As you can see, it's easy to understand that future treatment of hepatitis C could involve medications that target many different sites. There are now several clinical trials of the use of protease and polymerase inhibitors in the treatment of hepatitis C. Trials of other agents are being planned or soon to begin. One of the key clinical areas for research is determination of the absorption, disposition, activity, and interactions of the new therapies. Typical studies for determining these features of new drugs are called pharmacokinetic (PK) or pharmacodynamic (PD) studies. If you participate in a clinical trial of new drug therapy, often you will be asked to consider a substudy, or ancillary study, whereby additional samples of blood may be required to define the aspects of the new treatment.

Research Funding

It is my hope that we are entering a new era in the treatment of hepatitis C, where research may ultimately lead to discoveries of more effective treatments that benefit patients. Research into the basic mechanisms of hepatitis C replication and infection of the liver cell is absolutely essential, so that our understanding and treatment of this devastating disease may leap forward.

Funds for hepatitis C research at the National Institutes of Health increased from $34 million in 2000 to an estimated $130 million in 2005. This is a step in the right direction, but it's obvious that we do not yet understand the enormous financial—let alone emotional—scope of the HCV crisis. A report issued by Milliman & Robertson, Inc., developed an actuarial model to evaluate the economic impact of hepatitis C on the U.S. population. It found that without effective curative treatment (defined in the report as combination therapy, interferon-alfa plus ribavirin) total health care costs for patients infected with hepatitis C will peak at an estimated $26 billion (in current dollars) per year in about 2021."[1]

Clearly, research that results in better treatment ultimately saves money as well as lives. Hepatitis C patients, friends, and family members must focus attention on research. We must make it our top priority to confront, define, and eradicate this serious viral infection, chronic hepatitis C.

Where observation is concerned,
chance favors only the prepared mind.

Louis Pasteur

References

1. Dulworth, Sherrie, R.N., Sunit Patel, FSA, MAAA, Bruce S. Pyenson, FSA, MAAA. "The Hepatitis Epidemic: Looking at the Tip of the Iceberg," Milliman & Robertson, Inc. 2000:1.

2. Lanford RE, Matthew J. Evans, Volker Lohmann, Brett Lindenbach, Michael Gale Jr, Barbara Rehermann, Kyong-Mi Chang, Stanley M. Lemon. "The Accelerating Pace of HCV Research: A Summary of the 15th International Symposium on Hepatitis C Virus and Related Viruses." *Gastroenterology* 2009;136:9-16.

15

ADVANCES IN
TREATMENT

From Bench to Bedside:
Theory in Practice

I have been involved in the care and management of patients with chronic hepatitis C for over 30 years. Until 1989, the disease was called nonA, nonB hepatitis and there were few therapeutic options—only nonpegylated interferon, mainly through participation in clinical trials. Since the discovery of the hepatitis C virus, treatment options for patients with chronic hepatitis C have steadily improved—from nonpegylated interferon monotherapy to the current standard of pegylated interferon/ ribavirin. The two big steps in improving rates of SVR were the addition of ribavirin and the use of pegylated interferon. With the discovery and clinical development of inhibitors of the HCV protease and HCV polymerase, as well as other therapeutic advances, we should anticipate another big step forward in the treatment of chronic hepatitis C.

Dr. Everson

THE GOAL OF THIS chapter is to look to the future to give you an idea of the new treatments that may soon become clinical reality. Please understand that many of the treatments described in this chapter are in clinical trials and have not yet been approved by the Food and Drug Administration. Some are only in early phases of testing (Phase I) and others in later stages just prior to release for clinical use (Phase III) (see Chapter 14 for description of Phases of clinical trials).

Caution: There is no guarantee that any of the treatments discussed in this chapter will make the transition from research trials to use in the clinic.

In this final chapter, we'll cover latest information related to the following topics:

• New developments potentially impacting the management of pegylated interferon/ribavirin therapy and side effects
  Growth Factors
  Thrombopoeitin analogue
  Management of side effects

• Retreatment after an unsuccessful course of pegylated interferon/ribavirin
  Reduction in doses or discontinuation of pegylated interferon or ribavirin
  Retreatment Options based upon Virologic Response with Prior Therapy
    Breakthrough
    Relapse
    Slow Virologic Response
    Partial Response
    Null Response
    Indeterminate Response
    Treatment options

• Maintenance low-dose pegylated interferon monotherapy
  HALT-C Trial
  Other studies (COPILOT and EPIC)

• STAT-C Drugs
  Protease (NS3-4a) Inhibitors

Compounds in Phase III of Clinical Testing
Telaprevir
Boceprevir
Other Protease Inhibitors in Clinical Trials
Polymerase Inhibitors
Nucleoside Polymerase Inhibitors
Valopicitabine
R1626
R7128
Additional Nucleoside Polymerase Inhibitors under Development
Non-nucleoside Polymerase Inhibitors
HCV-796
NS5A Inhibitors
AZ12781194
BMS790052
Interferon-free STAT-C Treatment Regimens

• Nitazoxanide

• Summary

New Developments Potentially Impacting the Management of Pegylated Interferon/Ribavirin Therapy and Side Effects

GROWTH FACTORS

During pegylated interferon/ribavirin treatment, your white blood cell, red blood cell, and platelet counts typically decrease. Occasionally the decrease in blood cells and platelets may need treatment, especially if you and your treating physician or care provider wish to continue the pegylated interferon/ribavirin treatment. Treatment options are mainly twofold—reduce doses of pegylated interferon or ribavirin, or treat the reduced cell counts with drugs that stimulate the bone marrow to produce more blood cells. The three main groups of growth factors that are used in patients with chronic hepatitis C are synthetic analogues of naturally-occurring granulocyte-colony stimulating factor (G-CSF) for white cells, erythropoietin for red cells, and thrombopoeitin for platelets. Physicians with extensive experience in treating chronic hepatitis C will be familiar with both G-CSF and erythropoeitin analogue. Thrombopoeitin analogues are the newest addition to growth factor therapy and are currently under study in clinical trials.

Caution: Choosing one strategy over another is a complex clinical decision—you will need to work closely with your care providers to decide the best options for your specific case. The discussion below is meant to give you information about treatment options for low cell counts, but is not an endorsement or recommendation of a given strategy.

Granulocyte-colony stimulating factor (G-CSF). Pegylated interferon causes a reduction in white blood cells in nearly all patients—the decrease is greatest in a type of white blood cell called the neutrophil (as opposed to lymphocyte). Marked decreases in white blood cells may increase your risk of infection during pegylated interferon/ribavirin treatment and your doctor may advise reduction in pegylated interferon dose or treatment with G-CSF. Risk of infection is greatest when absolute neutophil count decreases below 250 neutrophils/µl. If pegylated interferon/ribavirin treatment reduces your neutrophil count to less than 500 neutrophils/µl, there are only two options—reduce the dose of pegylated interferon or treat with G-CSF. Reducing pegylated interferon may decrease your chances for SVR, but adding G-CSF is expensive and using G-CSF has not definitely been shown to increase your chance for SVR. The decision to dose reduce pegylated interferon or increase G-CSF will also depend upon other factors, including the rate of reduction in HCV RNA with treatment and other side effects that you might be experiencing that could be related to pegylated interferon. Your doctor will weigh all options when deciding the best strategy for your specific case.

Erythropoeitin analogues. Anemia, a decrease in your red blood cells, is mainly due to ribavirin. Ribavirin breaks down the older blood cells in your circulation (hemolysis)—this breakdown of the red blood cells not only lowers your red cell count, reducing your hematocrit, but also releases heme from the red cells that is then converted to bilirubin (the pigment in the blood that causes jaundice). The hemolysis from ribavirin is associated with a slight increase in your bilirubin; it should be noted that this increase is not due to worsening of your liver function, but simply reflects the red cell breakdown.

If the anemia is severe you can become fatigued and short of breath, or notice poor exercise tolerance. More serious complications of anemia can include limitation of delivery of oxygen to the heart causing chest pain or damage to other organs. Reduced supply of oxygen to the heart may place you at risk for a heart attack (myocardial infarction). If you develop significant anemia during pegylated interferon/ribavirin treatment, your doctor may advise reduction in ribavirin dose or treatment with erythropoeitin analogue. Risk of complications of anemia is greatest when the hemoglobin level in blood drops below 8 grams per deciliter. There are only two options—reduce the dose of ribavirin or treat with erythropoeitin analogue. Reducing ribavirin may reduce your chances for SVR, but adding erythropoeitin analogue is expensive and using erythropoeitin analogue has not definitely been shown to increase your chance for SVR. The decision to dose reduce ribavirin or use erythropoeitin analogue will also depend upon other factors, including the rate of reduction in HCV RNA with treatment and other side effects that you might be experiencing that could be related to pegylated interferon, ribavirin, or erythropoeitin analogue.

Caution: Erythropoeitin analogue has been associated with the very serious, but rare, complication of pure red cell aplasia, which is the loss of cells in the bone marrow that make red blood cells. The Food and Drug Administration has issued a warning that this adverse reaction can occur in patients with chronic hepatitis C who are treated with pegylated interferon/ribavirin and receive erythropoeitin analogue. Your doctor will need to weigh all options when deciding the best strategy for management of anemia in your specific case.

THROMBOPOEITIN ANALOGUE

Platelet count is reduced in patients with chronic hepatitis C, mainly in patients with advanced fibrosis or cirrhosis. The low platelet count in chronic liver disease results from portal hypertension, which enlarges the spleen where the platelets are trapped and destroyed. A second reason is reduction in the liver's production of thrombopoeitin—a growth factor produced by the liver that stimulates the bone marrow to make platelets. During pegylated interferon/ribavirin treatment, pegylated interferon may further reduce your platelet count by decreasing the rate of production of platelets by the bone marrow. The main consequence of significantly reduced platelet count is risk of bleeding, since platelets are the cellular elements in the blood that participate in initial clot formation. The lower limit of a normal platelet count is ~140,000 platelets/µl, but reduction in platelet count to as low as 30,000 platelets/µl is associated with only minimal risk for bleeding. Generally, to minimize risk of bleeding, the dose of pegylated interferon is reduced when platelet counts drop below 50,000 platelets/μl and held when the count is less than 30,000 platelets/μl.

Thrombopoeitin analogue may offer an alternative to dose reduction in patients experiencing significant thrombocytopenia (decrease in platelet count) during pegylated interferon treatment. Two drugs, romiplastin which is administered by injection and eltrombopag which is taken orally, are Food and Drug Administration approved for use in a rare disorder of the immune system called idiopathic thrombocytopenic purpura, which lowers platelet count. These two drugs, and a third, are currently under investigation in clinical trials for use in patients with liver disease. In the future, your care provider may be able to treat the decrease in your platelet count with one of the thrombopoeitin analogue in order to maintain doses of pegylated interferon in the therapeutic range.

MANAGEMENT OF SIDE EFFECTS

Current clinical research suggests that pegylated interferon/ribavirin will remain a component of the future treatment of chronic hepatitis C. The profile of side effects with pegylated interferon/ribavirin is considerable and discussed in Chapters 8 and 9. Most care providers are aware that patients with chronic hepatitis C treated with pegylated interferon/ribavirin may develop depression, mood instability, anxiety, and insomnia and require treatment with antidepressants, sedatives, and anxiolytics. The addition of another antiviral drug(s) may increase the intensity of typical pegylated interferon/ribavirin side effects or introduce new side effects that require additional management strategies. For example, ribavirin is associated with skin rash which improves or resolves with dose reduction of ribavirin. In the phase 2 trials of telaprevir administered with pegylated interferon/ribavirin, rash occurred with increased frequency and was more severe. The strategy for management included discontinuation of telaprevir, and use of topical therapy or systemic steroids. If rash persisted, ribavirin was either reduced or discontinued (rash management in patients taking telaprevir is discussed in greater detail below).

Retreatment After an Unsuccessful Course of Peginterferon/Ribavirin

You may have already had some type of interferon treatment yet, despite the treatment, you remain infected with hepatitis C virus. Prior to consideration of the future treatments, you and your physician may discuss the option of retreatment with peginterferon/ribavirin. If your prior therapy was interferon monotherapy, interferon plus ribavirin, or peginterferon monotherapy, retreatment with peginterferon/ribavirin has a reasonable chance for SVR (this topic is also discussed in greater detail in Chapter 9.) However, if your prior treatment was peginterferon/ribavirin, retreatment with peginterferon/ribavirin offers less chance for SVR. Retreatment should mainly be considered in patients whose first course of peginterferon/ribavirin was characterized by:

• Reduction in doses or discontinuation of pegylated interferon or ribavirin
• Breakthrough
• Relapse
• Slow virologic response

REDUCTIONS IN DOSES OR DISCONTINUATION OF PEGYLATED INTERFERON OR RIBAVIRIN.

Several studies have shown that both dose reductions and discontinuation of pegylated interferon or ribavirin reduce your chance for SVR. Highest rates of SVR are achieved by patients who are able to take 80% of the prescribed dose and duration of both pegylated interferon and ribavirin. In determining whether to retreat with pegylated interferon/ribavirin, you and your care provider must define the problems you experienced with the first course of pegylated interferon/ribavirin. And, importantly, whether options for managing or controlling the side effect(s) are available. For example, if reduced red blood cell count was a reason for dose reduction or discontinuation of ribavirin, perhaps erythropoeitin analogue could be used to maintain ribavirin dose. In another case, mood alteration may have lead to dose reduction. In this case, prophylaxis with antidepressant medications and psychological or social support may permit full-dose therapy. There are many factors causing dose reduction or discontinuation in pegylated interferon/ribavirin—the key is to identify an effective management strategy prior to initiating retreatment.

RETREATMENT OPTIONS BASED UPON VIROLOGIC RESPONSE WITH PRIOR THERAPY BREAKTHROUGH.

Breakthrough is defined by re-emergence of HCV RNA after achieving undetectable HCV RNA, despite ongoing treatment with pegylated interferon/ribavirin. In my experience, breakthrough is usually related to other factors or side effects that lead to dose reductions. Many studies include patients who have experienced breakthrough in the same category as patients who have experienced relapse.

Relapse. Relapse is defined by achieving undetectable HCV RNA during pegylated interferon/ribavirin and maintaining undetectable HCV RNA while completing the pegylated interferon/ribavirin course. Then, in post-treatment follow-up, HCV RNA re-emerges. Retreatment of patients experiencing relapse with a second course of pegylated interferon/ribavirin is associated with rates of SVR ranging from 30 to 40% (see below, and Chapter 9).

Slow Virologic Response. Slow virologic response is a term used to describe a slow rate of clearance of HCV RNA, not achieving undetectable HCV RNA until week 24 of treatment. Although this occurs mainly in patients infected with genotype 1 HCV, the principle applies to all genotypes. Patients with HCV genotype 1 and a slow virologic response to pegylated interferon/ribavirin have a characteristic treatment response:

- Week 4:   >1 log10 decrease from baseline HCV RNA
- Week 12:   >2 log10 decrease from baseline HCV RNA
- Week 24:   Negative HCV RNA
- Follow-up Rx: Increased risk for either Breakthrough or Relapse

Three studies have examined the impact of increasing duration of treatment in patients with a slow virologic response. In these trials, rates of SVR increased 13 to 28% by extension of the duration of treatment from 48 to 72 weeks. Extending duration of treatment is often recommended for patients with a slow virologic response.

Partial Response. Partial response on treatment is defined by >2 log_{10} (greater than 100 fold) decrease in HCV RNA from baseline but persistence of detectable HCV RNA. The patient with a partial response always tests positive for HCV RNA during and after therapy, despite marked reduction in HCV RNA during treatment. Patients with a partial virologic response who have detectable HCV RNA after 24 weeks of treatment have less than 5% chance for SVR. Retreatment with a second course of pegylated interferon/ribavirin is not likely to be effective in these patients.

Null Response. The patient with a null response fails to lower HCV RNA significantly at either 4 or 12 weeks of treatment. The usual definition is less than a 2 $\log_{10}$ (100-fold) decrease by week 12 of treatment relative to baseline HCV RNA level. Null responders are very unlikely to respond to another course of pegylated interferon/ribavirin and retreatment is not recommended.

Indeterminate Response. In some cases the response to the prior course of antiviral therapy is not well documented—the patient had a course of pegylated interferon/ribavirin and in follow-up after treatment remained positive for HCV RNA. These patients represent a mixture of responses including breakthrough, relapse, slow virologic response, partial response and null response. In the EPIC trial, SVR after retreatment of this group of patients with pegylated interferon/ribavirin was 14%.

Treatment Options. Patients whose prior course of treatment was pegylated interferon/ribavirin have only two options for re-treatment with currently available, FDA-approved therapy. These options include either a second course of pegylated interferon/ribavirin or interferon alfacon-1/ribavirin. Interferon alfacon-1 (consensus interferon or Infergen®), is discussed in some detail in Chapter 8. The results from studies of patients who relapsed or failed to respond to pegylated interferon/ribavirin, REPEAT, EPIC, and DIRECT, are given in the following table.

TABLE 15 A. RETREATMENT OF PATIENTS WHO RELAPSED OR FAILED TO RESPOND TO A PRIOR COURSE OF PEGYLATED INTERFERON/RIBAVIRIN

Prior Response	Study	Re-Treatment Regimen	SVR
Relapse	EPIC	PEG-2b + RBV, 48 wk	33%
Nonresponse	EPIC	PEG-2b + RBV, 48 wk	6%
	REPEAT	PEG-2a (360→180) + RBV, 48 wk	7%
		PEG-2a (180) + RBV, 48 wk	9%
		PEG-2a (360→180) + RBV, 72 wk	16%
		PEG-2a (180) + RBV, 72 wk	14%
	DIRECT	cIFN, 9μg/d + RBV, 48 wks	7%
		cIFN, 15μg/d + RBV, 48 wks	11%

Nonresponse includes both partial and null response–persistence of HCV RNA throughout the prior course of treatment and follow-up; SVR (sustained virologic response); PEG-2b (PEGINTRON); RBV (ribavirin); PEG-2a (PEGASYS); 360→180, µg administered in first 12 and subsequent weeks; cIFN (INFERGEN).

Retreatment of relapsers with another course of pegylated interferon/ribavirin yields a 33% chance for SVR. Retreatment of nonresponders is less favorable with only a 16% chance for SVR after 72 weeks of treatment and use of high dose pegylated interferon. With daily injections of high dose consensus interferon SVR was only 11%. Clearly, more effective options are needed for relapsers and nonresponders.

ARE THERE NEW INTERFERONS OR RIBAVIRIN SUBSTITUTES AVAILABLE THAT MIGHT INCREASE YOUR CHANCES FOR SVR?
New Interferons. Are there any new interferons on the horizon that might improve your chances for clearing hepatitis C? Other interferons, with less side effects, might yield higher rates of SVR with retreatment, especially if the prior course of treatment was complicated by dose reductions or discontinuations due to side effects or intolerance to pegylated interferon.

Albuferon is a synthetic protein made from the fusion of the gene for albumin with the gene for interferon and has recently completed two Phase III clinical trials in patients, unaware of treatment, with HCV genotype 1 (ACHIEVE 1) and HCV genotype 2/3 (ACHIEVE 2/3). The main advantage of Albuferon is longer duration of action, allowing dosing every 2 weeks instead of the weekly dosing required for pegylated interferon. In these trials, the combination of Albuferon, 900 ug administered every 2 weeks with ribavirin, was comparable to pegylated interferon/ribavirin in all measures of virologic response— rates of SVR were nearly identical. In HCV genotype 1, the SVR was 48% with Albuferon/ribavirin and 51% with pegylated interferon/ribavirin. In HCV genotype 2/3, the SVR was 80% with Albuferon/ribavirin and 85% with pegylated interferon/ribavirin. Not only were virologic responses similar, but incidence of side effects was also very similar.

If Albuferon is approved by the Food and Drug Administration and available, it is not clear that retreatment with Albuferon/ribavirin could improve the chances of prior nonresponders/relapsers to achieve SVR. Why? First, data using Albuferon/ribavirin to treat nonresponders/

relapsers is lacking. And, second, Albuferon is equivalent and not superior to pegylated interferon in terms of virologic response and the spectrum of side effects. Additional studies would be required to determine the role of Albuferon in this population of patients.

Caution. Albuferon remains under review and is not currently approved by the Food and Drug Administration.

Pegylated interferon–lambda is a type 3 interferon in early phases of testing (data presented at EASL 2009). Weekly and biweekly injections of pegylated interferon–lambda were given to 6 patients with HCV genotype 1 and who relapsed after a prior course of pegylated interferon-alfa therapy. This group of patients was chosen for study because they were known to be responsive to interferon-alfa treatment. HCV RNA declined by 2.3 to 4.9 $\log_{10}$ (100 to 100,000-fold decrease) by week 4 of re-treatment with pegylated interferon–lambda. These preliminary results suggest that it may be effective against HCV. In contrast to pegylated interferon-alfa, pegylated interferon–lambda had few side effects and did not decrease white blood cell or platelet counts. If proven to have potent antiviral effects, the low side effect profile could favor use of lambda interferon in retreatment protocols, especially in patients demonstrating intolerance of pegylated interferon-alfa during the initial course of treatment. Additional studies are needed to determine the role of pegylated interferon–lambda in the management of patients with chronic hepatitis C.

Ribavirin Substitutes. Another potential approach in retreatment could be the use of alternatives to ribavirin that have fewer side effects and adverse reactions. Unfortunately, effective ribavirin substitutes have not yet emerged.

Levovirin. One of the first ribavirin substitutes to be studied was L-ribavirin, the mirror image of R-ribavirin which is currently used in combination therapy. The huge advantage of L-ribavirin was its lack of side effects, specifically anemia. However, L-ribavirin was not active against hepatitis C and clinical development ceased.

Viramidine, a pro-drug of ribavirin, is taken orally, delivered to the liver via the portal circulation, and converted to ribavirin within the liver. Because viramidine is converted to ribavirin in the liver, concentrated in the liver, and delivers less ribavirin to the rest of the body, viramidine has the potential to mimick the effectiveness of ribavirin, but have less of ribavirin-related toxicity, such as anemia.

The safety and effectiveness of viramidine were compared to ribavirin in two large trials, VISER-1 and VISER-2. In these trials, combinations of pegylated interferons with viramidine were compared to pegylated interferons with ribavirin. In VISER-1 the pegylated interferon was Peg-Intron and in VISER-2 the pegylated interferon was Pegasys; otherwise, study designs between VISER-1 and VISER-2 were similar.

In VISER-1, anemia (hemoglobin less than or equal to 10 g/dL) occurred in only 5% of patients receiving viramidine compared to 24% receiving ribavirin. The perceived beneficial effect of viramidine, reduction of anemia, was realized. Unfortunately, rates of SVR were lower with viramidine (38 vs 52 percent). The lower rates of SVR to viramidine were consistent, regardless of genotype. Rates of SVR were 29 percent with viramidine compared to 42 percent with ribavirin for patients infected with HCV genotype 1. Rates of SVR were 62 percent with viramidine compared to 78 percent with ribavirin in patients infected with HCV genotypes 1, 2 and 3. Similar patterns of results were observed in VISER-2. Thus, although viramidine is less often associated with significant anemia, it is inferior to ribavirin in virologic responses.

Despite the lower rates of virologic response with viramidine that were observed in VISER trials, certain populations uniquely susceptible to adverse effects of ribavirin—such as transplant recipients, or patients with renal failure, chronic anemia, or cirrhosis—might still benefit from use of viramidine. However, these statements are speculative since there have been no studies examining viramidine in these patient populations.

There are no new ribavirin substitutes currently in clinical trials. In the absence of effective current measures to control HCV, could maintenance low-dose pegylated interferon halt the progression of liver disease? Should you take maintenance therapy?

Maintenance Low-Dose Pegylated Interferon Monotherapy HALT-C Trial

THE HEPATITIS C ANTIVIRAL LONG-TERM TREATMENT AGAINST CIRRHOSIS (HALT-C) TRIAL.

The National Institutes of Health (NIH), in conjunction with Roche as the industry partner, funded a multi-center trial to examine the ability of low-dose maintenance therapy with peginterferon alfa-a (PEGASYS), 90 µg/wk, to reduce the rate of progression of liver fibrosis to cirrhosis and prevent clinical deterioration. The full results of this trial have just recently been published in the New England Journal of Medicine (see references at end of this chapter).

The 1,050 patients enrolled in HALT-C had persistence of HCV RNA, despite a prior course of pegylated interferon/ribavirin, and had advanced fibrosis or cirrhosis on liver biopsy. Additional characteristics included 94% genotype 1 HCV, mean BMI 30 kg/m2, 70% male, and 41% had cirrhosis on liver biopsy. None of the patients with cirrhosis had had a prior clinical decompensation, meaning that these patients were clinically stable and had not had gastrointestinal bleeding, fluid retention, or changes in their mentation (mental status or cognition). Half of the patients received maintenance therapy and the other half were not treated but did undergo the clinical follow-up. Both groups were followed for 3.5 years or more and had frequent clinical assessments and laboratory tests. Ultrasonography was performed every 12 months, and endoscopy and liver biopsy performed at years 1.5 and 3.5 years after randomization.

The results were disappointing: low dose maintenance therapy did not slow disease progression or positively impact clinical outcomes in patients with either fibrosis or cirrhosis. The proportions of patients with an outcome were 34% in the treated group and 34% in the control untreated group—identical! Progression in fibrosis was defined as a two-point-increase in Ishak fibrosis score between baseline and follow-up liver biopsies. A two-point increase was observed in 28% of treated and 32% of untreated patients—again, nearly identical! Although not a primary objective of the study, maintenance pegylated interferon also failed to reduce risk for development of varices, enlargement of varices, and development of hepatocellular cancer.

In a subgroup analysis of the HALT-C patients, there was a suggestion that disease progression and development of clinical complications were less in patients on maintenance therapy who had complete viral suppression and had undetectable HCV RNA on treatment. But, the number of patients able to achieve complete viral suppression was very small and the significance of this finding is questionable.

OTHER STUDIES (COPILOT AND EPIC)

The final results of both COPILOT and EPIC, other studies of maintenance therapy using peginterferon alfa-2b, weekly 0.5 ug/kg, have not yet been published but they have been presented at several meetings.

Generally the results from these two trials confirm the results from HALT-C, which show that maintenance therapy fails to slow or prevent clinical complications. In contrast to the results in HALT-C, a subgroup of patients in COPILOT and EPIC who had cirrhosis and varices at baseline appeared to have lower rates of disease progression with maintenance therapy. In HALT-C, maintenance therapy had no impact on development of varices, progression in size of varices, bleeding from varices, or other measures of disease progression.

Although data are still under review, currently maintenance therapy is considered ineffective and not recommended for the prevention of clinical outcomes or disease progression in patients with chronic hepatitis C. Exceptions to this statement may be patients who exhibit complete viral suppression and undetectable HCV RNA, or, patients with compensated cirrhosis who have varices (portal hypertension). In addition, it should be appreciated that maintenance therapy has only been tested in relatively stable patients who had hepatitis C monoinfection. Maintenance therapy has not been examined in other populations characterized by rapid disease progression such as recipients of liver transplantation who develop recurrent hepatitis C or other patients with HCV/HIV coinfection. Maintenance therapy may still have a role in these populations. For more information about HALT C, visit the NIH website at www.nih.gov.

Retreatment with pegylated interferon/ribavirin, treatment with new interferons, treatment with ribavirin substitutes, and maintenance therapy are not the answer for a large number of patients. What's on the horizon? Can you anticipate new effective therapies?

STAT-C Drugs

Although development of specifically targeted antiviral therapy against hepatitis C (STAT-C) has been slow, we now are on the verge of an explosion of new treatment options for patients with chronic hepatitis C. Promising STAT-C drugs have emerged from preclinical laboratory studies, through Phase I and Phase II testing, and are now in Phase III clinical trials. First generation STAT-C drugs used in combination therapy are now being compared to the existing standard of care, to define clinical utility, and potentially gain approval by the US Food and Drug Administration.

The two main classes of STAT-C drugs presented in this chapter are HCV protease inhibitors and HCV polymerase inhibitors. Key to successful development of these drugs are strategies to reduce the risks for drug-resistance and side effects. Viral resistance is detected clinically by rebound in HCV RNA after initial suppression and viral variants are defined by sequence analysis (measurement of the HCV genes). The two main factors that increase risk for emergence of resistant variants are low potency of the STAT-C drug and use of monotherapy versus multi-drug treatment regimens. STAT-C drugs with low potency are associated with limited reduction in HCV RNA levels and maintenance of higher levels of viral replication. The latter factors favor mutational events which allow escape from suppression by the STAT-C drug. Multi-drug regimens inhibit viral replication at more than one locus of replication (point within the HCV life cycle)—variants resistant to one drug in a multidrug regimen are often sensitive to one or several of the other drugs in the regimen. The best strategy to prevent viral resistance is use of multiple drugs, each with a high potency against HCV. Tolerability is defined by the side effects of the drug and complexity of the treatment regimen. Efforts to improve tolerability ultimately lead to greater chance for SVR.

PROTEASE (NS3-4A) INHIBITORS
Compounds in Phase III of Clinical Testing
Optimum therapy for hepatitis C is under constant evaluation and reappraisal. One of the most exciting , and frustrating, parts of writing about emerging trends in research is that the current new treatments moving from the bench to bedside may be obsolete by the time you read this chapter. As of May 2009, two HCV-specific protease inhibitors, telaprevir and boceprevir, were in Phase III clinical trials. Others, listed below, were in earlier Phases, either I or II, of development.

Telaprevir
Telaprevir monotherapy, 750 mg by mouth three times a day for 14 days, demonstrated impressive inhibition of HCV, dropping blood levels nearly 50,000 fold (mean drop of 4.4 $\log_{10}$). The effects of this dose were compared to two other doses, 450 mg and 1250 mg, given twice daily. Interestingly, dosing three times a day with telaprevir was required for maximum suppression of HCV. Emergence of viral variants, escaping inhibition by telaprevir, was observed in the twice daily treatment arms; and, this effect was associated with increases in blood levels of HCV RNA. In both Phase II and Phase III trials, telaprevir is dosed every 8 hours.

Although monotherapy with a protease inhibitor, such as telaprevir, is certainly appealing both for patients and treating physicians, viral resistance limits the effectiveness of this approach. Currently, telaprevir and all other protease and polymerase inhibitors are being developed as "triple-therapy" in combination with pegylated interferon/ribavirin.

Three Phase II trials, PROVE 1, PROVE 2, and PROVE 3, have demonstrated the efficacy of telaprevir in combination with pegylated interferon/ribavirin in the treatment of patients infected with HCV genotype 1.

PROVE 1 was conducted in the US: 12 weeks of triple therapy, telaprevir/pegylated interferon/ribavirin, was followed by 0, 12, or 36 weeks of pegylated interferon/ribavirin. Patients who received only 12 weeks of triple therapy without additional pegylated interferon/ribavirin had a SVR of only 35%, which was lower than the SVR achieved with the standard of care, pegylated interferon/ribavirin only, of 41%. This regimen is no longer under consideration as a future treatment option. Rates of SVR in patients who received 24 and 48 week durations of total therapy were 61% and 67%, which compared favorably to standard of care. The increase in SVR above standard of care attributed to the addition of telaprevir was 20 to 26%.

Although a short 12 week course of triple therapy will not be an option for future treatment of HCV genotype 1, 24 weeks may. The data do suggest that 24 weeks of total treatment (12 weeks of triple therapy followed by 12 weeks of pegylated interferon/ribavirin) may yield results comparable to 48 weeks of total treatment (12 weeks of triple therapy followed by 36 weeks of pegylated interferon/ribavirin). SVR was similar (61% with 24 weeks vs 67% with 48 weeks) and relapse rates were very low (2 vs 6%). The two major side effects were skin rash, which was occasionally severe, and gastrointestinal complaints (nausea, diarrhea).

PROVE 2 was conducted at non-US sites: 12 weeks of triple (telaprevir/pegylated interferon/ribavirin) or dual (telaprevir/pegylated interferon, ribavirin-free) therapy followed by 0 or 12 weeks of pegylated interferon/ribavirin. SVR in the ribavirin-free dual therapy arm was only 36%, which was lower than the rate of 46% observed for standard of care, 48 weeks of pegylated interferon/ribavirin. SVR was 60% in patients receiving 12 weeks of triple therapy and 69% in patients receiving 12 weeks of triple therapy followed by 12 weeks of pegylated interferon/ribavirin. The results suggested that ribavirin was an important component of the treatment regimen, and that maximum efficacy of telaprevir requires the co-administration of both pegylated interferon and ribavirin.

PROVE 1 and PROVE 2 studied patients who were unaware of treatment. The results do not apply to patients who have had prior therapy and still have chronic hepatitis C. PROVE 3 was a study of relapsers and nonresponders—the results are very encouraging and suggest that triple therapy may be effective!

PROVE 3 was conducted at both US and non-US sites: A study of patients who remained infected with HCV genotype 1 despite a prior course of pegylated interferon/ribavirin. Three telaprevir treatment arms were compared to 48 weeks of pegylated interferon/ribavirin. The three telaprevir arms were 12 weeks triple therapy followed by 12 weeks pegylated interferon/ribavirin, 24 weeks triple therapy followed by 24 weeks pegylated interferon/ribavirin, and 24 weeks of telaprevir with pegylated interferon (ribavirin-free arm). SVR with standard of care, pegylated interferon/ribavirin for 48 weeks, was 14% overall. SVR was higher in patients treated in the ribavirin-free telaprevir arm, 23%. But, this result was inferior to the other two triple therapy arms. SVRs were 51% for 12 weeks triple therapy followed by 12 weeks pegylated interferon/ribavirin and 52% for 24 weeks triple therapy followed by 24 weeks pegylated interferon.

Several findings in PROVE 3 are particularly noteworthy. First, as in PROVE 2, ribavirin appears to be essential when telaprevir is applied in retreatment regimens. Second, extending triple therapy from 12 to 24 weeks offers little, if any, additional benefit. Third, prior relapsers enjoyed nearly a 75% rate of SVR, prior breakthroughs experienced nearly 55% SVR, and nonresponders nearly 40% SVR. To patients with ongoing chronic hepatitis C, who have failed a prior course of pegylated interferon/ribavirin, these results are very encouraging, and there is definitely hope that triple therapy can provide an effective new option!

Skin rash and anemia are the two most common adverse side effects of telaprevir. Five to 10% of patients may have to discontinue telaprevir due to rash. Rash typically occurs after 8 to 10 weeks of treatment, so even if rash occurs and treatment is discontinued, the patient has typically nearly completed the lead-in course of 12 weeks of triple therapy. Treatment of the rash involves topical lotions, steroid creams, antihistamines, in severe cases, systemic corticosteroids. Skin rash resolves and anemia improves after discontinuation of telaprevir.

The ongoing Phase III studies of telaprevir are examining not only the incremental benefit of the initial use of triple therapy, compared to standard peginterferon/ribavirin, but also optimal duration of dosing of both the triple therapy period and total period of treatment. In addition, use of a new formulation of telaprevir, that can be administered twice daily, is under investigation.

Boceprevir

The efficacy of boceprevir was examined in HCV SPRINT-1, a Phase II study using boceprevir in combination with peginterferon/ribavirin in patients unaware of treatment who were infected with HCV genotype 1 (presented at EASL 2009, unpublished data). In this trial, the SVR of the control, 48 weeks of peginterferon/ribavirin, was 38%. There were 5 boceprevir arms:

TABLE 15B. RATES OF SVR WITH BOCEPREVIR FROM HCV SPRINT—I TRIAL.

Arm	Lead-In	Weeks of Triple Therapy	Ribavirin Dose	SVR
1	Yes	28	Standard	56%
2	Yes	48	Standard	75%
3	No	28	Standard	54%
4	No	48	Standard	67%
5	No	48	Low Dose	36%

Lead-In, treatment with pegylated interferon/ribavirin for 4 weeks prior to triple therapy.

The key findings of this trial were once again the importance of ribavirin—arm 5 that included low-dose ribavirin had the lowest rate of SVR, only 36%. In addition, the arm with the highest response, arm 2 with SVR 75%, was characterized by a 4 week lead-in with peginterferon/ribavirin prior to institution of triple therapy and a total treatment duration of triple therapy of 48 weeks. My interpretation of these results is that the prolonged duration of triple therapy was more important than the 4 week peginterferon/ribavirin lead-in for maximizing SVR. In contrast to telaprevir, where prolonged use beyond 12 weeks added little additional benefit, prolonged exposure to boceprevir may be beneficial.

The main adverse side effects of boceprevir were anemia, fatigue, headache, and nausea. In the HCV SPRINT-1 trial approximately 50% of the patients treated with boceprevir received erythropoietin analogue to control anemia and maintain doses of boceprevir. Unlike telaprevir, boceprevir was not associated with skin rash.

The ongoing Phase III studies of boceprevir are examining not only the incremental benefit of the initial use of triple therapy, compared to standard peginterferon/ribavirin, but also lead-in strategies, and optimal duration of dosing of both the triple therapy period and total period of treatment.

Other Protease Inhibitors in Clinical Trials

Additional protease inhibitors are currently in or entering clinical trials. These include SCH900518 (Schering-Plough), MK7009 (Merck), and ITMN191/R7227 (Intermune/Roche). Early results in patients with chronic hepatitis C indicate potent antiviral activity and few side effects. All are progressing forward in clinical trials. The future of treatment of hepatitis C with these compounds appears to be very bright.

POLYMERASE INHIBITORS

Nucleoside Analogue vs. Non-Nucleoside Polymerase Inhibitors. Viral polymerase inhibitors are currently the largest class of antiviral drugs for the treatment of hepatitis B, HIV and herpes viruses and were some of the first drugs developed for the treatment of HCV. Nucleoside inhibitors are synthetic compounds that are analogues structurally similar to the natural building blocks of viral RNA and DNA. Nucleoside inhibitors of the HCV polymerase have similar activity against all HCV genotypes and exhibit high genetic barriers to development of viral resistance.

Non-nucleoside inhibitors inhibit HCV replication at different sites on the polymerase protein. HCV is more likely to develop resistance to these drugs. They have genotype-specific activity and potential for rapid selection of resistance. Due to their distinctive binding sites, different polymerase inhibitors could theoretically be used in combination to avoid development of resistance.

Several polymerase inhibitors have demonstrated clinical efficacy and advanced to clinical trials, but only R1728 (Pharmasset/Roche) remains under active clinical investigation at the time of this writing.

Nucleoside Polymerase Inhibitors

Valopicitabine: The efficacy and safety of valopicitabine alone and in combination with pegylated interferon were assessed in phase I and II clinical trials. High doses of valopicitabine were not well tolerated due to significant side effects, especially nausea and vomiting. Doses of 200 mg of valopicitabine were well tolerated in combination with peginterferon and effective. Studies in combination with ribavirin were not done due to increased gastrointestinal side effects.

One major Phase IIb trial examining the combination of valopicitabine with peginterferon failed to demonstrate improved efficacy over the standard of care of peginterferon/ribavirin. Side effects, primarily gastrointestinal, limited the patient's tolerance of this treatment—as a result, overall effectiveness was low. On review of the clinical data, the Food and Drug Administration revised the clinical trial of treating patients (unaware of treatment) by reducing the dose of valopicitabine from 800mg to 200 or 400mg/day. Subsequent analysis of the risk-benefit profile resulted in suspension of clinical development of valopicitabine.

R1626: Development of R1626 was terminated due to "new and unexpected safety findings" from the phase IIb study (POLI 1) (Roche earning report, October 21, 2008).

The initial experience with R1626 in 47 genotype 1 patients naïve to treatment was promising. Patients were randomized to receive R1626 orally at doses of 500 mg, 1500 mg, 3000 mg or 4500 mg or matched placebo twice daily for 14 days. Mean decreases in HCV RNA blood levels were 0.32, 1.2, 2.6, and 3.7 $\log_{10}$ for the respective treatment arms.

R1626 was generally well tolerated up to 3000 mg twice a day with only mild side effects. Gastrointestinal symptoms (diarrhea and nausea) were common, especially in the 4500 mg twice a day treatment group. In addition, there was depression of red cell, white cell, and platelet count with the 4500 mg bid dose. For these reasons, future clinical trials were limited to 3000 mg bid or less.

Dr. Pockros at Scripps Health examined the safety and efficacy of dosing R1626 for 28 days in combination with pegylated interferon or pegylated interferon/ribavirin. There were four treatment arms in this trial: DUAL 1500 (1500 mg bid R1626 + pegylated interferon), DUAL 3000 (3000 mg bid R1626 + pegylated interferon), TRIPLE 1500 (1500 mg bid R1626 + pegylated interferon + ribavirin), and standard of care (pegylated interferon/ribavirin).

The study randomized 107 patients to receive 28 days of R1626 (1500mg or 3000mg twice daily) with either pegylated interferon (DUAL arms) or pegylated interferon/ribavirin (TRIPLE arm). After day 28, all patients were treated for an additional 44 weeks with pegylated interferon/ribavirin to complete a 48 week course of treatment. Results were compared to standard of care. Growth factors were discouraged initially; however the study was amended such that investigators were advised to manage treatment-related adverse events according to their "best clinical judgment" which could have included growth factors (erythropoietin or granulocyte-colony stimulating factor). A strong antiviral effect for R1626 with pegylated interferon with and without ribavirin was observed; the mean reduction in HCV RNA was 2.4, 3.6, 4.5, and 5.2 $\log_{10}$ for standard of care, DUAL 1500, DUAL 3000, and TRIPLE 1500 arms, respectively.

Most adverse events were mild (80%) or moderate (16%). Most side effects were attributed to pegylated interferon (nausea, headache and fatigue). Gastrointestinal side effects were most commonly seen in the 3000 mg bid arm (diarrhea, 75%; nausea, 69%). Patients receiving R1626 were more likely to have hematological changes (neutropenia and anemia). Grade IV neutropenia occurred in 53% of patients in 3000 mg arm with 25% receiving G-CSF. This degree of neutropenia was not seen in the monotherapy study suggesting this observation was consequence of combining R1626 with pegylated interferon. The largest decrease in hemoglobin at 4 weeks was observed in the arm receiving R1626 and ribavirin (32% with Hb <10g/dL vs. 5% in standard of care arm). The authors state there was no evidence of hemolysis, therefore they postulate that it may be associated with reversible decreased red blood cell from bone marrow.

Unfortunately, despite the excellent viral suppression achieved during treatment, rates of SVR were not improved by R1626. SVRs were 50%, 24%, 53%, and 58% for standard of care, DUAL 1500, DUAL 3000, and TRIPLE 1500 arms, respectively.

R1626 has been withdrawn from further consideration for future drug development in the treatment of chronic hepatitis C. Two major factors led to this decision by the manufacturer (Roche)—namely suspicion for significant bone marrow suppression with even short courses of treatment and lack of superior efficacy with the studied regimens, compared to standard of care.

R7128: R7128, a pro-drug of the active molecule, is currently the most promising polymerase inhibitor in clinical development. In dose response studies, there was increase in virologic response with increasing dose, over a dose range from 750 mg daily qd to 1500 mg twice daily.

A phase 1b clinical study demonstrated mean HCV RNA reduction of 2.7 $\log_{10}$ IU/ml when administered as monotherapy at 1500 mg twice a day for two weeks in treatment experienced patients infected with genotype 1. In this study no serious adverse events were reported with more adverse events occurring in the placebo group.

In a phase IIa study, 81 genotype 1 patients, unaware of therapy, were randomized to either R7128 500mg bid, R7128 1000mg bid, or R7128 1500mg bid, each with pegylated interferon/ribavirin. Results were compared to patients treated with placebo and standard of care. Baseline characteristics were similar in each group. Subjects receiving 1000 mg or 1500 mg twice a day and standard of care achieved a rapid virologic response (HCV RNA <15 IU/ml at week 4) in 88% and 85%, respectively vs. 19% for placebo and standard of care. There were no apparent differences in HCV RNA reduction across race/ethnicity with respect to R7218 1000 or 1500mg bid dosing. No dose-related changes in terms of safety and tolerability were noted. No serious adverse events were noted and a majority of side effects were mild. The SVR results from this trial have not yet been presented or published.

Because R7128 is a nucleoside polymerase inhibitor, activity against HCV genotypes, other than just genotype 1, is expected. Preliminary data (up to day 56 in all) are available in 25 HCV genotype 2 and 3 patients (10 non-responders, 15 relapsers to standard of care) receiving R7128 1500mg bid and standard of care (n=20) compared to placebo and standard of care (n=5) for 28 days. Plasma HCV RNA levels decreased a mean of 5.0 $\log_{10}$ IU/ml (90% RVR) in the treatment group compared to 4.3 $\log_{10}$ IU/ml (60% RVR) in the placebo group. Again, no serious adverse events or dose-related side effects were reported with many side effects brought on by peginterferon (fatigue, malaise and headache). The SVR results from this trial have not yet been presented or published.

R7128 is moving forward into Phase II clinical trials. The anticipated study will enroll 400 treatment-naïve, genotype 1 or genotype 4 HCV-infected patients. Primary efficacy endpoint will be sustained virological response and will involve 5 arms (24 and 48 weeks of total treatment, 500mg and 1000mg twice a day of R7128 for 8 weeks or 12 weeks and control arm of pegylated interferon and ribavirin for 48 weeks).

Additional Nucleoside Polymerase Inhibitors under Development: *IDX184.* In January 2009, Idenix announced that it will study its polymerase inhibitor, IDX184, in HCV genotype 1 treatment-naive patients who will receive one of four doses (25 to 100 mg once-per-day). Unlike first generation HCV nucleoside inhibitors (valopicitabine, R7128 and R1626), IDX184 is a "liver-targeted" pro-drug, which theoretically may provide comparatively greater anti-HCV efficacy and safety.

MK-0608. MK-0608 (Merck) is a potent nucleoside analogue in preclinical trials.

Non-Nucleoside NSB5 Polymerase Inhibitors: *HCV-796.* In the replicon system HCV-796 effectively suppressed HCV RNA levels. Although preliminary results in patients with chronic hepatitis C were promising, development was halted due to an increased incidence of elevated liver enzymes in patients treated with HCV-796. The drug has been removed from further consideration by the manufacturer, Wyeth.

Other non-nucleoside NS5B polymerase inhibitors are in development and may be effective in genotype-1 HCV. These include BILB 1941 (Boehringer Ingelheim), PF-00868554 (Pfizer), GS9190 (Gilead), VCH-759 (ViroChem Pharma), VCH-916 (ViroChem Pharma), GSK625433 (GlaxocoSmithKline), ANA598 (Anadys Pharmaceuticals), and ABT-333 (Abbott).

NS5A Inhibitors: The exact function of NS5A is not completely understood. This viral protein may participate in a number of essential functions important to the viral life cycle, including inhibition of the response to interferon, facilitation of replication of HCV RNA, and viral assembly and secretion. Given the potential involvement of NS5A in a number of key viral processes, inhibition of NS5A might be expected to exert potent antiviral activity.

AZ12781194. The first drug in this class was developed by Arrow Therapeutics. A new class of inhibitor, AZ12781194 (Arrow), is more potent—50% inhibition of HCV genotype 1b replication is achieved at 7 nM. One drawback of this compound is the apparent lower sensitivity of HCV genotype 1a (versus 1b) and the limited activity against other genotypes. The drug is just beginning the early phases of clinical trials.

BMS790052. BMS790052 is extremely potent—50% inhibition of HCV genotype 1b replication is achieved at drug concentrations of 9 pM (potentially 1000-fold more potent than AZ12781194, although there has been no direct head-to-head comparison). In addition, BMS790052 is active against all subtypes of HCV genotype 1 and all genotypes of HCV. A single dose of BMS790052 decreases HCV RNA by 3.6 $\log_{10}$. The drug is just beginning the early phases of clinical trials.

INTERFERON-FREE STAT-C TREATMENT REGIMENS

In November 2008, Pharmasset, Roche and InterMune initiated INFORM-1 trial to investigate the combination of R7128 with Inter-Mune's protease inhibitor (ITMN-191). The first study, a Phase I study called INFORM-1, to examine the use of 14 days of a combination of an inhibitor of HCV polymerase (R7128) with an inhibitor of HCV protease (R7227/ITMN191) was just presented this year, 2009. There were no drug interactions and treatment was well tolerated. HCV RNA decreased dramatically, with just 14 days of therapy and no interferon or ribavirin!

TABLE 15C. COMBINATION THERAPY OF INHIBITORS OF HCV PROTEASE AND POLYMERASE, AN INTERFERON-FREE, RIBAVIRIN-FREE PILOT STUDY EXAMINING EARLY VIROLOGY RESPONSE.

Dose R7128	Dose R7227	% of Patients with HCV RNA <LOQ
500 mg	100 mg	13%
1000 mg	100 mg	63%
500 mg	200 mg	71%
1000 mg	200 mg	63%

LOQ, limit of quantification.

The results are exciting and raise the possibility that future treatments might include regimens that exclude interferon, and possibly even ribavirin, which would reduce side effects and improve the tolerability of the treatment regimen. Obviously these results are extremely preliminary and require longer term treatment and follow-up and confirmation in larger Phase I, Phase II, and Phase III trials.

The emergence of STAT-C drugs makes this an exciting time for patients with chronic HCV infection and those who care for them. Polymerase inhibitors, given their potent antiviral effects, represent a major contribution to the future of HCV treatment. Despite the enthusiasm these drugs have created, numerous questions regarding safety, tolerability, efficacy and resistance profiles remain to be answered by ongoing and future clinical trials. The low genetic barrier for non-nucleoside inhibitors will likely require their combination with protease inhibitors and other polymerase inhibitors as well as pegylated interferon and ribavirin. Whether these new drugs will have a role in the treatment of the difficult patient (non-responders, those co-infected with HIV, decompensated liver disease and liver transplant recipients) remains to be determined.

Nitazoxanide

Nitazoxanide was developed originally as an antiparasitic drug, and is licensed in the United States as Alinia (Romark Laboratories) for treatment of intestinal parasitic diseases. An antiviral effect was first suspected when patients with AIDS, coinfected with HIV/HCV or HIV/HBV, experienced reduction in ALT during treatment of an intestinal parasite, cryptosporidium, with nitazoxanide. Subsequent studies in an HCV replicon system confirmed potent inhibition of replication of HCV when administered alone, and especially when administered in combination with interferon.

Initial studies were conducted in Egypt in patients infected with HCV genotype 4. A small study of nitazoxanide was conducted in 47 patients, 23 treated and 24 placebo controls. Seven had undetectable HCV RNA (30.4%) and four achieved SVR (17.4%) with nitazoxanide treatment. This study suggested that nitazoxanide has activity against HCV and could potentially affect treatment of chronic hepatitis C in patients.

The above results prompted performance of another Egyptian study in patients infected with HCV genotype 4—a randomized controlled trial of nitazoxanide in combination with peginterferon or peginterferon/ribavirin. There were 3 study groups: standard of care (peginterferon/ribavirin) for 48 weeks (N=40), 12 weeks of nitazoxanide followed by 36 weeks of nitazoxanide/peginterferon (N=28), and 12 weeks of nitazoxanide followed by 36 weeks of nitazoxanide/peginterferon/ribavirin (N=28). Rates of SVR were 50%, 61%, and 79%, respectively. The higher SVR with nitazoxanide/peginterferon (p=NS) and nitazoxanide/peginterferon/ribavirin (p=0.023) have encouraged investigators to explore the therapy in other patients, including patients with HCV genotype 1.

A placebo-controlled trial of 4 weeks of nitazoxanide followed by 44 weeks of nitazoxanide/peginterferon/ribavirin was conducted in 112 treatment-naïve patients with chronic hepatitis C, HCV genotype 1 and the on-treatment results were reported at EASL 2009.

TABLE 15D. VIROLOGIC RESPONSE IN PATIENTS WITH HCV GENOTYPE 1 RECEIVING NITAZOXANIDE.

	N	RVR	cEVR	EVR
Nitazoxanide Arm	75	12%	60%	80%
Placebo Arm	37	19%	49%	68%

RVR, undetectable HCV RNA at week 4; cEVR, undetectable HCV RNA at week 12; EVR, >2log10 decrease in HCV RNA at week 12 of treatment.

The results suggest a slightly higher virologic response in the nitazoxanide-treated patients, and differences were greatest in patients with HCV RNA levels >600,000 IU/mL (data not shown). Adverse events were similar, except for discolored yellow urine noted with nitazoxanide. Serious adverse events were reported in 6 nitazoxanide-treated and 4 placebo-treated patients. There were two deaths due to pneumonia and respiratory failure in patients treated with nitazoxanide and one death due to cardiac arrest in patients treated with placebo. The role of nitazoxanide in treatment of chronic hepatitis C remains to be determined by additional prospective trials.

Summary

We are on the verge of a new era in the treatment of chronic hepatitis C with the introduction of STAT-C drugs into the arsenal for treating and hopefully curing patients infected with HCV. Pegylated interferon/ribavirin will likely remain a backbone of future treatment regimens and the lessons learned by providers using this combination will enhance and facilitate the application of new regimens to treat patients with chronic hepatitis C. The immediate attention and excitement is focused on two emerging protease inhibitors, telaprevir and boceprevir, both of which are in Phase III clinical trials. Assuming at least one of these two achieves the goal of Food and Drug Administration approval, new triple therapy regimens might be available as soon as the year 2011. As a result, rates of SVR in HCV genotype 1 infection could approximate 70% in patients unaware of treatment, 70% in prior relapsers, and 40% in prior nonresponders. Several additional therapies, including other protease inhibitors, polymerase inhibitors, and inhibitors of NS5A, may further modify the treatment landscape and enhance the chances to be cured of hepatitis C. The final results from HALT-C, COPILOT, and EPIC were disappointing—maintenance therapy with low dose pegylated interferon for patients who remain infected with HCV after courses of antiviral therapy is ineffective. New maintenance strategies will be required. Finally, the guideline for future management of patients with chronic hepatitis C will be tailoring treatment to the rate and nature of the virologic response with the end result to improve the chance for an individual with chronic hepatitis C to be cured.

Do not go gentle into that good night.

Dylan Thomas

References

1. JG McHutchison, Everson GT, Gordon SC, Jacobson IM, Sulkowski M, Kauffman R, McNair L, Alam J, Muir AJ, PROVE1 Study Team. Telaprevir with Peginterferon and Ribavirin for Chronic HCV Genotype 1 Infection. N Engl J Med 2009;1827-1838.
2. C Hezode, Forestier N, Dusheiko G, Ferenci P, Pol S, Goeser T, Bronowicki JP, Bourliere M, Gharakhanian S, Bengtsson L, McNair L, George S, Kieffer T, Kwong A, Kauffman RS, Alam J, Pawlotsky JM, Zeuzem S, PROVE2 Study Team. Telaprevir and Peginterferon with or without Ribavirin for Chronic HCV Infection. N Engl J Med 2009; 360:1839-1850.
3. JH Hoofnagle. A Step Forward in Therapy for Hepatitis C. N Engl J Med 2009;360:1899-1901.

4. Di Bisceglie AM, Shiffman ML, Everson GT, Lindsay KL, Everhart JE, Wright EC, Lee WM, Lok AS, Bonkovsky HL, Morgan TR, Ghany MG, Morishima C, Snow KK, Dienstag JL; HALT-C Trial Investigators. Prolonged therapy of advanced chronic hepatitis C with low dose peginterferon. N Engl J Med 2008;359:2429-2441.

Resources

Organizations

American Liver Foundation (ALF)
75 Maiden Lane, Suite 603
New York, NY 10038-4810
800-GO-LIVER
888-4-HEP-ABC
888-4-HEP-USA
Website: www.liverfoundation.org
Email: webmail@liverfoundation.org

The Hep C Connection
1177 Grant Street
Suite 200
Denver, CO 80203
303-860-0800
HepC Hotline: 800-522-HEPC
Website: www.hepc-connection.org
Email: info@hepc-connection.org

Hepatitis C Awareness Project
P.O. Box 41803
Eugene, OR 97404
541-607-5725
Website: www.hcvinprison.org
Email: hepcaware@aol.com

Hepatitis C Global Foundation
1404 Madison Avenue
Redwood City, CA 94061
650-369-0330
www.hepcglobal.org
Email: jtranchina@hepcglobal.org

Hepatitis C Support Project
P.O. Box 427037
San Francisco, CA 94142
415-978-2400
Website: www.hcvadvocate.org
Email: sfhepcat@pacbell.net

Hepatitis Education Project
4603 Aurora Avenue North
Seattle, WA 98103
800-218-6932
206-732-0311
Website: www.scn.org/health/hepatitis
Email: hep@scn.org

Hepatitis Foundation International (HFI)
30 Sunrise Terrace
Cedar Grove, NJ 07009
800-891-0707
Website: www.hepfi.org
Email: HFI@intac.com

Latino Organization for Liver Awareness (LOLA)
P.O. Box 842, Throgs Neck Station
Bronx, NY 10465
888-367-LOLA
Website: www.lola-national.org
Email: mdlola@aol.com

National Hepatitis C Advocacy Council (NHCAC)
Website: www.hepcnetwork.org

Parents of Kids with Infectious Diseases (PKIDs)
P.O. Box 5666
Vancouver, WA 98668
877-55-PKIDS
360-695-0293
Website: www.pkids.org
Email: pkids@pkids.org

Veterans Aimed Towards Awareness
111 West Main Street
Middletown, DE 19709
302-633-5357
Website: www.veteranshepaware.com
Email: bakfield@aol.com

Government Agencies

Centers for Disease Control and Prevention (CDC)

Hepatitis Branch, Mailstop G37
1600 Clifton Road N.E.
Atlanta, GA 30333
404-639-3311
CDC Hepatitis Hotline: 1-888-443-7232
CDC Public Inquiries: 1-800-311-3435
Website: http: www.cdc.gov/ncidod/diseases/hepatitis/
Email: dvd1hep@cdc.gov

Departments of Public Health
For information about hepatitis C in your state, call your State Department of Public Health, Epidemiology Division.

The National Institutes of Health (NIH) is the largest biomedical research center in the world. It's the research arm of the Public Health Service, U.S. Department of Health and Human Services.
Visitor Information Center: 301-496-1776
Website: www.nih.gov.
A helpful resource is CHID Online (Combined Health Information Database)
Website: www.chid.nih.gov.

Among its institutes that conduct and support research on hepatitis viruses are the National Institute of Allergy and Infectious Diseases (NIAID) and the National Institute of Diabetes & Digestive & Kidney Diseases (NIDDK):

National Institute of Allergy and Infectious Diseases (NIAID)
The NIAID has the largest budget for research into viral hepatitis. For an informational packet on hepatitis C, write to:
NIAID Office of Communications
Building 31
Room 7A50
Bethesda, MD 20892
301-496-5717
Press releases, fact sheets, and other materials are available on the Internet via the NIAID home page: www.niaid.nih.gov.

National Institute of Diabetes & Digestive & Kidney Diseases (NIDDK)
For a packet of materials on hepatitis C, write to:
National Digestive Diseases Information Clearinghouse (NDDIC)
2 Information Way
Bethesda, MD 20892-3570
Website: www.niddk.nih.gov
Email: nddic@info.niddk.nih.gov

Transplant Organizations and Agencies

Children's Liver Alliance
3835 Richmond Avenue
Box 190
Staten Island, NY 10312
718-987-6200
Website: http://livertx.org
Email: livers4kids@earthlink.net

Transplant Recipients International Organization, Inc. (TRIO)
Nationwide support group for patients and families
1000 16th Street N.W.
Suite 602
Washington, DC 20036-5705
800-TRIO-386
202-293-0980
Website: www.trioweb.org

United Network for Organ Sharing (UNOS)
1100 Boulders Parkway
Suite 500
P.O. Box 13770
Richmond, VA 23225-8770
804-330-8500
Patient services: 888-TX INFO1 (888-894-6361)
Website: www.unos.org

U.S. Department of Health and Human Services
Division of Transplantation
5600 Fishers Lane
Room 481
Rockville, MD 20857
301-443-7577
888-ASK-HRSA
TTY/TTD: 877-4TY-HRSA
Website: www.hrsa.gov
Website: www.organdonor.gov

Note: Multiple Internet sites with information on hepatitis C exist. Although many have important information, we do not specifically endorse any of these sites although we have used resources from government-based websites in the production of this book.

Selected Bibliography

Chapter 1

Alter, H.J., R.H. Purcell, J.W. Shih, J.C. Melpolder, M. Houghton, Q.L. Choo, G. Kou. 1989. Detection of Antibody to Hepatitis C Virus in Prospectively Followed Transfusion Recipients with Acute and Chronic Non-A, Non-B Hepatitis. *New England Journal of Medicine.* 321:1494-1500.

Alter, M.J., H.S. Margolis, K. Krawczynski, F.N. Judson, A. Mares, W.J. Alexander, P.Y. Hu, J.K. Miller, M.A. Gerber, R.E. Sampliner, E.L. Meeks, M.J. Beach. 1992. The Natural History of Community-Acquired Hepatitis C in the United States. *New England Journal of Medicine.* 327:1899-905.

Everhart JE, Ruhl CE. Burden of Digestive Diseases in the United States Part III: Liver, Biliary Tract, and Pancreas. 2009. Gastroenterology 136:1134-1144.

Everson, G.T. 2001. "Natural History of Hepatitis C." *Chronic Viral Hepatitis: Diagnosis and Management.* R.S. Koff, G.Y. Wu, eds. Totowa: Humana Press. (160 refs)

Kou, G., Q.L. Choo, H.J. Alter, G.L. Gitnick, A.G. Redeker, R.H. Purcell, T. Miyamura, J.L. Dienstag, M.J. Alter, C.E. Stevens, G.E. Tegtmeier, F. Bonino, M. Colombo, W.S. Lee, C. Kou, K. Berger, J.R. Shuster, L.R. Overby, D.W. Bradley, M. Houghton. 1989. An Assay for Circulating Antibodies to a Major Etiologic Virus of Human Non-A, Non-B Hepatitis. *Science.* 244:362-364.

Mandell, G.L., J.E. Bennett, R. Dolin, eds. 1995. *Principles and Practice of Infectious Diseases,* Vol.2. New York: Churchill Livingstone.

National Center for Infectious Diseases. Centers for Disease Control and Prevention. 16 Aug 2005. "Frequently Asked Questions about Hepatitis C." http://www.cdc.gov/ncidod/diseases/hepatitis/c/faq.htm. 7 Sept 2005.

National Institutes of Diabetes and Digestive and Kidney Diseases. Feb. 2003. Chronic Hepatitis C: Current Disease Management. NIH Publication No. 03-4230. http://digestive.niddk.nih.gov/ddiseases/pubs/chronichepc/index.htm. 15 Sept 2005.

Nguyen GC, Segev DL, Thuluvath PJ. Nationwide Increase in Hospitalizations and Hepatitis C Among Inpatients with Cirrhosis and Sequelae of Portal Hypertension. 2007. Clinical Gastroenterology and Hepatology 5:1092-1099.

Radetsky, P. 1994. *The Invisible Invaders: Viruses and the Scientists Who Pursue Them.* Boston: Little, Brown and Co.

Rodriguez-Torres M. Latinos and Chrónic Hepatitis C: A Singular Population. 2008. Clinical Gastroenterology and Hepatology 6:484-490.

Strader, D.B., Wright, T., Thomas, D.L., Seeff, L.B. AASLD Practice Guidelines: Diagnosis, Management, and Treatment of Hepatitis C. 2004. Hepatology 39:1147-1171.

"Viral Hepatitis C Fact Sheet." 16 August 2005. *National Center for Infectious Diseases. Centers for Disease Control and Prevention.* http://www.cdc.gov/ncidod/diseases/hepatitis/c/fact.htm. 7 Sept 2005.

Wise M, Bialek S, Finelli L, Bell BP, Sorvillo F. Changing Trends in Hepatitis C-Related Mortality in the United States, 1995-2004. 2008. Hepatology 47:1128-1135.

World Health Organization. "Hepatitis C/Fact Sheet No. 164." Oct. 2000. http://www.who.int/inf-fs/en/fact164.html. 17 May 2001.

World Health Organization. "Global Distribution of Hepatitis A, B, and C". 2002. Weekly Epidemiological Record. No. 6, 77. http://www.who.int/wer. 8 Feb, 47.

Chapter 2

Bren, Linda. "Hepatitis C: An Update." Food and Drug Administration. *FDA Consumer.* July–Aug. 2001. Vol. 35. No. 4:24–29.

"FDA Approves First Home Test for Hepatitis C Virus. 29 April 1999. Food and Drug Administration. http://www.fda.gov/bbs/topics/ANSWERS/ANS00952.html. 1 June 2001.

Fried MW. Hepatitis C Infection with Normal Liver Chemistry Tests. 2008. Clinical Gastroenterology and Hepatology 6:503–505.

Ghany, M.G., Strader, D.B., Thomas, D.L., Seeff, L.B. Diagnosis, Management, and Treatment of Hepatitis C: An Update. 2009. Hepatology 49:1335–1374.

Kato, N., O. Yokosuka, M. Omata, K. Hosoda, M. Ohto. 1990. Detection of Hepatitis C Virus Ribonucleic Acid in the Serum by Amplification with Polymerase Chain Reaction. *Journal of Clinical Investigation.* 86:1764–1767.

Lau, J.Y.N., G.L. Davis, L.E. Prescott, G. Maertens, K.L. Lindsay, K.P. Qian, M. Mizokami, P. Simmonds, and Hepatitis Interventional Therapy Group. 1996. Distribution of Hepatitis C Virus Genotypes Determined by Line Probe Assay in Patients with Chronic Hepatitis C Seen at Tertiary Referral Centers in the United States. *Annals of Internal Medicine.* 124:868–76.

Ohno, T., J.Y.N. Lau. 1996. The "Gold-Standard," Accuracy, and the Current Concepts: Hepatitis C Virus Genotype and Viremia (editorial). *Hepatology.* 24:1312-1315.

Pawlotsky, J-M, M. Bouvier-Alias, C. Hezode, F. Darthuy, J. Remire, D. Dhumeaux. 2000. Standardization of Hepatitis C Virus RNA Quantitation. *Hepatology.* 32:654-659.

Rockey, D.C., Caldwell, S.H., Goodman, Z.D., Nelson, R.C., Smith, A.D. Liver Biopsy. 2009. Hepatology 49:1017-1044.

Saadeh, S., G. Cammell, W. D. Carey, Z. Younossi, D. Barnes, K. Easley. 2001. The Role of Liver Biopsy in Chronic Hepatitis C. *Hepatology.* 33:196-200.

Sarrazin, C., G. Teuber, R. Kokka, H. Rabenau, S. Zeuzem. 2000. Detection of Residual Hepatitis C Virus RNA by Transcription-Mediated Amplification in Patients with Complete Virologic Response According to Polymerase Chain Reaction-Based Assays. *Hepatology.* 32:818-823.

Zein, N.N., J. Rakela, E. Krawitt, K.R. Reddy, T. Tominaga, D. Persing, and the Collaborative Study Group. 1996. Hepatitis C Virus Genotypes in the United States: Epidemiology, Pathogenicity, and Response to Interferon Therapy. *Annals of Internal Medicine.* 125:634-640.

Chapter 3

Alter, H. J., C. Conry-Cantilena, J. Melpolder, D. Tan, M. Van Raden, D. Herion, D. Lau, J. H. Hoofnagle. 1997. Hepatitis C in Asymptomatic Blood Donors. *Hepatology:*26 (Suppl 1):29S-33S.

Alter, M.J., D. Kruszon-Moran, O.V. Nainan, G.M. McQuillan, F. Gao, L.A. Moyer, R.A. Kaslow, H.S. Margolis. 1999. The Prevalence of Hepatitis C Virus Infection in the United States, 1988 through 1994. *New England Journal of Medicine.* 341:556-562.

"Basic Guidelines for Getting a Tattoo." *Alliance of Professional Tattoists.* http://www..safetattoos.com/faq.htm. 30 May 2001.

Benamouzig, R.,V. Ezratty, S. Chaussade. 1990. Risk for Type C Hepatitis Through Sexual Contact (editorial*). Annals of Internal Medicine.* 113:638.

Bourliere, M., P. Halfon,Y. Quentin, P. David, C. Mengotti, I. Portal, H. Khiri, S. Benali, H. Perrier, C. Boustiere, M. Jullien, G. Lambot. 2000. Covert Transmission of Hepatitis C Virus During Bloody Fisticuffs. *Gastroenterology.* 119:507-511.

Busch, M.P., S.A. Glynn, S.Stamer. et al. 2005. A New Strategy for Estimating Risks of Transfusion-Transmitted Viral Infections Based on Rates of Detection of Recently Infected Donors. Transfusion. 45:254-264.

Castrone, L. 2 July 1996. Piercing and Tattooing, Body Language of 90s Worries Health Experts. *Rocky Mountain News.* 3D.

Department of Health and Human Services, Substance Abuse and Mental Health Services Administration Office of Applied Studies. Revisions as of 9/8/2005. "Results from the 2004 National Survey on Drug Use and Health: National Findings". http://www.oas.samha.gov/NSDUH/2k4NSDUH/2k4results/2k 4results.htm. 25 Oct 2005.

Donahue, J.G., A. Munoz, P.M. Ness, D.E. Brown, D.H.Yawn, H.A. McAllister, B.A. Reitz, K.E. Nelson. 1992. The Declining Risk of Post-transfusion Hepatitis C Virus Infection. *New England Journal of Medicine.* 327:369-73.

Esteban, J.I., A. González, J.M. Hernández, L.Viladomiu, C. Sánchez, J.C. López-Talavera, D. Lucea, C. Martin-Vega, X.Vidal, R. Esteban, J. Guardia. 1990. Evaluation of Antibodies to Hepatitis C Virus in a Study of Transfusion-Associated Hepatitis. *New England Journal of Medicine.* 323:1107-1112.

Everhart, J.E., A.M. Di Bisceglie, L.M. Murray, H.J. Alter, J.J. Melpolder, G. Kuo, J. Hoofnagle. 1990. Risk for Non-A, Non-B (Type C) Hepatitis Through Sexual or Household Contact with Chronic Carriers. *Annals of Internal Medicine.* 112:544-545.

Goodenough, L.T., A. Shander, M.E. Brecher. 2003. Transfusion Medicine: Looking into the future. Lancet 361:161-169.

"Government Urges Safer Needles." Food and Drug Administration. *FDA Consumer.* March–April 2000:2.

Haley, R.W., R.P. Fischer. 2001. Commercial Tattooing as a Potentially Important Source of Hepatitis C Infection: Clinical Epidemiology of 626 Consecutive Patients Unaware of Their Hepatitis C Serologic Status. *Medicine.* 80:134-151.

Hollinger, F.B., J.L. Hsiang. 1992. Community-Acquired Hepatitis C Virus Infection (editorial). *Gastroenterology.* 102:1425-29.

Kelen, G.D., G.B. Green, R.H. Purcell, D.W. Chan, B.F. Qaqish, K.T. Sivertson, T.C. Quinn. 1992. Hepatitis B and Hepatitis C in Emergency Department Patients. *New England Journal of Medicine.* 326:1399-404.

Koff, R.S. 1992. The Low Efficiency of Maternal-Neonatal Transmission of Hepatitis C Virus: How Certain Are We? (editorial). *Annals of Internal Medicine.* 117:967-969.

Long, G.E., L.S. Rickman. 1994. Infectious Complications of Tattoos. *Clinical Infectious Diseases.* 18:610-9.

Mannucci, P.M., K. Schimpf, B. Brettler, N. Ciavarella, M. Colombo, F. Haschke, K. Lechner, J. Lusher, G. Weissbach, and the International Study Group. 1990. Low Risk for Hepatitis C in Hemophiliacs Given a High-Purity, Pasteurized Factor VIII Concentrate. *Annals of Internal Medicine.* 113:27-32.

McCashland,T.M.,T.L.Wright,J.P. Donovan, D.F. Schafer, M.F. Sorrell, T.G. Heffron, A.N. Langnas, I.J. Fox, B.W. Shaw, Jr., R.K. Zetterman. 1995. Low Incidence of Intraspousal Transmission of Hepatitis C Virus after Liver Transplantation. *Liver Transplantation and Surgery.* 1:358-361.

Mitsui,T., K. Iwano, K. Masuko, C.Yamazaki, H. Okamoto, F.Tsuda,T. Tanaka, S. Mishiro. 1992. Hepatitis C Virus Infection in Medical Personnel After Needlestick Accident. *Hepatology.* 16:1109-1114.

"Needle Safety Jabs World's Attention." Hepatitis Foundation International. *Hepatitis Alert.* Summer 2000: 6.

Ohto, H., S.Terazawa, N. Sasaki, N. Sasaki, K. Hino, C. Ishiwata, M. Kako, N. Ujiie, C. Endo, A. Matsui, H. Okamoto, S. Mishiro, and the Vertical Transmission of Hepatitis C Virus Collaborative Study Group. 1994.Transmission of Hepatitis C Virus from Mothers to Infants. *New England Journal of Medicine.* 330:744-50.

Pereira, B.J.G., E.L. Milford, R.L. Kirkman, A.S. Levey. 1991.Transmission of Hepatitis C Virus by Organ Transplantation. *New England Journal of Medicine.* 325:454-60.

Pereira, B.J.G., E.L. Milford, R.L. Kirkman, S. Quan, K.R. Sayre, P.J. Johnson, J.C.Wilber, A.S. Levey. 1992. Prevalence of Hepatitis C Virus RNA in Organ Donors Positive for Hepatitis C Antibody and in the Recipients of Their Organs. *New England Journal of Medicine.* 327:910-5.

Roth, D., J.A. Fernandez, S. Babischkin, A. De Mattos, B.E. Buck, S. Quan, L. Olson, G.W. Burke, J.R. Nery,V. Esquenazi, E.R. Schiff, J. Miller. 1992. Detection of Hepatitis C Virus Infection among Cadaver Organ Donors: Evidence for Low Transmission of Disease. *Annals of Internal Medicine.* 117:470-475.

Roudot-Thoraval, F., J. Pawlotsky, V. Thiers, L. Deforges, P. Girollet, F. Guillot, C. Huraux, P. Aumont, C. Brechot, D. Dhumeaux. 1993. Lack of Mother-to-infant Transmission of Hepatitis C Virus in Human Immunodeficiency Virus-seronegative Women: A Prospective Study with Hepatitis C Virus RNA Testing. *Hepatology.* 17:772-777.

Rumi, M.G., M. Colombo, A. Gringeri, P.M. Mannucci. 1990. High Prevalence of Antibody to Hepatitis C Virus in Multitransfused Hemophiliacs with Normal Transaminase Levels. *Annals of Internal Medicine.* 112:379-380.

Schiff, E.R. 1992. Hepatitis C Among Health Care Providers: Risk Factors and Possible Prophylaxis (editorial). *Hepatology.* 16:1300-1301.

Schreiber, G.B., M.P. Busch, S.H. Kleinman, J.J. Korelitz, for the Retrovirus Epidemiology Donor Study. 1996. The Risk of Transfusion-Transmitted Viral Infections. *New England Journal of Medicine.* 334:1685-90.

Seeff, L.B., H.J. Alter. 1994. Spousal Transmission of the Hepatitis C Virus? (editorial). *Annals of Internal Medicine.* 120:807-809.

Seeff, L.B., Z. Buskell-Bales, E.C. Wright, S.J. Durako, H.J. Alter, F.L. Iber, F.B. Hollinger, G. Gitnick, R.G. Knodell, R.P. Perrillo, C.E. Stevens, C.G. Hollingsworth, and National Heart, Lung, and Blood Institute Study Group. 1992. Long-term Mortality after Transfusion-Associated Non-A, Non-B Hepatitis. *New England Journal of Medicine.* 327:1906-11.

Shakil, A.O., C. Conry-Cantilena, H.J. Alter, P. Hayashi, D.E. Kleiner, V. Tadeschi, K. Krawczynski, H.S. Conjeevaram, R. Sallie, A.M. Di Bisceglie, and Hepatitis C Study Group. 1995. Volunteer Blood Donors with Antibody to Hepatitis C Virus: Clinical, Biochemical, Virologic, and Histologic Features. *Annals of Internal Medicine.* 123:330-337.

Tong, M.J., N.S. El-Farra, A.R. Reikes, R.L. Co. 1995. Clinical Outcomes after Transfusion-Associated Hepatitis C. *New England Journal of Medicine.* 332:1463-6.

U.S. Department of Health and Human Services, Food and Drug Administration, Center for Biologics Evaluation and Research. March 1998. *Supplemental Testing and the Notification of Consignees of Donor Test Results for Antibody to Hepatitis C Virus (Anti-HCV).* Rockville: Office of Communication, Training and Manufacturers Assistance (HFM-40).

Van de Laar T, Pybus O, Bruisten S, Brown D, Nelson M, Bhagani S, Vogel M, Baumgarten A, Chaix M-L, Gotz H, Matthews GV, Neifer S, White P, Rawlinson W, Pol S, Rockstroh J, Coutinho R, Dore GJ, Dusheiko GM, Danta M. Evidence of a Large, International Network of HCV Transmission in HIV-Positive Men Who Have Sex With Men. 2009. Gastroenterology 136:1609-1617.

Chapter 4

Hamilton, E. 1940, reprint 1989. *Mythology, Timeless Tales of Gods and Heroes.* Reprint. New York: Meridian.

Hanouneh IA, Feldstein AE, Lopez R, Yerian L, Pillai A, Zein CO, Zein NN. Clinical Significance of Metabolic Syndrome in the Setting of Chronic Hepatitis C Virus Infection. 2008. Clinical Gastroenterology and Hepatology 6:584-589.

Lauer, G. M., B. C. Walker. 2001. Hepatitis C Virus Infection. *New England Journal of Medicine.* 345:41-52.

Lyons, A.S., J.R. Petrucelli, II. 1978. *Medicine, An Illustrated History.* New York: Harry N. Abrams.

Mehta, S. H., F. L. Brancati, M. S. Sulkowski, S. A. Strathdee, M. Szklo, D. L. Thomas. 2000. Prevalence of Type 2 Diabetes Mellitus among Persons with Hepatitis C Virus Infection in the United States. *Annals of Internal Medicine.* 133:592-599.

Neruda, Pablo. 1977. *Nuevas Odas Elementales, Cuarta Edicion.* Buenos Aires; Editorial Losada.

"Sculpture in Spain Salutes the 'Silent, Unselfish' Liver." *Austin-American Statesman* 28 June 1987: A2.

Vigano M, Lampertico P, Rumi MG, Folli C, Maggioni L, Morabito A, del Ninno E, Cicardi M, Colombo M. Natural History and Clinical Impact of Cryoglobulins in Chronic Hepatitis C: 10-Year Prospective Study of 343 Patients. 2007. Gastroenterology 133:835-842.

Chapter 5

Angell, M., J.P. Kassirer. 1998. Alternative Medicine – The Risks of Untested and Unregulated Remedies. *New England Journal of Medicine.* 339:839-841.

Boigk, G., L. Stroedter, H. Herbst, J. Waldschmidt, E. O. Riecken, D. Schuppan. 1997. Silymarin Retards Collagen Accumulation in Early and Advanced Biliary Fibrosis Secondary to Complete Bile Duct Obliteration in Rats. *Hepatology.* 26:643-649.

Breidenbach, T.H., M.W. Hoffman, T.H. Becker, H. Schlitt, J. Klempnauer. 27 May 2000. Drug Interaction of St. John's Wort with Cyclosporine. *Lancet.* 355:1912.

Caregaro, L., F. Alberino, P. Amodio, C. Merkel, M. Bolognesi, P. Angeli, A. Gatta. 1996. Malnutrition in Alcoholic and Virus-Related Cirrhosis. *American Journal of Clinical Nutrition.* 63:602-9.

Coppes, M.J., R.A. Anderson, R.M. Egeler, J.E.A. Wolff. 1998. Alternative Therapies for the Treatment of Childhood Cancer. *New England Journal of Medicine.* 339:846.

Cowley, J., 1996. Herbal Warning. *Newsweek.* 6 May, 63.

DiPaola, R.S., H. Zhang, G.H. Lambert, R. Meeker, E. Licitra, M.M. Rafi, B.T. Zhu, H. Spaulding, S. Goodin, M.B. Toledano, W.N. Hait, M.A. Gallo. 1998. Clinical and Biologic Activity of an Estrogenic Herbal Combination (PC-SPES) in Prostate Cancer. *New England Journal of Medicine.* 339:785-791.

Eisenberg, D.M. 1997. Advising Patients Who Seek Alternative Medical Therapies. *Annals of Internal Medicine.* 127:61-69.

Greenwald, John. 1998. Herbal Healing. *Time*, 23 November, 60-69.

Gugliotta, Guy. "Supplements Aren't So Healthy." *Denver Post.* 19 March 2000: 5A.

Henkel, John. "fda.gov/A Look at Medical Alternatives." *FDA Consumer.* May-June 2001: 34.

Ko, R.J. 1998. Adulterants in Asian Patent Medicines. *New England Journal of Medicine.* 339:847.

Kurtzweil, Paula. 1998. An FDA Guide to Dietary Supplements. *FDA Consumer.* Vol.32 No.5:28-35.

Larrey, D., F. P. Pageaux. August 1995. Hepatotoxicity of Herbal Remedies and Mushrooms. *Seminars in Liver Disease.* 15:183-188.

Limonick, Michael D. 2004. "How We Grew So Big. *Time.* 7 June, 163, No.23.

"Medicines and Your Liver." Hepatitis Foundation International. *Hepatitis Alert.* Summer 2000. 5.

Munoz, S.J. 1991. Nutritional Therapies in Liver Disease. *Seminars in Liver Disease.* 11:278-291.

Nompleggi, D.J., H.L. Bonkovsky. 1994. Nutritional Supplementation in Chronic Liver Disease: An Analytical Review. *Hepatology.* 19:518-533.

"Research Funding Up for Alternative Medicine." Hepatitis Foundation International. *Hepatitis Alert.* Spring 2000, Vol. VI, No. 2: 6.

Schuppan, D., J.D. Jia, B. Brinkhaus, E.G. Hahn. 1999. Herbal Products for Liver Disease: A Therapeutic Challenge for the New Millennium. *Hepatology.* 30:1099–1104.

Slifman, N.R., W.R. Obermeyer, S.M. Musser, W.A. Correll, S.M. Cichowicz, J.M. Betz, L.A. Love. 1998. Contamination of Botanical Dietary Supplements by Digitalis Lanata. *New England Journal of Medicine.* 339:806–811.

U.S. Department of Agriculture, U.S. Department of Health and Human Services. 2005. *Dietary Guidelines for Americans.* Washington – 2005.

Woolf, G.M., L.M. Petrovic, S.E. Rojter, S. Wainwright, F.G. Villamil, W.N. Katkov, P. Michieletti, I.R. Wanless, F.R. Stermitz, J.J. Beck, J.M. Vierling. 1994. Acute Hepatitis Associated with the Chinese Herbal Product Jin Bu Huan. *Annals of Internal Medicine.* 121:729–735.

Chapter 6

Anderson, Greg. 1993. *50 Essential Things to Do When the Doctor Says It's Cancer.* New York: Plume/Penguin.

Benson, Herbert with Marg Stark. 1996. *Timeless Healing, the Power and Biology of Belief.* New York: Scribner.

Benson, Herbert with Miriam Z. Klipper. 1975. *The Relaxation Response.* New York: Avon.

Brennan M.R., Z.M. Younassi, R.D. Hays, D. Revicki, S. Robbins, F. Kanwal. April 2005. Impact of Hepatitis C on Health Related Quality of Life: A Systemic Review and Quantitative Assessment. *Hepatology* 41:790–800.

LeShan, Lawrence. 1994. *Cancer As a Turning Point.* New York. Plume/Penguin.

Moyers, Bill. 1993. *Healing and the Mind.* New York/Doubleday.

Spiegel, David, M.D. 1993. *Living Beyond Limits.* New York: Random House.

Topf, Linda Noble with Hal Z. Bennett. 1995. *You Are Not Your Illness.* New York: Fireside.

Chapter 7

Beam, Jr., Burton T. and Kenn B. Tacchino. Jan. 1997. *The Health Insurance Portability and Accountability Act of 1996.* Journal of the American Society of CLU & ChFC. 14+.

Centers for Medicare and Medicaid Services. Sept. 2005. *Medicare & You 2006.* Publication No. CMS-10050-09.

Social Security Administration. Aug 2005. *Social Security Supplemental Security Income.* SSA Publication No. 05-11000.

Social Security Administration. Jan. 2005. *Social Security Disability Benefits.* SSA Publication No. 05-10029.

U.S. Department of Labor Employment Standards Administration, Wage and Hour Division. Dec. 1996. Publication 1421. *Compliance Guide to the Family and Medical Leave Act.* Washington: U.S. Government Printing Office.

U.S. Department of Labor Employment Standards Administration, Wage and Hour Division. April 1995. WH Publication 1419. Federal Regulations Part 825. *The Family and Medical Leave Act of 1993.* Washington: U.S. Government Printing Office.

U.S. Department of Labor Employment Standards Administration, Wage and Hour Division. June 1993. WH Publication 1420. *Your Rights Under the Family and Medical Leave Act of 1993.* Washington: U.S. Government Printing Office.

U.S. Department of Labor Program. 1993. *The Family and Medical Leave Act of 1993.* Highlights Fact Sheet No. ESA 93-2. Washington: U.S. Government Printing Office.

U.S. Equal Employment Opportunity Commission, U.S. Department of Justice, Civil Rights Division. 1992. *The Americans with Disabilities Act, Questions and Answers.* Washington.

U.S. Equal Employment Opportunity Commission. 1991. *The Americans With Disabilities Act.* Washington.

United Network for Organ Sharing (UNOS). 2004. *What Every Patient Needs to Know.*

Chapter 8

Bonkovsky, H.L., B.F. Banner, A.L. Rothman. 1997. Iron and Chronic Viral Hepatitis. *Hepatology.* 25:759-767.

Brillanti S., F. Levantesi, L. Masi, M. Foli, L. Bolondi. 2000. Triple Antiviral Therapy as a New Option for Patients With Interferon Nonresponsive Chronic Hepatitis C. *Hepatology.* 32:630-634.

Causse, X., H. Godinot, M. Chevallier, P. Chossegros, F. Zoulim, D. Ouzan, J.P. Heyraud, T. Fontanes, J. Albrecht, C. Meschievitz, C. Trepo. 1991. Comparison of 1 or 3 MU of Interferon Alfa-2b and Placebo in Patients with Chronic Non-A, Non-B Hepatitis. *Gastroenterology.* 101:497-502.

Cheng, S.J., P.A.L. Bonis, J. Lau, N.Q. Pham, J.B. Wong. 2001. Interferon and Ribavirin for Patients with Chronic Hepatitis C Who Did Not Respond to Previous Interferon Therapy: A Meta-Analysis of Controlled and Uncontrolled Trials. *Hepatology.* 33:231-240.

Chemello, L., P. Bonetti, L. Cavallettoi, F. Talato, V. Donadon, P. Casarin, F. Belussi, M. Fezza, F. Noventa, P. Pontisso, L. Benvegnu, C. Casarin, A. Alberti, the TriVeneto Viral Hepatitis Group. 1995. Randomized Trial Comparing Three Different Regimens of Alpha-2a-Interferon in Chronic Hepatitis C. *Hepatology.* 22:700-706.

Davis, G.L., L.A. Balart, E.R. Schiff, K. Lindsay, H.C. Bodenheimer, R.P. Perrillo, W. Carey, I.M. Jacobson, J. Payne, J.L. Dienstag, D.H. VanThiel, C. Tamburro, J. Lefkowitch, J. Albrecht, C. Meschievitz, T.J. Ortego, A. Gibas, and the Hepatitis Interventional Therapy Group. 1989. Treatment of Chronic Hepatitis C, with Recombinant Interferon Alfa. A Multicenter Randomized, Controlled Trial. *New England Journal of Medicine.* 321:1501-1506.

Davis, G.L., R. Esteban-Mur, V. Rustgi, J. Hoefs, S.C. Gordon, C. Trepo, M.L. Shiffman, S. Zeuzem, A. Craxi, M-H. Ling, J. Albrecht, for the International Hepatitis Interventional Therapy Group. 1998. Interferon Alfa-2b Alone Or In Combination With Ribavirin For The Treatment of Relapse of Chronic Hepatitis C. *New England Journal of Medicine.* 339:1493-9.

Di Bisceglie, A.M., P. Martin, C. Kassianides, M. Lisker-Melman, L. Murray, J. Waggoner, Z. Goodman, S.M. Banks, J. Hoofnagle. 1989. Recombinant Interferon Alfa Therapy for Chronic Hepatitis C. A Randomized, Double-blind, Placebo-controlled Trial. *New England Journal of Medicine.* 321:1506-1510.

Di Bisceglie, A.M., J. Thompson, N. Smith-Wilkaitis, E.M. Brunt, B.R. Bacon. 2001. Combination of Interferon and Ribavirin in Chronic Hepatitis C: Re-Treatment of Nonresponders to Interferon. *Hepatology.* 33:704-707.

Dusheiko, G.M., J.A. Roberts. 1995. Treatment of Chronic Type B and C Hepatitis with Interferon Alfa: an Economic Appraisal. *Hepatology.* 22:1863-1873.

Everson, G.T. 2000. Maintenance Interferon for Chronic Hepatitis C: More Issues than Answers? *Hepatology.* 32:436-438.

Hasan, F., L.J. Jeffers, M. DeMedina, K.R. Reddy, T. Parker, E.R. Schiff, M. Houghton, Q. Choo, G. Kuo. 1990. Hepatitis C-associated Hepatocellular Carcinoma. *Hepatology.* 12:589-591.

Hoofnagle, J.H., A.M. Di Bisceglie. 1997. The Treatment of Chronic Viral Hepatitis. *New England Journal of Medicine.* 336:347-356.

Hoofnagle, J.H., K.D. Mullen, D.B. Jones, V. Rustgi, A. Di Bisceglie, M. Peters, J.G. Waggoner, Y. Park, E.A. Jones. 1986. Treatment of Chronic Non-A, Non-B Hepatitis with Recombinant Human Alpha Interferon. *New England Journal of Medicine.* 315:1575-1578.

Koff, R.S., L.B. Seeff. 1995. Economic Modeling of Treatment in Chronic Hepatitis B and Chronic Hepatitis C: Promises and Limitations. *Hepatology.* 22:1880-82.

Lampertico, P., M. Rumi, R. Romeo, A. Craxi, R. Soffredini, D. Biassoni, M. Colombo. 1994. A Multicenter Randomized Controlled Trial of Recombinant Interferon-a2b in Patients with Acute Transfusion-associated Hepatitis C. *Hepatology.* 19:19-22.

Liang, T.J. 1998. Combination Therapy for Hepatitis C Infection. *New England Journal of Medicine.* 339:1549-50.

Lindsay, K.L., G.L. Davis, E.R. Schiff, H.C. Bodenheimer, L.A. Balart, J.L. Dienstag, R.P. Perrillo, C.H. Tamburro, J.S. Goff, G.T. Everson, M. Silva, W.N. Katkov, Z. Goodman, J.Y.N. Lau, G. Maertens, J. Gogate, B. Sanghvi, J. Albrecht, and the Hepatitis Interventional Therapy Group. 1996. Response to Higher Doses of Interferon Alfa-2b in Patients with Chronic Hepatitis C: A Randomised Multicenter Trial. *Hepatology.* 24:1034-1040.

Marcellin, P., N. Boyer, E. Giostra, C. Degott, A.M. Courouc, F. Degos, H. Coppere, P. Cales, P.K. Couzigou, J.P. Benhamou. 1991. Recombinant Human a-Interferon in Patients with Chronic Non-A, Non-B Hepatitis: a Multicenter Randomized Controlled Trial from France. *Hepatology.* 13:393-397.

Marcellin, P., M. Pouteau, M. Martinot-Peignoux, F. Degos, V. Duchatelle, N.M. Boyer, C. Lemonnier, C. Degott, S. Erlinger, P. Benhamou. 1995. Lack of Benefit of Escalating Dosage of Interferon Alfa in Patients with Chronic Hepatitis C. *Gastroenterology.* 109:156-165.

McHutchison, J.G., S.C. Gordon, E.R. Schiff, M.L. Shiffman, W.M. Lee, V.K. Rustgi, Z.D. Goodman, M-H. Ling, S. Cort, J. K. Albrecht, for the Hepatitis Interventional Therapy Group. 1998. Interferon Alfa-2b Alone Or In Combination With Ribavirin As Initial Treatment For Chronic Hepatitis C. *New England Journal of Medicine.* 339:1485-92.

Poynard, T., P. Bedossa, M. Chevallier, P. Mathurin, C. Lemonnier, C. Trepo, P. Couzigou, J.L Payen, M. Sajus, J.M. Costa, M. Vadaud, J.C. Chaput, the Multicenter Study Group. 1995. A Comparison of Three Interferon Alfa-2b Regimens for the Long-term Treatment of Chronic Non-A, Non-B Hepatitis. *New England Journal of Medicine.* 332:1457-62.

Poynard, T., V. Leroy, M. Cohard, T. Thevenot, P. Mathurin, P. Opolon, J.P. Zarski. 1996. Meta-Analysis of Interferon Randomized Trials in the Treatment of Viral Hepatitis C: Effects of Dose and Duration. *Hepatology.* 24:778-789.

Poynard, T., J. McHutchison, G.L. Davis, R. Esteban-Mur, Z. Goodman, P. Bedossa, J. Albrecht for the FIBROVIRC Project Group. 2000. Impact of Interferon Alfa-2b and Ribavirin on Progression of Liver Fibrosis in Patients with Chronic Hepatitis C. *Hepatology.* 32:1131-1137.

Reichard, O., H. Glaumann, A. Fryden, G. Norkrans, R. Schvarcz, A. Soonerborg, Z.B. Yun, O. Weiland. 1995. Two Year Biochemical, Virological, and Histological Follow-Up in Patients with Chronic Hepatitis C Responding in a Sustained Fashion to Interferon Alfa-2b Treatment. *Hepatology.* 21:918-922.

Serfaty, L., O. Chazouilleres, J.M. Pawlotsky, T. Andreani, C. Pellet, R. Poupon. 1996. Interferon Alfa Therapy in Patients with Chronic Hepatitis C and Persistently Normal Aminotransferase Activity. *Gastroenterology.* 5110:291–295.

Shiffman, M.L., C.M. Hofmann, V.A. Luketic, A.J. Sanyal, M.J. Contos, A.S. Mills. 1996. Improved Sustained Response Following Treatment of Chronic Hepatitis C by Gradual Reduction in the Interferon Dose. *Hepatology.* 24:21–26.

Shiffman, M.L., C.M. Hofmann, J. Gabbay, V.A. Luketic, R.K. Sterling, A.J. Sanyal, M.J. Contos, M.J. Ryan, C.Yoshida, V. Rustgi. 2000. Treatment of Chronic Hepatitis C in Patients Who Failed Interferon Monotherapy: Effects of Higher Doses of Interferon and Ribavirin Combination Therapy. *American Journal of Gastroenterology.* 95:2928–2935.

Simon, D.M., S.C. Gordon, M.M. Kaplan, R.S. Koff, F. Regenstein, G. Everson, Y.M. Lee, F. Weiner, A. Silverman, T. Plasse, D. Fedorczyk, M. Liao. 1997. Treatment of Chronic Hepatitis C with Interferon Alfa-n3: A Multicenter, Randomized, Open-Label Trial. *Hepatology.* 25:445–448.

Viladomiu, L., J. Genesca, J.I. Esteban, H. Allende, A. Gonzalez, J.C. Lopez-Talavera, R. Esteban, J. Guardia. 1992. Interferon-a in Acute Posttransfusion Hepatitis C: A Randomized, Controlled Trial. *Hepatology.* 15:767–769.

Woolf, G.M., L.M. Petrovic, S.E. Rojter, S. Wainwright, F.G. Villamil, W.N. Katkov, P. Michieletti, I.R. Wanless, F.R. Stermitz, J.J. Beck, J.M. Vierling. 1994. Acute Hepatitis Associated with the Chinese Herbal Product Jin Bu Huan. *Annals of Internal Medicine. 121:729–735.*

Chapter 9

Andriulli A, Mangia A. Peginterferon Alfa-2a and Ribavirin for 16 or 24 Weeks in HCV. 2007. N Engl J Med 357:1660–1662.

Backus LI, Boothroyd DB, Phillips BR, Mole LA. Predictors of Response of US Veterans to Treatment for the Hepatitis C Virus. 2007. Hepatology 46:37-47.

Bacon BR, Shiffman ML, Mendes F, Ghalib R, Hassanein T, Morelli G, Joshi S, Rothstein K, Kwo P, Gitlin N. Retreating Chronic Hepatitis C with Daily Interferon Alfacon-1/Ribavirin After Nonresponse to Pegylated Interferon/Ribavirin: DIRECT Results. 2009. Hepatology 49:Epub only, in Press.

Ferenci P, Laferl H, Scherzer T-M, Gschwantler M, Maieron A, Brunner H, Stauber R, Bischof M, Bauer B, Datz C, Loschenberger K, Formann E, Staufer K, Steindl-Munda P for the Austrian Hepatitis Study Group. Peginterferon alfa-2a and Ribavirin for 24 Weeks in Hepatitis C Type 1 and 4 Patients with Rapid Virologic Response. 2008. Gastroenterology 135:451-458.

Fried, M.W., M.L. Shiffman , R.K. Reddy, C. Smith, G. Marinos, F.L. Goncales, D. Haeussinger, M. Diago, G. Carosi, D. Dhumeaux, A. Craxi, A. Lin, J. Hoffman, J.Yu. Peginterferon Alfa-2a Plus Ribavirin for Chronic Hepatitis C Virus infection. 2001. Pegylated (40 kDa) Interferon Alfa-2a in Combination with Ribavirin: Efficacy and Safety Results from a Phase III, Randomized, Actively-Controlled, Multicenter Study. *Gastroenterology.* 120 (suppl):A55.

George SL, Bacon BR, Brunt EM, Mihindukulasuriya KL, Hoffmann J, DiBisceglie AM. Clinical, Virologic, Histologic, and Biochemical Outcomes After Successful HCV Therapy: A 5-Year Follow-up of 150 patients. 2009. Hepatology 49:729-738.

Glue, P., R. Rouzier-Panis, C. Raffanel, R. Sabo, S.K. Gupta, M. Salfi, S. Jacobs, R.P. Clement, and the Hepatitis C Intervention Therapy Group. 2000. A Dose Ranging Study of Pegylated Interferon Alfa-2b and Ribavirin in Chronic Hepatitis C. *Hepatology* 32:647-653.

Hadziyannis SJ, Sette H Jr, Morgan TR, Balan V, Diago M, Marcellin P, Ramadori G, Bodenheimer H, Bernstein D, Rizzetto M, Zeuzem S, Pockros PJ, Lin A, Ackrill AM, for the PEGASYS International Study Group. Peginterferon-α2a and Ribavirin Combination Therapy in Chronic Hepatitis C: A Randomized Study of Treatment Duration and Ribavirin Dose. 2004. Ann Intern Med 140:346-355.

Harrison SA. Insulin Resistance Among Patients With Chronic Hepatitis C: Etiology and Impact on Treatment. 2008. Clinical Gastroenterology and Hepatology 6:864-876.

Heathcote, E.J., M.L. Shiffman, G.E. Cooksley, G.M. Dusheiko, S.S. Lee, L. Balart, R Reindollar, R.K. Reddy, T.L. Wright, A. Lin, J. Hoffman, J. DePamphilis. 2000. Peginterferon Alfa-2a in Patients with Chronic Hepatitis C and Cirrhosis. *New England Journal of Medicine.* 343:1673-1680.

Howell CD, Dowling TC, Paul M, Wahed AS, Terrault NA, Taylor M, Jeffers L, Hoofnagle JH for the VIRAHEP-C Study Group. Peginterferon Pharmacokinetics in African American and Caucasian American Patients with Hepatitis C Virus Genotype 1 Infection. 2008. Clinical Gastroenterology and Hepatology 6:575-583.

Jensen DM, Marcellin P, Freilich B, Andreone P, DiBisceglie AM, Brandao-Mello C, Reddy KR, Craxi A, Martin AO, Teuber G, Messinger D, Thommes JA, Tietz A. Re-treatment of Patients with Chronic Hepatitis C Who Do Not Respond to Peginterferon-α2b: A Randomized Trial. 2009. Ann Intern Med 150:528-540

Lindsay, K.L., C. Trepo, T. Hentges, M.L. Shiffman, S.C. Gordon, J.C. Hoefs, E.R. Schiff, Z.D. Goodman, M. Laughlin, R. Yao, J.K. Albrecht for the Hepatitis Interventional Therapy Group. 2001. A Randomized, Double-Blind Trial Comparing Pegylated Interferon Alfa-2b to Interferon Alfa-2b as Initial Treatment for Chronic Hepatitis C. *Hepatology.* 34:395-403.

Mangia A, Minerva N, Bacca D, Cozzolongo R, Ricci GL, Carretta V, Vinelli F, Scotto G, Montalto G, Romano M, Cristofaro G, Mottola L, Spirito F, Andriulli A. Individualized Treatment Duration for Hepatitis C Genotype 1 Patients: A Randomized Controlled Trial. 2008. Hepatology 47:43-50.

Manns, M.P., J.G. McHutchison, S. Gordon, V. Rustgi, M.L. Shiffman, W.M. Lee, M.L. Ling, S. Cort, J. Albrecht. 2000. Peginterferon alfa-2b plus ribavirin compared with interferon alfa-2b plus ribavirin for initial treatment of chronic hepatitis C: a randomized trial. 2001. Lancet 358:958-965.

McHutchison JG, Dusheiko G, Shiffman ML, Rodriguez-Torres M, Sigal S, Bourliere M, Berg T, Gordon SC, Campbell FM, Theodore D, Blackman N, Jenkins J, Afdhal NH for the TPL102357 Study Group. Eltrombopag for Thrombocytopenia in Patients with Cirrhosis Associated with Hepatitis C. 2007. N Engl J Med 357:2227-2236.

Nelson DR, Davis GL, Jacobson IM, Everson GT, Fried MW, Harrison SA, Hassanein T, Jensen DM, Lindsay KL, Terrault N, Zein N. Hepatitis C Virus: A Critical Appraisal of Approaches to Therapy. 2009. Clinical Gastroenterology and Hepatology 7:397-414.

Poordad F, Reddy KR, Martin P. Rapid Virologic Response: A New Milestone in the Management of Chronic Hepatitis C. 2008. Clinical Infectious Disease 46:78-84.

Poynard T, Colombo M, Bruix J, Schiff E, Terg R, Flamm S, Moreno-Otero R, Carrilho F, Schmidt W, Berg T, McGarrity T, Heathcote EJ, Goncales F, Diago M, Craxi A, Silva M, Brass C, Albrecht J for the EPIC Study Group. Peginterferon alfa-2b and Ribavirin: Effective in Patients with Hepatitis C Who Failed Interferon alfa/Ribavirin Therapy. 2009. Gastroenterology 136:1618-1628.

Reddy, K.R., T.L. Wright, P.J. Pockros, M. Shiffman, G. Everson, R. Reindollar, M.W. Fried, P.P. Purdum, D. Jensen, C. Smith, W.M. Lee, T.D. Boyer, A. Lin, S. Pedder, J. DePamphilis. 2001. Efficacy and Safety of Pegylated (40 kD) Interferon alfa-2a Compared with Interferon alfa-2a in Noncirrhotic Patients with Chronic Hepatitis C. *Hepatology.* 33:433–438.

Shiffman, M.L. 2001. PEGylated Interferons: What Role Will They Play in the Treatment of Chronic Hepatitis C? *Current Gastroenterology Reports.* 3:30–37.

Shiffman ML, Salvatore J, Hubbard S, Price A, Sterling RK, Stravitz RT, Luketic VA, Sanyal AJ. Treatment of Chronic Hepatitis C Virus Genotype 1 with Peginterferon, Ribavirin, and Epoetin alpha. 2007. Hepatology 46:371–379.

Shiffman ML, Suter F, Bacon BR, Nelson D, Harley H, Sola R, Shafran SD, Barange K, Lin A, Soman A, Zeuzem S for the ACCELERATE Investigators. 2007. N Engl J Med 357:124–134.

Sulkowski, M.S., R. Reindollar, J. Yu. 2000. Pegylated Interferon Alfa-2a (PEGASYS) and Ribavirin Combination Therapy for Chronic Hepatitis C: A Phase II Open-Label Study. *Gastroenterology.* 188 (suppl 2):A950.

Zeuzem, S., S.V. Fienman, J. Raseneck, E.J. Heathcote, M-Y. Lai, E. Gane, J. O'Grady, J. Reichen, M. Diago, A. Lin, J. Hoffman, M.J. Brunda. 2000. Peginterferon Alfa-2a in Patients with Chronic Hepatitis C. *New England Journal of Medicine.* 343:1666–1672.

Chapter 10

Burroughs, A.K. 2000. Posttransplantation Prevention and Treatment of Recurrent Hepatitis C. *Hepatology.* 6 (Suppl 2): S35–S40.

Chazouilleres, O., M. Kim, C. Combs, L. Ferrell, P. Bacchetti, J. Roberts, N.L. Ascher, P. Neuwald, J. Wilber, M. Urdea, S. Quan, R. Sanchez-Pescador, T.L. Wright. 1994. Quantitation of Hepatitis C Virus RNA in Liver Transplant Recipients. *Gastroenterology.* 106:994-999.

Dienstag, J.L. 1997. The Natural History of Chronic Hepatitis C and What We Should Do About It. *Gastroenterology.* 112:651-655.

Everhart, J.E., Y. Wei, H. Eng, M.R. Charlton, D.H. Persing, R.H. Weisner, J.J. Germer, J.R. Lake, R.K. Zetterman, J.H. Hoofnagle. 1999. Recurrent and New Hepatitis C Infection after Liver Transplantation. *Hepatology.* 29:1220-1226.

Everson, G.T., I. Kam. 1996. Liver Transplantation: Current Status and Unresolved Controversies. *Advances in Internal Medicine.* Vol. 42. London: Mosby-Year Book, Inc. pp. 505-553.

Everson, G.T., I. Kam. 2001. Immediate Postoperative Care. In *Transplantation of the Liver.* Editors Maddrey, W. C., E. R. Schiff, M. F. Sorrell. Lippincott Williams & Wilkins, Philadelphia. pp 131 – 162.

Fattovich, G., G. Giustina, F. Degos, F. Tremolada, G. Diodati, P. Almasio, F. Nevens, A. Solinas, D. Mura, J.T. Brouwer, H. Thomas, C. Njapoum, C. Casarin, P. Bonetti, P. Fuschi, J. Basho, A. Tocco, A. Bhalla, R. Galassini, F. Noventa, S.W. Schalm, G. Realdi. 1997. Morbidity and Mortality in Compensated Cirrhosis Type C: A Retrospective Follow-up Study of 384 Patients. *Gastroenterology.* 112:463-472.

Ferrell, L.D., T.L. Wright, J. Roberts, N. Ascher, J. Lake. 1992. Hepatitis C Viral Infection in Liver Transplant Recipients. *Hepatology.* 16:865-876.

Gane, E.J., N.V. Naoumov, K.P. Qian, M.U. Mondelli, G. Maertens, B.C. Portmann, J.Y.N. Lau, R. Williams. 1996. A Longitudinal Analysis of Hepatitis C Virus Replication Following Liver Transplantation. *Gastroenterology*. 110:167–177.

Gane, E.J., B.C. Portmann, N. Naoumov, H.M. Smith, J.A. Underhill, P.T. Donaldson, G. Maertens, R. Williams. 1996. Long-term Outcome of Hepatitis C Infection after Liver Transplantation. *New England Journal of Medicine*. 334:815–20.

Rosen, H.R. 2000. Retransplantation for Hepatitis C: Implications of Different Policies. *Hepatology*. 6 (Suppl 2):S41–S46.

Terrault, N.A. 2000. Hepatitis C and Liver Transplantation. *Seminars in Gastrointestinal Disease*. 11:96–114.

Testa, G., J.S. Crippin, G.J. Netto, R..M. Goldstein, L.W. Jennings, B.S. Brkic, B K. Brooks, M. F. Levy, T.A. Gonwa, G.B. Klintmalm. 2000. Liver Transplantation for Hepatitis C: Recurrence and Disease Progression in 300 Patients. *Liver Transplantation*. 6:553–561.

UNOS OPTN and Scientific Registry Data. From the Organ Procurement and Transplantation Network and the US Scientific Registry of Transplant Recipients, www.unos.org, May, 2009.

Chapter 11

Achkar, J-P., V. Araya, R.L. Baron, J.W. Marsh, I. Dvorchik, J. Rakela. 1998. Undetected Hepatocellular Carcinoma: Clinical Features and Outcome After Liver Transplantation. *Liver Transplantation and Surgery*. Vol. 4, No. 6 (Nov.):477–482.

Bruix, J. 1997. Treatment of Hepatocellular Carcinoma. *Hepatology*. 25:259–261.

Collier, J., M. Sherman. 1998. Screening for Hepatocellular Carcinoma. *Hepatology*. 27:273–278.

Di Bisceglie, Adrian M., R.L. Carithers, Jr., G.J. Gores. 1998. Hepatocellular Carcinoma. *Hepatology.* 28:1161-1165.

Di Bisceglie, A.M., S.E. Order, J.L. Klein, J.G. Waggoner, M.H. Sjogren,
G. Kuo, M. Houghton, Q-L. Choo, J.H. Hoofnagle. 1991. The Role
of Chronic Viral Hepatitis in Hepatocellular Carcinoma in the
United States. *American Journal of Gastroenterology.* 86:335-338.

El-Serag, H.B., A.C. Mason. 1999. Rising Incidence of Hepatocellular
Carcinoma in the United States. *New England Journal of Medicine.*
340:745-50.

Everson, G.T. 2000. Increasing Incidence and Pretransplantation
Screening of Hepatocellular Carcinoma. *Liver Transplantation.* Vol. 6,
No. 6, Suppl. 2 (Nov.):S2-S10.

Gordon, S.C., N. Bayati, A.L. Silverman. 1998. Clinical Outcome of
Hepatitis C as a Function of Mode of Transmission. *Hepatology.*
28:562-567.

Imai, Yasuharu, S. Kawata, S. Tamura, I. Yabuuchi, S. Noda, M. Inada, Y.
Maeda, Y. Shirai, T. Fukuzaki, I. Kaji, H. Ishikawa, Y. Matsuda, M.
Nishikawa, K. Seki, Y. Matsuzawa. 1998. Relation of Interferon
Therapy and Hepatocellular Carcinoma in Patients with Chronic
Hepatitis C. *Annals of Internal Medicine.* 129:94-99.

Llovet, J.M., M. Sala, J. Bruix. 2000. Nonsurgical Treatment of Hepatocellular Carcinoma. *Hepatology.* 6 (Suppl 2):S11-S15.

Lok AS, Seeff LB, Morgan TR, DiBisceglie AM, Sterling RK, Curto
TM, Everson GT, Lindsay KL, Lee WM, Bonkovsky HL, Dienstag
JL, Ghany MG, Morishima C, Goodman ZD, and the HALT-C
Trial Group. Incidence of Hepatocellular Carcinoma and Associ-
ated Risk Factors in Hepatitis C-Related Advanced Liver Disease.
2009. Gastroenterology 136:138-148.

Mazzaferro, V., E. Regalia, R. Doci, S. Andreola, A. Pulvirenti, F. Bozzetti, F. Montalto, M. Ammatuna, A. Morabito, L. Gennari. 1996. Liver Transplantation for the Treatment of Small Hepatocellular Carcinomas in Patients With Cirrhosis. *New England Journal of Medicine.* 334:693–699.

McMahon, B.J., T. London. 1991. Workshop on Screening for Hepatocellular Carcinoma. *Journal of the National Cancer Institute.* Vol. 83, No. 13 (July 3):916–919.

Penn, I. 1991. Hepatic Transplantation for Primary and Metastatic Cancers of the Liver. *Surgery.* 110:726–734.

Schalm, Solko W., G. Fattovich, J.T. Brouwer. 1997. Therapy of Hepatitis C: Patients With Cirrhosis. *Hepatology;* The National Institutes of Health Consensus Development Conference: Management of Hepatitis C. 26 (Suppl 1):128S–132S.

Serfaty, Lawrence, H. Aumaître, O. Chazouillères, A. Bonnand, O. Rosmorduc, R.E. Poupon, R. Poupon, 1998. Determinants of Outcome of Compensated Hepatitis C Virus-Related Cirrhosis. *Hepatology.* 27:1435–1440.

Sherman M. Hepatitis C and Hepatocellular Carcinoma: Grist for the Mill. 2009. Gastroenterology 136:39–42.

Takayama, T., M. Makuuchi, S. Hirohashi, M. Sakamoto, J. Yamamoto, K. Shimada, T. Kosuge, S. Okada, K. Takayasu, S. Yamasaki. 1998. Early Hepatocellular Carcinoma as an Entity with a High Rate of Surgical Cure. *Hepatology.* 28:1241–1246.

Tanaka H, Imai Y, Hiramatsu N, Ito Y, Imanaka K, Oshita M, Hijioka T, Katayama K, Yabuuchi I, Yoshihara H, Inoue A, Kato M, Takehara T, Tamura S, Kasahara A, Hayashi N, Tsukuma H. Declining Incidence of Hepatocellular Carcinoma in Osaka, Japan, from 1990 to 2003. 2008. Ann Intern Med 148:820–826.

Wall, W.J., P.J. Marotta. 2000. Surgery and Transplantation for Hepatocellular Cancer. *Hepatology.* 6 (Suppl 2):S16–S22.

Williams, R., P. Rizzi. 1996. Treating Small Hepatocellular Carcinomas. *New England Journal of Medicine.* Vol. 334, No. 11:728–729.

Wong, L.L., W.M. Limm, R. Severino, L.M. Wong. 2000. Improved Survival with Screening for Hepatocellular Carcinoma. *Liver Transplantation.* Vol. 6, No. 3 (May):320–325.

World Health Organization. *Prevention of Liver Cancer.* Technical Report Series 691. Geneva: WHO, 1983.

Yuen, M–F, C–C. Cheng, I.J. Lauder, S–K. Lam, C. G–C. Ooi, C–L. Lai. 2000. Early Detection of Hepatocellular Carcinoma Increases the Chance of Treatment: Hong Kong Experience. *Hepatology.* 31:330–335.

Chapter 12

Abramowicz, M., Ed. 1995. Drugs for AIDS and Associated Infections. *The Medical Letter on Drugs and Therapeutics.* Vol. 37 (Issue 959):87–94.

Berger, A., M. v. Depka Prondzinski, H.W. Doerr, H. Rabenau, B. Weber. 1996. Hepatitis C Plasma Viral Load Is Associated With HCV Genotype But Not With HIV Coinfection. *Journal of Medical Virology.* 48:339–343.

Boyer, N., P. Marcellin, C. Degott, F. Degos, A. G. Saimot, S. Erlinger, J. P. Benhamou, and the Comite´ des Anti-Viraux. 1992. Recombinant Interferon–alpha for Chronic Hepatitis C in Patients Positive for Antibody to the Human Immunodeficiency Virus. *The Journal of Infectious Diseases.* 165:723–726.

Cacciola, I., T. Pollicino, G. Squadrito, G. Cerenzia, M.E. Orlando, G. Raimondo. 1999. Occult hepatitis B Virus Infection in Patients with Chronic Hepatitis Liver Disease. *New England Journal of Medicine.* 341:22–26.

Chang, C.J., Y.C. Ko, H.W. Liu. 2000. Serum Alanine Aminotransferase Levels in Relation to Hepatitis B and C Virus Infections among Drug Abusers in an Area Hyperendemic for Hepatitis B. *Digestive Disease and Science.* 45:1949-1952.

Chamot, E., B. Hirschel, J. Wintsch, C.F. Robert, V. Gabriel, J.J. Déglon, S. Yerly, L. Perrin. 1990. Loss of Antibodies Against Hepatitis C Virus in HIV-Seropositive Intravenous Drug Users. *AIDS.* 4:1275-1277.

Cribier, B., D. Rey, C. Schmitt, J.M. Lang, A. Kirn, F. Stoll-Keller . 1995. High Hepatitis C Viraemia and Impaired Antibody Response in Patients Coinfected with HIV. *AIDS.* 9, no. 10: 1131-1136.

Danner, S.A., A. Carr, J.M. Leonard, L.M. Lehman, F. Gudiol, J. Gonzales, A. Raventos, R. Rubio, E. Bouza, V. Pintado, A.G. Aguado, J.G. De Lomas, R. Delgado, J.C.C. Borleffs, A. Hsu, J. M. Valdes, C.A.B. Boucher, D.A. Cooper, for the European-Australian Collaborative Ritonavir Study Group. 1995. A Short-Term Study of the Safety, Pharmacokinetics, and Efficacy of Ritonavir, an Inhibitor of HIV-1 Protease. *New England Journal of Medicine.* 333:1528-33.

DenBrinker, M., F.W.N.M. Witt, P.M.E. Wertheim-VanDillen, S. Jurriaans, J. Weel, R. Van Leeuwen, N.G. Pakkor, P. Reiss, S.A. Danner, G.J. Weverling, J.M.A. Lange. 2000. Hepatitis B and C Virus Co-Infection and the Risk for Hepatotoxicity of Highly Active Antiretroviral Therapy in HIV-1 Infection. *AIDS.* 14:2895-2902.

Dove, L.M., J. Alonzo, T.L. Wright. 2000. Clinicopathological Conference: Hepatitis C in a Patient with Human Immunodeficiency Virus Infection. *Hepatology.* 32:147-152.

Eyster, M.E., L.S. Diamondstone, J-M Lien, W.C. Ehmann, S. Quan, J.J. Goedert for the Multicenter Hemophilia Cohort Study. 1993. Natural History of Hepatitis C Virus Infection in Multitransfused Hemophiliacs Effect of Coinfection with HIV. *Journal of Acquired Immune Deficiency Syndrome.* 602-10.

Fong, T.L., A.M. DiBisceglie, J.G. Waggoner, S.M. Banks, J.H. Hoofnagle. 1991. The Significance of Antibody to Hepatitis C Virus in Patients with Chronic Hepatitis B. *Hepatology.* 14:64-67.

García-Samaniego, J., V. Soriano, J. Castilla, R. Bravo, A. Moreno, J. Carbó, A. Iñiguez, J. González, F. Muñoz, and The Hepatitis/HIV Spanish Study Group. 1997. Influence of Hepatitis C Virus Genotypes and HIV Infection on Histologic Severity of Chronic Hepatitis C. *The American Journal of Gastroenterology.* 92:7:1130-34.

Gostin, L.O., J.W. Ward, A.C. Baker. 1997. National HIV Case Reporting for the United States: A Defining Moment in the History of the Epidemic. *New England Journal of Medicine.* 337:1162-67.

Hayashi, P.H., N. Flynn, S.A. McCurdy, I..K. Kuramoto, P.V. Holland, J.B. Zeldis. 1991. Prevalence of Hepatitis C Virus Antibodies Among Patients Infected with Human Immunodeficiency Virus. *Journal of Medical Virology.* 33:177-80.

Kazemi-Shirazi, L., D. Petermann, C. Muller. 2000. Hepatitis B Virus DNA in Sera and Liver Tissue of HBsAg Negative Patients with Chronic Hepatitis C. *Journal of Hepatology.* 33:785-790.

Marriott, E., S. Navas, J. del Romero, S. Garcia, I. Castillo, J.A. Quiroga, V. Carreño. 1993. Treatment with Recombinant alpha-Interferon of Chronic Hepatitis C in Anti-HIV-Positive Patients. *Journal of Medical Virology.* 40:107-111.

Markowitz, M., M. Saag, W.G. Powderly, A.M. Hurley, A. Hsu, J.M. Valdes, D. Henry, F. Sattler, A. La Marca, J.M. Leonard, D.D. Ho. 1995. A Preliminary Study of Ritonavir, an Inhibitor of HIV-1 Protease, to Treat HIV-1 Infection. *New England Journal of Medicine.* 333:1534-9.

Pol, S., N. Trinh Thi, V. Thiers, F. Jaffredo, F. Camot, B. Lamorthe, H. Zylberberg, P. Bethelot, C. Bréchot, B. Nalpas. 1995. Chronic Hepatitis C of Drug Users: Influence of HIV Infection, Abstract No. 933. *Hepatology.* 22:340A.

Quan, C. M., M. Krajden, G.A. Grigoriew, I.R. Salit. 1993. Hepatitis C Virus Infection in Patients Infected with the Human Immunodeficiency Virus. *Clinical Infectious Diseases.* 17:117-9.

Ragni, M.V., O.K. Ndimbie, E.O. Rice, F.A. Bontempo, S. Nedjar. 1993. The Presence of Hepatitis C Virus HCV Antibody in Human Immunodeficiency Virus-Positive Hemophiliac Men Undergoing HCV "Seroreversion." *Blood.* 82:1010-15.

Remis, R.S., A. Dufour, M. Alary, J.Vincelette, J. Otis, B. Masse, B. Turmel, R. LeClerc, R. Parent, R. Lavoie. 2000. Association of Hepatitis B Virus Infection with Other Sexually Transmitted Infections in Homosexual Men. *American Journal of Public Health.* 90:1570-1574.

Rumi, M.G., M. Colombo, A. Gringeri, P.M. Mannucci. 1990. High Prevalence of Antibody to Hepatitis C Virus in Multitransfused Hemophiliacs with Normal Transaminase Levels. *Annals of Internal Medicine.* 112:379-380.

Sagnelli, E., N. Coppola, C. Scolastico, P. Filippini, T. Santantonio, T. Stroffolini, F. Piccinino. 2000. Virologic and Clinical Expressions of Reciprocal Inhibitory Effect of Hepatitis B, C, and Delta Viruses in Patients with Chronic Hepatitis. *Hepatology.* 32:1106-1110.

Selik, R.M., et al. April 2000. Increases In the Percentage with Liver Disease Among Deaths with HIV Infection. 10th International Symposium on Viral Hepatitis and Liver Disease; Atlanta, Georgia. (http://www.hivandhepatitis.com/hepb/bo4240002.html).

Sherman, K.E., S. Freeman, S. Harrison, L. Andron. 1991. Prevalence of Antibody to Hepatitis C Virus in Patients Infected with the Human Immunodeficiency Virus. *Journal of Infectious Diseases.* 163:414-415.

Soto, B., L. Rodrigo, J.A. del Olmo, M. Garcia-Begoechea, J. Hernandez-Quero, E. Lissen. 1994. Influence of Human Immunodeficiency Virus Type I Infection on the Natural History of Chronic Parenteral-Acquired Hepatitis C: A Multicenter Study on 547 Patients. Abstract No. 10. *Journal of Hepatology.* 21 S25.

Chapter 13

Alter, M. 1996. Epidemiology and Disease Burden of Hepatitis B and C. *Antiviral Therapy.* 1 (suppl 3): 9-14.

American Academy of Pediatrics, Committee on Infectious Diseases. 1998. Hepatitis C Virus Infection. *Pediatrics.* 101:481-485.

Bortolotti, F., M. Resti, R. Giacchino, C. Azzari, N. Gussetti, C. Crivellaro, C. Barbera, F. Mannelli, L. Zancan, A. Bertolini. 1997. Hepatitis C Virus Infection and Related Liver Disease in Children of Mothers with Antibodies to the Virus. *Journal of Pediatrics.* 130:990-993.

Centers for Disease Control and Prevention. 1998. Recommendations for Prevention and Control of Hepatitis C Virus (HCV) Infection and HCV-Related Chronic Disease. *Morbidity and Mortality Weekly Report.* 47 (No. RR-19):22-25, 28-31.

Gibb, D.M., R.L. Goodall, D.T. Dunn, M. Healy, P. Neave, M. Cafferkey, K. Butler. 2000. Mother-to-Child Transmission of Hepatitis C Virus: Evidence for Preventable Peripartum Transmission. *Lancet.* 356:904-07.

Jonas, Maureen M. 1998. Viral Hepatitis. *Pediatric Gastrointestinal Disease,* Vol. II, 2nd Edition. Walker, W. A., P. R. Durie, J. R. Hamilton, J. A. Walker-Smith, J. B. Watkins, eds. St. Louis: Mosby. 1028-1041.

Kage, M., T. Fujisawa, K. Shiraki, T. Tanaka, T. Fujusawa, A. Kimura, K. Shimamatsu, E. Nakashima, M. Kojiro, M. Koike, Y. Tazawa, D. Abukawa, M. Okaniza, H. Takita, A. Matsui, T. Hayashi, T. Etou, S. Terawawa, K. Sugiyama, H. Tajiri, A. Yoden, Y. Kajiwara, M. Sata, Y. Uchimura, and the Child Liver Study Group of Japan. 1997. Pathology of Chronic Hepatitis C in Children. *Hepatology.* 26:771–775.

Zein, N. 1997. Vertical Transmission of Hepatitis C: To Screen or Not to Screen. *Journal of Pediatrics.* 130:859–861.

Chapter 14

Belli, L.S., C. Zavaglia, A.B. Alberti, F. Poli, G. Rondinara, E. Silini, E. Taioli, L. DeCarlis, M. Scalamogna, D. Forti, G. Pinzello, G. Ideo. 2000. Influence of Immunogenetic Background on the Outcome of Recurrent Hepatitis C after Liver Transplantation. Hepatology 31:1345–1350.

Bekkering, F.C., C. Stalgis, J.G. McHutchison, J.T. Brouwer, A.S. Perelson. 2001. Estimation of Early Hepatitis C Viral Clearance in Patients Receiving Daily Interferon and Ribavirin Therapy Using a Mathematical Model. *Hepatology.* 33:419–423.

Department of Health and Human Services, Food and Drug Administration. March 1990. From Test Tube to Patient: New Drug Development in the United States. *An FDA Consumer Special Report,* DHHS Publication No. 90-3168. Rockville: Jan. 1998, Rev.

Dulworth, Sherrie, S. Patel, B.S. Pyenson. 2000. "The Hepatitis Epidemic: Looking at the Tip of the Iceberg." New York: Milliman & Robertson, Inc.

Fanning, L.J., J. Levis, E. Kenny-Walsh, F. Wynne, M. Whelton, F. Shanahan. 2000. Viral Clearance in Hepatitis C (1b) Infection: Relationship with Human Leukocyte Antigen Class II in a Homogeneous Population. *Hepatology.* 31:1334–1337.

Ferenci P, Scherzer T-M, Kerschner H, Rutter K, Beinhardt S, Hofer H, Schoniger-Hekele M, Holzmann H, Steindl-Munda P. Sililbinin Is a Potent Antiviral Agent in Patients with Chronic Hepatitis C Not Responding to Pegylated Interferon/Ribavirin Therapy. 2008. Gastroenterology 135:1561-1567.

Grakoui, A., H.L. Hanson, C..M. Rice. 2001. Bad Time for Bonzo? Experimental Models of Hepatitis C Virus Infection, Replication, and Pathogenesis. *Hepatology.* 33:489-495.

Hepatitis B Foundation. "Do Dollars Equal Concern?". *B Informed.* Winter 2005. No. 42, 5.

Honda, M., S. Kaneko, H. Kawai, Y. Shirota, K. Kobayashi. 2001. Differential Gene Expression between Chronic Hepatitis B and C Hepatic Lesion. *Gastroenterology.* 120:955-966.

Howell, C., L. Jeffers, J.H. Hoofnagle. 2000. Hepatitis C in African Americans: Summary of a Workshop. *Gastroenterology.* 119:1385-1396.

Kim, W.R., J.B. Gross, J.J. Poterucha, G.R. Locke III, E.R. Dickson. 2001. Outcome of Hospital Care of Liver Disease Associated with Hepatitis C in the United States. *Hepatology.* 33:201-206.

Lanford RE, Evans MJ, Lohmann V, Lindenbach B, Gale M Jr, Rehermann B, Chang K-M, Lemon SM. The Accelerating Pace of HCV Research: A summary of the 15th International Symposium on Hepatitis C Virus and Related Viruses. 2009. Gastroenterology 136:9-16.

Layden, J.E., T.J. Layden. 2001. How can Mathematics Help Us Understand HCV? *Gastroenterology.* 120:1546-1549.

Lee, P.A., L. M. Blatt, K. S. Blanchard, K. S. Bouhana, P.A. Pavco, L. Bellon, J.A. Sandberg. 2000. Pharmacokinetics and Tissue Distribution of a Ribozyme Directed Against Hepatitis C Virus RNA Following Subcutaneous or Intravenous Administration in Mice. *Hepatology.* 32:640-646.

McHutchison, J.G., T. Poynard, S. Pianko, S.C. Gordon, A.E. Reid, J. Dienstag, T. Morgan, R. Yao, J. Albrecht, for the International Hepatitis Interventional Therapy Group (HIT). 2000. The Impact of Interferon Plus Ribavirin on Response to Therapy in Black Patients with Chronic Hepatitis C. *Gastroenterology.* 119:1317-1323.

Orland, J.R., T.L. Wright, S. Cooper. 2001. Acute Hepatitis C. *Hepatology.* 33:321-327.

Pawlotsky, J.-M. 2000. Hepatitis C Virus Resistance to Antiviral Therapy. *Hepatology.* 32:889-896.

Sakamoto, N., C.H. Wu, G.Y. Wu. 1996. Intracellular Cleavage of Hepatitis C Virus RNA and Inhibition of Viral Protein Translation by Hammerhead Ribozymes. *Journal of Clinical Investigation.* 98:2720-8.

Sarnow, P. 1995. *Current Topics in Microbiology and Immunology.* Volume 203; Berlin Heidelberg: Springer-Verlag. pp: 99-112.

Sherman, K.E., M. Sjogren, R.L. Creager, M.A. Damiano, S. Freeman, S. Lewey, D. Davis, S. Root, F.L. Weber, K.G. Ishak, Z.D. Goodman. 1998. Combination Therapy With Thymosin a1 and Interferon for the Treatment of Chronic Hepatitis C Infection: A Randomized, Placebo-Controlled Double-Blind Trial. *Hepatology.* 27:1128-1135.

Taylor, D.R. Hepatitis C Virus and Interferon Resistance: It's More Than Just PKR. 2001. *Hepatology.* 33:1547-1549.

Wu, C.H., G.Y. Wu. 1998. Targeted Inhibition of Hepatitis C Virus-Directed Gene Expression in Human Hepatoma Cell Lines. *Gastroenterology.* 114:1304-1312.

Zeuzem, S., E. Herrmann, J-H Lee, J. Fricke, A.U. Neumann, M. Modi, G. Colucci, W.K. Roth. 2001. Viral Kinetics in Patients with Chronic Hepatitis C Treated with Standard or Peginterferon alfa-2a. *Gastroenterology.* 120:1438-1447.

Chapter 15

Ali S, Leveque V, Le Pogam S, Ma H, Philipp F, Inocencio N, Smith M, Alker A, Kang H, Najera I, Klumpp K, Symons J, Cammack N, Jiang W-R. Selected Replicon Variants with Low-Level In Vitro Resistance to the Hepatitis C Virus NS5B Polymerase Inhibitor PSI-6130 Lack Cross-Resistance with R1479. 2008. Antimicrobial Agents and Chemotherrapy 52:4356-4369.

Bacon B, et al. Phase 2 Randomized, Double-Blind, Placebo-Controlled Study of Nitazoxanide Plus PegIFN/RBV in HCV Gt 1 Patients. 2009. Presented at the 44th Annual Meeting of the European Association for the Study of the Liver. Copenhagen, Denmark.

Bacon BR, Shiffman ML, Mendes F, Ghalib R, Hassanein T, Morelli G, Joshi S, Rothstein K, Kwo P, Gitlin N. Retreating Chronic Hepatitis C with Daily Interferon Alfacon-1/Ribavirin After Nonresponse to Pegylated Interferon/Ribavirin: DIRECT Results. 2009. Hepatology 49:Epub only, in Press

Bruix, J, Poynard T, Colombo M, Schiff E, Reichen J, Burak K, Heathcote EJ, Berg T, Poo J-L, Brandao-Mello C, Guenther R, Niederau C, Terg R, Boparai N, Harvey J, Griffel LH, Burroughs M, Brass CA, Albrecht JK for the EPIC[3] Study Group. Peginterferon Maintenance Therapy in Cirrhotic (METAVIR F4) HCV Patients Who Failed to Respond to Interferon/Ribavirin (IR) Therapy: Final Results of the EPIC[3] Cirrhosis Maintenance Trial. 2009. Presented at the 44th Annual Meeting of the European Association for the Study of the Liver. Copenhagen, Denmark.

Burton JR Jr., Everson GT. *"HCV NS5B Polymerase Inhibitors"*. 2009. In Clin Liver Dis (in Press).

Darling JM, Fried MW. Nitazoxanide: Beyond Parasites Toward a Novel Agent for Hepatitis C. 2009. Gastroenterology 136:760-763.

DiBisceglie AM, Shiffman ML, Everson GT, Lindsay KL, Everhart JE,
    Wright EC, Lee WM, Lok AS, Bonkovsky HL, Morgan TR, Ghany
    MG, Morishima C, Snow K, Dienstag JL for the HALT-C Investi-
    gators. Prolonged Therapy of Advanced Chronic Hepatitis C with
    Low-Dose Peginterferon. 2008. N Engl J Med 359:2429-2441.

Everson GT, Hoefs JC, Seeff LB, Bonkovsky HL, Naishadham D, Shiff-
    man ML, Kahn JA, Lok ASF, DiBisceglie AM, Lee WM, Dienstag
    JL, Ghany MG, Morishima C, and the HALT-C Trial Group. Im-
    pact of Disease Severity on Outcome of Antiviral Therapy for
    Chronic Hepatitis C: Lessons from the HALT-C Trial. 2006.
    Hepatology 44:1675-1684.

Forns X, Marcellin P, Goeser T, Ferenci P, Nevens F, Carosi G, Drenth
    JP, De Backer K, van Heeswijk R, Vangeneugden T, Picchio G,
    Beumont-Mauviel M. Phase 2 Study of Telaprevir Administered
    q8h or q12h with Peginterferon Alfa-2a or Alfa-2b and Ribavirin
    in Treatment-Naïve Patients with Genotype 1 Hepatitis C: Week
    12 Interim Results. 2008. Presented at the 59th Annual Meeting
    of the American Association for the Study of Liver Diseases, San
    Francisco, CA, USA.

Gane EJ, et al. First-in-Man Demonstration of Potent Antiviral Activ-
    ity with a Nucleoside Polymerase (R7128) and Protease Inhibitor
    (R7227/ITMN-191) Combination in HCV. 2009. Presented at
    the 44th Annual Meeting of the European Association for the
    Study of the Liver. Copenhagen, Denmark.

Gish RG, Arora S, Reddy KR, Nelson DR, O'Brien C, Xu Y, Murphy
    B. Virologic response and safety outcomes in therapy-naïve pa-
    tients treated for chronic hepatitis C with taribavirin or ribavirin in
    combination with pegylated interferon alfa-2a: A randomized,
    phase 2 study. 2007. J Hepatology 47:51-59.

Hezode C, Forestier N, Dusheiko G, Ferenci P, Pol S, Goeser T, Bronowicki J-P, Bourliere M, Gharakhanian S, Bengtsson L, Mc-Nair L, George S, Kieffer T, Kwong A, Kauffman RS, Alam J, Pawlotsky J-M, Zeuzem S for the PROVE2 Study Team. Telaprevir and Peginterferon with or without Ribavirin for Chronic HCV Infection. 2009. N Engl J Med 360:1839-1850.

Kieffer TL, Sarrazin C, Miller JS, Welker MW, Forestier N, Reesink HW, Kwong AD, Zeuzem S. Telaprevir and Pegylated Interferon-alpha-2a Inhibit Wild-Type and Resistant Genotype 1 Hepatitis C Virus Replication in Patients. 2007. Hepatology 46:631-639.

Hoofnagle JH. A Step Forward in Therapy for Hepatitis C. 2009. N Engl J Med 360:1899-1901.

Kwo P, Lawitz EJ, McCone J, Schiff ER, Vierling JM, Pound D, Davis M, Galati JS, Gordon SC, Ravendhran N, Rossaro L, Anderson FH, Jacobsen IM, Rubin R, Koury K, Pedicone L, Chaudhri E, Albrecht JK. HCV SPRINT-1: Final Results SVR 24 Boceprevir plus PegIFN α-2b/Ribavirin HCV 1 Treatment Naïve Patients. 2009. Presented at the 44th Annual Meeting of the European Association for the Study of the Liver. Copenhagen, Denmark.

Jensen DM, Marcellin P, Freilich B, Andreone P, DiBisceglie AM, Brandao-Mello C, Reddy KR, Craxi A, Martin AO, Teuber G, Messinger D, Thommes JA, Tietz A. Re-treatment of Patients with Chronic Hepatitis C Who Do Not Respond to Peginterferon-α2b: A Randomized Trial. 2009. Ann Intern Med 150:528-540

Manns M, et al. Telaprevir in Hepatitis C Gt 1 Infected Patients with Prior Non-Response, Viral Breakthrough, or Relapse to PegIFN alfa-2a/b and RBV Therapy (PROVE3). 2009. Presented at the 44th Annual Meeting of the European Association for the Study of the Liver. Copenhagen, Denmark.

Marcello T, Grakoul A, Barbra-Spaeth G, Machlin ES, Kotenko SV, MacDonald MR, Rice CM. Interferons alpha and lambda inhibit hepatitis C virus replication with distinct signal transduction and gene regulation kinetics. 2006. Gastroenterology 131:1887-1898.

McCown MF, Rajyaguru S, Le Pogam S, Ali S, Jiang W-R, Kang H, Symons J, Cammack N, Najera I. The Hepatitis C Replicon Presents a Higher Barrier to Resistance to Nucleoside Analogs than to Nonnucleoside Polymerase or Protease Inhibitors. 2008. Antimicrobial Agents and Chemotherapy 52:1604-1612.

McHutchison JG, Everson GT, Gordon SC, Jacobson IM, Sulkowski M, Kauffman R, McNair L, Alam J, Muir AJ. Telaprevir with Peginterferon and Ribavirin for Chronic HCV Genotype 1 Infection. 2009. N Engl J Med 360:1827-1838.

McHutchison JG, Bacon BR, Gordon SC, Lawitz E, Shiffman M, Afdhal NH, Jacobson IM, Muir A, Al-Adhami M, Morris ML, Lekstrom-Himes JA, Efler SM, Davis HL. Phase 1B, Randomized, Double-Blind, Dose-Escalation Trial of CPG 10101 in Patients with Chronic Hepatitis C Virus. 2007. Hepatology 46:1341-1349.

Modi AA, Hoofnagle JH. New Therapies for Hepatitis C. 2007. Hepatology 46:615-617.

Pockros PJ, Nelson D, Godofsky E, Rodriguez-Torres M, Everson GT, Fried MW, Ghalib, R, Harrison S, Nyberg L, Shiffman ML, Najera I, Chan A, Hill G. R1626 Plus Peginterferon Alfa-2a Provides Potent Suppression of Hepatitis C Virus RNA and Significant Antiviral Synergy in Combination with Ribavirin. 2008. Hepatology 48:385-397.

Pockros PJ, Nelson D, Godofsky E, Rodriguez-Torres M, Everson GT, Fried MW, Ghalib, R, Harrison S, Nyberg L, Shiffman ML, Najera I, Chan A, Hill G. High Relapse Rate Seen at Week 72 for Patients Treated with R1626 Combination Therapy. 2008. Hepatology 48:1349-1350.

Poynard T, Colombo M, Bruix J, Schiff E, Terg R, Flamm S, Moreno-Otero R, Carrilho F, Schmidt W, Berg T, McGarrity T, Heathcote EJ, Goncales F, Diago M, Craxi A, Silva M, Brass C, Albrecht J for the EPIC Study Group. Peginterferon alfa-2b and Ribavirin: Effective in Patients with Hepatitis C Who Failed Interferon alfa/Ribavirin Therapy. 2009. Gastroenterology 136:1618-1628.

Reesink HW, Bergmann JF, deBruijne J, Weegink CJ, van Lier J, van Vliet A, Keung A, Li J, O'Mara E, Treitel MA, Hughes EA, Janssen HLA, deKnegt RJ. Safety and Antiviral Activity of SCH 900518 Administered as Monotherapy and in Combination with Peginterferon Alfa-2b to Naïve and Treatment-Experienced HCV-1 Infected Patients. 2009. Presented at the 44th Annual Meeting of the European Association for the Study of the Liver. Copenhagen, Denmark.

Roberts SK, Cooksley G, Dore GJ, Robson R, Shaw D, Berns H, Hill G, Klumpp K, Najera I, Washington C. Robust Antiviral Activity of R1626, a Novel Nucleoside Analog: A Randomized, Placebo-Controlled Study in Patients with Chronic Hepatitis C. 2008. Hepatology 48:398-406.

Rossignol J-F, Elfert A, El-Gohary Y, Keefe EB. Improved Virologic Response in Chronic Hepatitis C Genotype 4 Treated with Nitazoxanide, Peginterferon, and Ribavirin. 2009. Gastroenterology 136:856-862.

Shiffman ML, Berg T, Poordad F, Bronowicki J-P, Muir AJ, Gordon SC, George S, Adda N, McHutchison JG. A Study of Telaprevir Combined with Peginterferon Alfa-2a and Ribavirin in Patients with Well-documented Non-response or Relapse after Previous Peginterferon Alfa-2a and Ribavirin Treatment: Interim Analysis. 2008. Presented at the 59th Annual Meeting of the American Association for the Study of Liver Diseases, San Francisco, CA, USA.

Shiffman ML, et al. PegIFN-lambda: Antiviral Activity and Safety Profile in a 4-Week Phase 1B Study in Relapsed Gt 1 Hepatitis C Infection. 2009. Presented at the 44th Annual Meeting of the European Association for the Study of the Liver. Copenhagen, Denmark.

van Wolleghem T, Meuleman P, Libbrecht L, Roskams T, de Vos R, Leroux-Roels G. Ultra-Rapid Cardiotoxicity of the Hepatitis C Virus Protease Inhibitor BILN 2061 in the Urokinase-Type Plasminogen Activator Mouse. 2007. Gastroenterology 133:1144-1155.

Zhang EZ, Bartels DJ, Sullivan JC, Adiwijara B, Marcial M, Dorrian JL, Tigges A, Kwong AD, Kieffer TL. No Compensatory Fitness Mutations Selected in NS3/4a Protease Cleavage Sites During Treatment with Telaprevir, Peg-IFN Alfa-2a, and Ribavirin in Phase 2 Studies (PROVE1 and PROVE2) in Treatment Naïve HCV Genotype 1-infected Patients. 2008. Presented at the 59th Annual Meeting of the American Association for the Study of Liver Diseases, San Francisco, CA, USA.

Index